Controlled Epidemiological Studies

This book covers classic epidemiological designs that use a reference/control group, including case-control, case-cohort, nested case-control and variations of these designs, such as stratified and two-stage designs. It presents a unified view of these sampling designs as representations of an underlying cohort or target population of interest. This enables various extended designs to be introduced and analysed with a similar approach: extreme sampling on the outcome (extreme case-control design) or on the exposure (exposure-enriched, exposure-density, countermatched), designs that re-use prior controls and augmentation sampling designs. Further extensions exploit aggregate data for efficient cluster sampling, accommodate time-varying exposures and combine matched and unmatched controls. Self-controlled designs, including case-crossover, self-controlled case series and exposure-crossover, are also presented. The test-negative design for vaccine studies and the use of negative controls for bias assessment are introduced and discussed.

This book is intended for graduate students in biostatistics, epidemiology and related disciplines, or for health researchers and data analysts interested in extending their knowledge of study design and data analysis skills.

This book

1. Bridges the gap between epidemiology and the more mathematically oriented biostatistics books.
2. Assembles the wealth of epidemiological knowledge about observational study designs that is scattered over several decades of scientific publications.
3. Illustrates the performance of methods in real research applications.
4. Provides guidelines for implementation in standard software packages (Stata, R).
5. Includes numerous exercises, covering simple mathematical proofs, consideration of proposed or published designs, and practical data analysis.

Chapman & Hall/CRC Biostatistics Series

Recently Published Titles

Advanced Statistics in Regulatory Critical Clinical Initiatives
Edited By Wei Zhang, Fangrong Yan, Feng Chen, Shein-Chung Chow

Medical Statistics for Cancer Studies
Trevor F. Cox

Real World Evidence in a Patient-Centric Digital Era
Edited by Kelly H. Zou, Lobna A. Salem, Amrit Ray

Data Science, AI, and Machine Learning in Pharma
Harry Yang

Model-Assisted Bayesian Designs for Dose Finding and Optimization
Methods and Applications
Ying Yuan, Ruitao Lin and J. Jack Lee

Digital Therapeutics: Strategic, Scientific, Developmental, and Regulatory Aspects
Oleksandr Sverdlov, Joris van Dam

Quantitative Methods for Precision Medicine
Pharmacogenomics in Action
Rongling Wu

Drug Development for Rare Diseases
Edited by Bo Yang, Yang Song and Yijie Zhou

Case Studies in Bayesian Methods for Biopharmaceutical CMC
Edited by Paul Faya and Tony Pourmohamad

Statistical Analytics for Health Data Science with SAS and R
Jeffrey Wilson, Ding-Geng Chen and Karl E. Peace

Design and Analysis of Pragmatic Trials
Song Zhang, Chul Ahn and Hong Zhu

ROC Analysis for Classification and Prediction in Practice
Christos Nakas, Leonidas Bantis and Constantine Gatsonis

Controlled Epidemiological Studies
Marie Reilly

For more information about this series, please visit: https://www.routledge.com/Chapman--Hall-CRC-Biostatistics-Series/book-series/CHBIOSTATIS

Controlled Epidemiological Studies

By

Marie Reilly

CRC Press
Taylor & Francis Group
Boca Raton London New York

CRC Press is an imprint of the
Taylor & Francis Group, an **informa** business
A CHAPMAN & HALL BOOK

Designed cover image: © Shutterstock 1967534398, edited by Marie Reilly, and © Marie Reilly

First edition published 2023
by CRC Press
6000 Broken Sound Parkway NW, Suite 300, Boca Raton, FL 33487-2742

and by CRC Press
4 Park Square, Milton Park, Abingdon, Oxon, OX14 4RN

CRC Press is an imprint of Taylor & Francis Group, LLC

Library of Congress Cataloging-in-Publication Data

Names: Reilly, Marie (Professor of biostatistics), author.
Title: Controlled epidemiological studies / by Marie Reilly.
Description: First edition. | Boca Raton : CRC Press, 2023. | Series:
Chapman & Hall/CRC Press biostatistics series | Includes bibliographical
references and index. | Identifiers: LCCN 2022055389 (print) | LCCN 2022055390 (ebook) | ISBN
9780367186784 (hardback) | ISBN 9781032458182 (paperback) | ISBN
9780429197574 (ebook)
Subjects: LCSH: Epidemiology--Statistical methods. | Case-control method. |
Epidemiology--Research--Methodology.
Classification: LCC RA652.2.M3 R45 2023 (print) | LCC RA652.2.M3 (ebook)
| DDC 614.4--dc23/eng/20230313
LC record available at https://lccn.loc.gov/2022055389
LC ebook record available at https://lccn.loc.gov/2022055390

ISBN: 978-0-367-18678-4 (hbk)
ISBN: 978-1-032-45818-2 (pbk)
ISBN: 978-0-429-19757-4 (ebk)

DOI: 10.1201/9780429197574

Typeset in Latin Modern font
by KnowledgeWorks Global Ltd.

Publisher's note: This book has been prepared from camera-ready copy provided by the authors.

Table of Contents

Preface

This book presents a unified view of sampling designs for addressing questions concerning the health of a population. Whether an investigator has followed up a group for their health events over time (in a cohort study), sampled them at a single point in time (in a cross-sectional study), or compared cases of a disease to a subsample of non-diseased individuals (in a case-control study), each of these classic sampling strategies is an effort to describe the health of the background population from which the data were drawn. Most epidemiologists and biostatisticians are familiar with matched and unmatched cohort and case-control designs and the appropriate statistical methods for valid analysis. However, numerous other designs have been developed that are useful, and often more efficient, when a sample is selected from a well-defined cohort or population, such as an electronic register.

Despite their long history, the case-cohort, counter-matched and case-crossover/case-series designs have not been widely adopted. Many other creative designs continue to appear, some as a novel approach to study a specific health outcome and others proposed as more general methodology. Despite all these developments, simple cohort and case-control designs predominate in epidemiology and biostatistics textbooks and in the epidemiological and medical literature. This book aims to establish familiar and less familiar designs as simply different strategies for sampling from a population to address a research question of interest. Recognising how classic designs can be made to represent the underlying study base, opens the way to more extensive and informative data analysis and a rich collection of other designs.

Even where software is available for their implementation, the wide adoption of useful new designs is hampered by the lack of sufficient 'showcasing' in a range of real applications. This book hopes to bridge this gap, by combining the unified view of sampling strategies with real examples from substantive research, to illustrate the important contribution of epidemiology as a tool in medical research. The vision, represented by the cover image, is that in any application, the design is "a piece of the puzzle" of how to best choose and use the comparison (control) group in order to reconstruct the experience of the source population.

Use of this book

The material in this book has grown out of many years of teaching biostatistics: (i) introductory course in an undergraduate medical program, (ii) core courses for PhD students of epidemiology and (iii) advanced courses for PhD students, post-doctoral scientists and health professionals. The book is a suitable text for students of epidemiology and biostatistics, primarily aimed at masters and PhD students. The preliminary chapters cover basic epidemiology, before progressing through extensions to familiar designs and methods of analysis, to the final chapters that introduce more sophisticated designs of interest in specific areas of health research. Pre-requisites for a course of study using this book should include some understanding of basic statistics, discrete and continuous probability distributions, the concept of sampling distribution and simple linear regression. The following are suggested chapters, that, together with the extensive exercises (and associated datasets at `https://www.meb.ki.se/biostat/CES.htm`, could be used as teaching or learning material at different levels:

- Introduction to epidemiology and public health: Chapters 1 and 2, Sections 6.1-6.2
- Biostatistics for master's level: Chapters 1 and 2, Sections 4.1-4.4, Chapter 5, Sections 6.1, 6.2, 10.1
- PhD-level core training: Chapters 1-5, Sections 6.1, 6.2, 10.1
- PhD advanced courses: Chapters 2, 5, 6-10

Acknowledgements

Many of the illustrative examples in the early chapters arose from the interaction with students during their first encounter with epidemiological ideas. In later chapters, the data applications include several real research problems from my own work or that of colleagues who presented challenging epidemiological "puzzles": I am grateful to them for sharing their knowledge and data, and for their trust that a solution could be found, with particular mention of Kamila Czene. These solutions owe much to the fruitful and enjoyable collaboration with my biostatistics colleagues, particularly Agus Salim, Chuen Seng Tan, Nathalie Støer and Yilin Ning. My apologies to anyone that I may have forgotten to mention.

The presentation of the book owes a large debt of gratitude to Anastasia Lam, whose dedication to data, display and detail were critical in helping to transform the collection of accumulated material into a coherent manuscript, typeset with her remarkable skills in Overleaf. She worked tirelessly with the large volume of research papers and data, implementing numerous examples in Stata and R. Thanks is also due to Yilin Ning and Jay Achar for their excellent work on specific illustrative examples, and to Zihan Dong for patiently 'pilot testing' all the exercises and improving many of the plots. Much of this work was supported by a grant from the Swedish Cancer Society, *Cancerfonden*, to whom I am also grateful for the years of support for the methodological work that laid the foundation for the book.

Finally, the decision to embark on this project owes much to the encouragement, and to the intellectual and gastronomic support, of 'mo fhear-chéile', Yudi Pawitan, who understood that the distillation of many years of work into this textbook would bring much reward and fulfilment.

List of Figures

List of Tables

List of Abbreviations

APOE Apolipoprotein E

ARI Absolute Risk Increase

BMI Body Mass Index

CBC Contralateral Breast

CHD Coronary Heart Disease

CI Confidence Interval

CIN Case Impact Number

CLR Conditional Logistic Regression

COPD Chronic Obstructibe Pulmonary Disease

CT Chlamydia Trachomatis

CVD Cardiovascular Disease

ECC Extreme Case-control

EIN Exposure Impact Number

HLA Human Leukocyte Antigen

HPV Human Papilloma Virus

HR Hazard Ratio

HRT Hormone Replacement Therapy

IPW Inverse Probabiity Weighting

IRR Incidence Rate Ratio

ln Natural log (log_e)

MECC More Extreme Case-control

MMR Measles, Mumps, Rubella

NCC Nested Case-control

NHL Non-Hodgkins Lymphoma

NNE Number Needed to Expose

NNEB Number Needed to Expose for Benefit

NNEH Number Needed to Expose for Harm

NNT Number Needed to Treat

OR Odds Ratio

PAF Population Attributable Fraction

PAR Population Attributable Risk

PE Preeclampsia

PIN Population Impact Number

PSA Prostate Specific Antigen

RBC Red Blood Cells

RD Risk Difference

RR Relative Risk

SBP Systolic Blood Pressure

SE Standard Error

SES Socio-Economic Status

SIDS Sudden Infant Death Syndrome

VTE Venous Thromboembolism

WHO World Health Organisation

1

Classic Epidemiological Designs

The science of epidemiology is concerned with the study of the distribution and determinants of health and disease in a population. Although theoretical concepts have made important contributions, epidemiology at its heart is a practical, data-driven science, where the information collected from a population provides evidence concerning a research question of interest. There are rigorous methods or designs for data collection and analysis that ensure the validity of such evidence. The power of these underlying principles has been manifest in a number of triumphs of epidemiology since it became established as a scientific discipline.

In contrast to experimental studies, where the investigator assigns a treatment or intervention to the participants, in observational epidemiological studies the investigator simply observes the participants without any attempt to modify their condition or behaviour. A familiar experimental study is a clinical trial , where volunteers are invited to participate in the assessment of the effect of a new drug or procedure. By comparing two groups of volunteers, only one of which was assigned to the intervention of interest, a measure of the effectiveness of the intervention is obtained. The individuals who did not receive the treatment will be offered some control intervention (such as standard treatment or inactive placebo), which will depend on the state of knowledge concerning the research question. In such comparison studies, known as controlled trials, participants will often be randomly assigned to treatment, to ensure a fair comparison. These randomised controlled trials were long regarded as the 'gold standard' in terms of study design and placed at the top of the evidence pyramid. However, observational studies that involve the comparison of a group of individuals of interest with some reference group are also controlled studies, and like controlled experiments, the validity of the comparison depends crucially on a systematic and rigorous methodology for the selection of subjects to be observed and an appropriate method of analysis. The quality of evidence from such studies is no longer thought to be inferior just because of the study's observational nature [217, 157], and for questions concerning how whole populations are affected by real-life health interventions, promotions, services or treatments, well-controlled observational studies are clearly superior.

The widely accepted approaches to epidemiological investigation are usually presented in standard textbooks as belonging to three major designs: cross-sectional (or survey), cohort, or case-control, which we will return to later in the chapter. However, this classification loses sight of the fact that *all* these designs, and more, are simply methods for investigating questions concerning the health of a population or group of individuals (a 'cohort') followed over a period of time, where the question of interest may result in a more astute choice of design. This view was expressed by one of the pioneers of epidemiology, Olli Miettinen [147], and a recent elegant presentation from Neil Pearce [168] noting that all studies of a population followed over a period of time, regardless of the design used, are directed at just two measures of disease occurrence – prevalence or incidence. This realisation not only simplifies the teaching of students and researchers who are new to epidemiological concepts, but it also has an unexpected power to sharpen the focus on the research question that has been posed and consequently on the choice of an appropriate study design.

1.1 Review of Measures of Disease Occurrence and Risk

The purpose of an epidemiological investigation is to convey information about the presence or risk of disease in a population. For a single individual, the current state of health can be described simply as the presence or absence of disease, and for those who acquire the disease, the duration and severity provide measures of the magnitude of disease burden for the patient. The current state of health of a population with respect to a specific disease can be simply described as the number (or proportion) of individuals with the disease. However, susceptibility to disease varies from one individual to another depending on their age, socioeconomic status, genetics and other factors. The risk of disease may also change with calendar time due to short-term (seasonal) or long-term (societal) factors. Thus, to describe the current disease burden or the risk of future disease in a population, we need measures of the presence, onset and duration of disease, whose magnitude can be meaningfully compared across different groups of individuals or populations.

1.1.1 Prevalence

The simplest measure of the occurrence of disease in a population is the **prevalence**, which describes the proportion of the population with the disease *at a specified time*, such as the proportion of persons absent from work on a specific day due to winter flu, or the proportion of persons living with HIV who currently have access to anti-retroviral medication. We can represent prevalence as simply π, or if we wish to emphasise the time aspect, $\pi(t)$. Since much of epidemiology is concerned with conditions that affect only a small minority of individuals in the population, alternatives to proportions or percentages are often used to express prevalence. For quantifying the prevalence of chronic diseases in the general population, it is common to report the number of cases per 100,000 persons. For example, the World Cancer Research Fund's Continuous Update Project reports that Australia has 468.0 cancer cases per 100,000 persons (men and women combined) [19]. For studies of special susceptible populations, such as patient cohorts, other denominators, such as 10,000 or 1000, are often used to provide clearer information.

It can be useful to present a prevalence (or indeed any proportion) as an **odds** , which is the number of affected persons per unaffected person, or the ratio of the proportions (or numbers) affected and unaffected:

$$\frac{\pi}{1-\pi} \quad \text{or} \quad \frac{\pi(t)}{1-\pi(t)}$$

For a disease with a prevalence of 10%, the odds of 10/90 or 1/9 indicates that for every affected person there are nine unaffected. For example, the Global Health Observatory data provided by the WHO estimates that there are 21,000 people living with HIV in The Gambia and that 6800 have access to antiretroviral therapy [237]. Thus, the prevalence of antiretroviral therapy among persons living with HIV is 6800/21,000 or 32.4%, which is equivalent to an odds of 6800/14,200 or 142 persons untreated for every 68 treated.

Figure 1.1a provides a simple illustration of the prevalence of a simulated infectious disease in a small community. The prevalence varies during the one-year period, with no cases in the first month, a prevalence of 6.7% (2/30) in month 3, 16.7% (5/30) in month 6, and no cases after month 9, a pattern that could be seen for winter flu if the start of observation (month '0') was July.

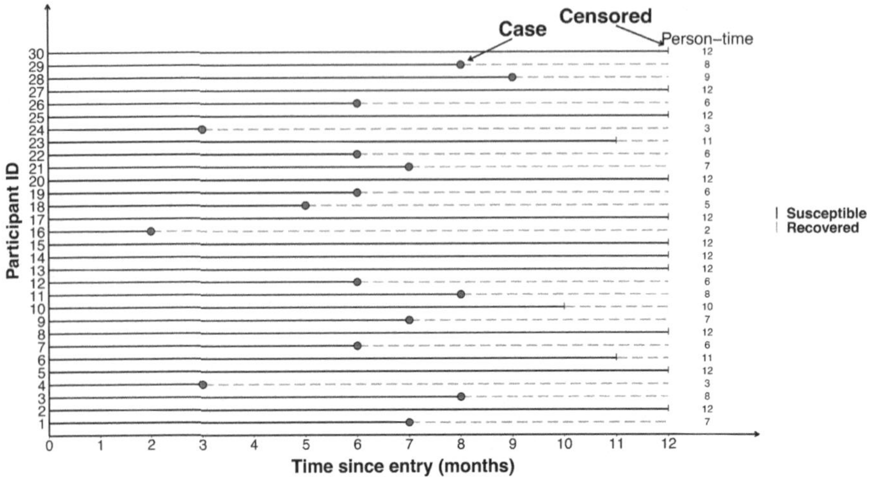

(a) *30 participants followed up for an infectious disease for 12 months 261 total person-months (or 21.75 total person-years).*

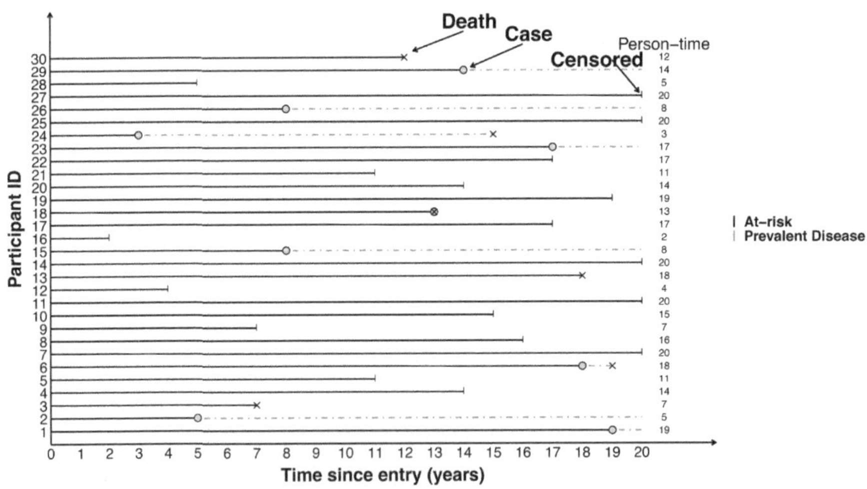

(b) *30 participants followed up for a chronic disease for 20 years 394 total person-years at risk.*

FIGURE 1.1: *Simulated infectious disease and chronic disease cohorts followed up over time.*

1.1.2 Incidence

The **incidence** of a disease is a measure of the *rate* at which the disease occurs. It describes the probability (or risk) that a person who is currently free of the disease will develop it in a specified time. Incidence is often reported as the number of new cases per 100,000 persons per year, but for acute conditions such as winter flu, the number of new cases per 100 persons per day may be more appropriate. To calculate the incidence of a specific disease in a given time period, we need to know the number of new cases diagnosed during the period, as well as the number of persons in the population who could have developed the disease during that period, whom we refer to as the 'population at risk' .

$$\text{incidence} = \frac{\text{number of new cases in a specified time period}}{\text{population at risk}} \times 100000$$

In the example of an infectious disease in Figure 1.1a, let us suppose that the disease confers immunity, so that individuals who get the disease and recover are not at risk of a second episode. In month 6, there are only 26 individuals at risk since the other 4 have recovered and are assumed immune. Thus, the incidence is $5/26 = 0.192$ per person-year, or 19.2 cases per 100 person-years .

Incidence is a measure routinely used by cancer registries around the world to report the annual rates of various types of cancer in the populations they cover . The overall and site-specific cancer incidence is usually reported as the number of new cases per 100,000 persons per year. For example, the Swedish Childhood Cancer Foundation reported that between 1984 and 2010, the annual incidence of cancer in children (under 15 years) was 16.0 per 100,000 [72]. A reasonable interpretation of such a rate is that for every 100,000 children residing in the country and cancer-free at the start of any year, an average of 16 were diagnosed by the end of the year. Even if one could know the exact number of children (without cancer) in the population on Jan 1st, there are several other issues that complicate the seemingly-simple incidence rate: new children will be born into the population, and other children will reach 15 years of age and should no longer be considered either in the numerator (if they develop cancer) or in the child population in the denominator . There will also be changes in the population due to immigration, emigration and deaths. The usual method of computing an approximate incidence rate is to use the mid-year population count (or an estimate of this count) as the number of individuals at risk in the denominator, assuming that this is approximately equal to the total person-years accumulated during the year by all individuals.

A more precise measure of incidence called the **incidence density** or **person-time incidence rate** can be obtained if complete information is available over time for the status of each individual in the population being studied. In this situation, the exact time contributed by each individual can be calculated, so we do not need to assume a number of persons, all of whom contribute a full year (a 'person-year') to the denominator. This is illustrated for the small cohort of 30 individuals in Figure 1.1b, who are followed-up for 20 years for the occurrence of a chronic disease. The number of person-years contributed by each individual varies, ranging from just 2 years for participant 16, whose disease status is unknown after that time (i.e. they are 'censored') , to the entire 20 years follow-up contributed by a few participants, who are censored at the end of the study period. The other participants contribute to the person-time as long as they are 'at risk' , i.e. free of disease and under observation. The total person-time from all 30 individuals is 394 person-years, and so the 9 cases occurring during this time represent an incidence of $(9/394) * 100 = 2.28$ cases per 100 person-years.

A quantity related to incidence is the proportion of disease-free individuals who develop the disease at *any* time during a specified follow-up. This is not a rate, but a simple proportion called the **cumulative incidence**, or occasionally the **incidence proportion**. In the illustration in Figure 1.1a, the cumulative incidence of the infectious disease is $16/30 = 53.3\%$ for the 12-month period, but in the period after month 6, it is $7/21$ as the recovered (and assumed immune) individuals in the population are no longer at risk. As mentioned above, any proportion can be reported as an odds, so in this case, the incidence odds and cumulative odds are $16/14$ and $7/14$, respectively. For the chronic disease scenario depicted in Figure 1.1b, the interpretation of cumulative risk over the 20-year period is complicated by the many individuals who are lost to follow-up due to censoring or death. For such settings, the cumulative incidence is only meaningful over a shorter time interval, and a more meaningful representation of the occurrence over the entire follow-up would be provided by the incidence.

The concept of incidence rate in a shorter time-interval is central to another important measure of risk known as the **hazard rate** or **instantaneous incidence rate** . The hazard rate of a disease is the risk that a person who is disease-free prior to a specific time t will develop the disease at that time (or to be more realistic, in the next instant, which is sometimes stated as 'in the time between t and $t + \delta t$' where δt is an infinitesimally small increment of time). To provide a clear definition, it is useful to introduce some simple notation. We will denote the disease outcome of interest as Y, and define $Y = 1$ as disease and $Y = 0$ as non-disease, and the status of a specific individual i with respect to the outcome at time t as $Y_i(t)$. Thus in Figure 1.1b, individual 2 would be described as:

$$Y_2(t) = 0 \quad \text{for} \quad t < 5$$
$$Y_2(5) = 1$$

For the simple scenario in Figure 1.1b, the hazard rate at 5 years is the probability that an individual who is still at risk *just before* 5 years becomes a case at the 5-year time point, which is 1/27: note that only 27 of 30 participants in that example are still at risk at 5 years. Of course, this example would be more accurately referred to as an *instantaneous* incidence rate if instead of the large time increments (one year) we had the exact dates of events to enable a representation of the daily risk. However, it is not uncommon to work with data that has recorded cruder time intervals, either for logistical convenience or to ensure the anonymity of the individuals in the study.

In the following definition, we will assume that the exact times of events in the study population are recorded. For a dichotomous outcome Y, defined as above, the hazard rate at a specific time t_e is:

$$h(t_e) = \text{probability}(Y(t_e) = 1|Y(t) = 0 \text{ for } t \leq t_e)$$

which is the probability of the event at time t_e for an individual who has not had the event before t_e.

1.1.3 Relative measures of disease occurrence: risks and ratios

Much of epidemiological research is concerned not only with the distribution of disease but with the determinants, commonly referred to as 'risk factors' or 'exposures' . A simple measure of the impact of a suspected risk factor for a disease can be obtained by comparing the prevalence or incidence of the disease in those exposed and unexposed to the factor. If a simple proportion is compared, such as the prevalence or cumulative incidence in the two groups, the ratio is called a **relative risk**, while a comparison of the odds or cumulative odds in the two groups is an **odds ratio**. Likewise, the ratio between the incidence rate in two groups is an

incident rate ratio, and a comparison of hazard rates is a **hazard ratio**. In the medical literature, any of these ratios might be loosely called a **relative risk**, and they are often understood to be a ratio of two risks (i.e. proportions), which has an intuitive appeal. When the disease under investigation is rare, referring to (and understanding) an odds ratio as a relative risk is only a matter of semantics, as the two quantities are very similar in magnitude: when most individuals in the population do not have the disease, then it makes little difference whether one expresses the number of individuals with the disease relative to the total population (risk) or relative to the number without the disease (odds). It is generally accepted that for a prevalence of 10% or lower, one can interpret the odds ratio as a relative risk. However, since the odds ratio is more frequently reported from epidemiological investigations (for reasons that will become clear in subsequent chapters), it is important to recognise how it differs from the relative risk when the disease is not rare. Since the odds ratio uses the number of non-diseased individuals in the denominator, it is larger than the relative risk (which uses the total population), and this difference in the two measures will be greater for diseases with higher prevalence [180].

A close reading of the study methods in a scientific report should make it clear if a simple proportion was estimated in each of the groups, and if not, which risk measure was compared. If the authors have compared two groups of individuals for the prevalence or cumulative incidence of disease, then the ratio of these simple proportions is rightly called a relative risk. However, for a study where the two groups have been followed over time and their contributed person-years recorded, a comparison of incidence rates will likely be of primary interest: whether an incidence rate ratio or hazard ratio is presented depends on how the authors chose to analyse and interpret their data. If the study compared a group of patients with a disease to a group without the disease and determined the proportions in these two groups that have been exposed to some risk factor, then it is clear that these proportions are not the risks of interest since they represent the prevalence of exposure (among diseased and non-diseased), not of disease (among exposed and unexposed). However, if instead of proportion, the odds is used to describe how common the exposure is among the diseased and non-diseased, then the odds ratio provides a meaningful comparison since the odds ratio of exposure in the diseased and non-diseased persons is equivalent to the odds ratio of disease in the exposed and unexposed persons. This can be made clear by a simple example.

The Physicians' Health Study [170] was conducted in the 1980s to investigate the potential benefit of low-dose aspirin for the prevention of cardiovascular disease. Approximately 22,000 male physicians between the ages of 40 and 84, who had no history of stroke or myocardial infarction (MI), agreed to be randomised to low-dose aspirin or placebo. After 5 years of follow-up [170], the risk of MI in the two groups was compared:

The cumulative risk of MI in the placebo group was $189/11{,}034 = .01713$, while in the aspirin group the risk was $104/11{,}037 = .00942$. Thus, the individuals taking placebo had almost twice the risk (relative risk $= .01713/.00942 = 1.818$) of having an MI at some time during the 5-year follow-up, or equivalently, the individuals taking aspirin had approximately half the risk (relative risk $= .00942/.01713 = 0.5499$) of those taking placebo.

The occurrence of MI in the two groups could also be compared using the odds ratio, which we would expect to be very similar to the relative risk as the disease is rare: the odds of MI was $104/10933$ in the aspirin group and $189/10845$ in the placebo group, yielding an odds ratio of $(104/10933)/(189/10845) = 0.5458$. If the investigators instead chose to compare the odds of aspirin exposure between MI cases and non-cases, then the ratio of the odds of exposure to aspirin in the MI cases compared to non-cases is: $(104/189)/(10933/10845) = 0.5458$, exactly as before. Thus, we can compare individuals with and without a disease outcome (in this example, MI) for their exposure *prior to the disease*, and from this comparison obtain the same odds ratio as would be obtained from comparing the exposed and unexposed group for their disease occurrence during follow-up. Thus, epidemiological investigators can use a *retrospective* comparison to address a question concerning *prospective* disease risk since the odds ratios are identical. Furthermore, if the disease is rare, the retrospective odds ratio will be of similar magnitude to the relative risk that would have been obtained from the prospective data so that one obtains not just a valid (prospective) odds ratio but a good estimate of the (prospective) relative risk. These simple properties of the odds ratio have led to numerous important developments in the design and analysis of epidemiological studies, many of which are part of standard research practice. Thus, a clear understanding of what the odds ratio measures and its relationship to other measures of relative risk is a fundamental component of epidemiological literacy and will be discussed in detail in the subsequent sections of this chapter.

1.2 Study Population, Study Base

In the words of Miettinen [147], an epidemiological design is 'a vision of the end product of a study on one hand and a scheme for carrying out a study on the other'. Estimates of disease occurrence or risk in a population are end products of an epidemiological study and the previous sections discussed various measures of these, such as prevalence, incidence and relative risk. If data are available for the entire population, then the 'scheme' for carrying out a study involves how these data are analysed to provide estimates of the health experience of the population that are valid and meaningful. However, in many research studies, only a sample of selected individuals are available, and these are assumed to represent the general background population of interest. In such studies, the 'scheme' involves how the subjects are sampled (the sampling design) and how the collected data are analysed, in order for the generalisations to be valid. In other words, the estimates of disease occurrence or risk obtained from the sampled individuals should provide valid estimates of these measures in the population from which the sample was drawn.

It is worth distinguishing here between the population of interest to the researcher (the **target population**) and the population from which the study subjects are actually selected (the **study population**). Occasionally these could be the same, but typically they will differ due to logistical and practical constraints. For example, in a study of the prognosis in patients undergoing a specific surgical procedure, the target population consists of all such patients (or at least those in the researcher's country). However, if the conduct of the study involves the review of non-computerised patient records (such as scans, patient charts, clinician notes or other documents) it may be much more efficient to conduct the study in a few larger hospitals or even in the researcher's own hospital. If the study population is representative of the target population so that the findings can be generalised to the (wider) target population, we say that the study has 'external validity' . Randomised clinical trials provide some extreme examples of the difference between target and study populations: inclusion and exclusion criteria may limit the participants in the trial to a much narrower group than those for whom the intervention or drug is ultimately intended. For this reason, many drugs found to be effective in a clinical trial are subject to post-marketing surveillance in order to assess the risk of adverse effects in the total population of users.

There are a number of useful terms for describing a study population, whether it is to be studied in its entirety or a sample selected. For a **closed population**, once membership is defined, no new members enter, and all individuals identified as belonging to the population contribute to the description of any characteristic of the population. Such populations are common in national registers, such as the population of all individuals recorded in the most recent census, the population of all persons on the electoral register on voting day, or the population of 'millennium' infants (born in the year 2000) in a specific country. For a closed population, prevalence is readily calculated provided information is available on the health indicator of interest. However, a measure of incidence can only be obtained if there is some follow-up of the population so that the experience over time can be quantified, as illustrated in the simple examples in Figure 1.1.

Although a closed population is simplest to imagine, it is likely that most people associate the word *population* with a real, geographic population that changes over time as individuals are born into the population, immigrate, emigrate or die. In contrast to the closed population, the members of this **open** or **dynamic population** are not always the same individuals but can change over time. For example, the cancer registers maintained by many countries around the world publish annual reports of cancer in their (dynamic) populations. While the number of persons diagnosed with cancer in a given year will be explicitly recorded, the number of individuals in the population is estimated as the mid-year count or the average of the population at the beginning and end of the year. The total number of person-days lived by members of the population is simply this estimated number multiplied by 365, equivalent to a constant number of persons actually present in the population each day for the entire year. This provides the total person-time that is required for the computation of incidence. Further details are provided in an expository paper by Vandenbroucke and Pearce [221]. The ability to estimate incidence in an open population is important since it enables real populations to be compared for their disease occurrence.

Since the focus of an epidemiological investigation is the health experience of the study population over the time period of the study, the term **study base** is sometimes used to distinguish this concept from the usual understanding of the term *population* as simply a specific group of individuals. For example, the population of women with a diagnosis of breast cancer recorded in the Stockholm cancer register from 1976 to 2008 were studied for two outcomes subsequent to their initial diagnosis: contralateral breast cancer (i.e. a new breast cancer in the opposite breast) and metastases [48]. Thus the background population consists of all breast cancer patients registered in the region during a 32-year period. The study base for the investigation of contralateral breast cancer consisted of the follow-up (hospitalisations, outpatient visits, cause of death register) of these women from the time of their initial diagnosis and treatment to the diagnosis of contralateral breast cancer or the end of 2008. However, for the metastases study, only the women with an initial diagnosis between 1997 and 2005 were followed for subsequent metastases, so the study base in this setting consisted of the follow-up of women from the time of their initial breast cancer diagnosis (from 1997) to a diagnosis of metastases or the end of 2005. This study base included a wide range of person-times, from at most nine years to perhaps some days. In contrast, the study base for the contralateral study included not only more individuals from the population (those diagnosed from 1976 to 1996 and from 2006 to 2008), together with their experience following diagnosis, but also more person-time for those diagnosed between 1997 and 2005.

1.2.1 Primary and secondary study base

In the discussion above, we are implicitly assuming a well-defined study base where the health events of individuals, such as hospitalisations, outpatient visits or other health-care contacts, are recorded and accessible to an investigator. In such a setting, where one can first define the study base and subsequently identify events such as disease or death in those individuals, the target population or study base is referred to as *primary*. Such is the case for studies conducted using electronic registers, as the total regional, national, or patient population registered during the study period constitutes the primary study base, and the occurrence of disease among these individuals can be described. In contrast, a 'case-referent' epidemiological study begins by identifying cases of a disease of interest, for example in a hospital or clinic. The background population whose disease experience is represented by these cases is then called a *secondary* study base since its definition depends on how the cases were ascertained, and this is the study base that should be represented by the controls selected for a case-control study. In a hospital-based study, the most general and accurate description of the secondary study base is the population of individuals who, had they developed the disease in question, would have been among the cases identified for the study. In other words, the secondary study base should include all those individuals at risk of the disease and whose diagnosis would be captured by the hospital. In practice, the exact secondary study base might be very difficult to describe, and various simplifications are used, such as the population resident in the catchment area of the hospital.

1.3 Sampling Designs

Once the study population has been decided, the focus of epidemiological research is some measure of health or disease in this population. This may be a population in the usual sense of the word (for example, all persons residing in a specific geographic area) but could also be some well-defined cohort of individuals, such as patients with a specific diagnosis or who have undergone a medical procedure and are being actively followed up. The availability of national registers of populations and their health events, such as the Swedish population databases maintained by Statistics Sweden (`https://scb.se/en/`), the health registers maintained by the National Board of Health and Welfare (`https://www.socialstyrelsen.se/en/`) and the 'quality registers' of patient groups (`https://skr.se/en/kvalitetsregister/forskning.43894.html`) enable the investigation of health in an entire population of individuals or patients, provided the data sources have recorded all details of interest to the researcher. However, when there are no suitable registers available, or the information is inadequate, a sample of individuals is selected from the study population, and the results from this study sample are used to make generalisations about the population. For these generalisations to be valid, it is important that the sample provides a valid representation of the population. There are various prescribed ways of choosing a representative sample for an epidemiological study, which will be presented in the following sections. These all have a common objective: the estimation of some measure of health or disease in the underlying population. The appropriate sampling design will depend on the measure (i.e. *parameter*) of interest.

1.3.1 Cross-sectional study (survey)

To estimate a prevalence, or any proportion, in a well-defined population at a specified time point, the study sample consists of a selection of the individuals in the population at that time, from whom information is gathered by means of interviews, postal or electronic questionnaires, or other internet tools. This is known as survey sampling or cross-sectional sampling, and Figure 1.2 represents such a sample taken from a population at present ('right now'). The simplest and most easily understood sampling scheme is random sampling, where each individual in the population has an equal chance of being selected. This is intuitively 'fair' and is the method used to choose the winner in a national lottery or to ascertain the voting preferences in a population prior to an election. But for an epidemiological study, it is common to select random samples from each of a number of categories of individuals (called *strata*), in order to ensure that all these groups are represented. The most familiar example is random sampling stratified on sex and further stratified on age group, to overcome any imbalances in the population. While such sampling allows estimation of sex- and age-specific characteristics, it can be very inefficient if the purpose is to study the effect of a rare exposure on disease risk in the population: the sample of individuals may yield very few (or no) exposed persons. In this case, if it is possible to identify the exposed and unexposed individuals in the population (for example, an environmental exposure associated with area of residence or type of job), then the problem of low prevalence of the exposure could be overcome by a simple modification to the sampling, where an equal number of exposed and unexposed persons are (randomly) sampled.

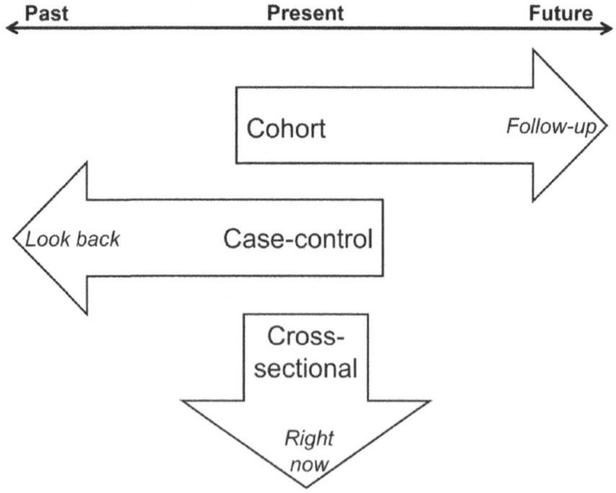

FIGURE 1.2: *Diagram of study designs.*

1.3.2 Cohort study

If the population parameter of interest is an incidence rate, then the experience of the population over time is required. Where the individuals in the population are followed up in national registers, then the required information may be readily available electronically. However, in the absence of such resources, the population, or a representative sample from it, needs to be followed up in real time for the outcome(s) of interest. For example, if the 'Child of the New Century' (https://childnc.net/about/) study had enrolled all infants born in the UK in 2000 - 2001, then this would constitute a closed population of all children born in the millennium year. However, the study follows the lives of approximately 19,000 individuals, and is known to epidemiologists as the Millennium Cohort Study [231].

In contrast to a cross-sectional study, which provides a snapshot of a population at a given time point, a cohort study is more like a video recording, as it identifies individuals and follows them over time for their health outcomes (see Figure 1.2). There are several well-known large cohort studies conducted from the mid-1900s that have established the place of epidemiology in medical research, especially public health. The British Doctors Study investigated the effect of smoking on lung cancer at a time when smoking was not considered to have any ill effects on health. All doctors in Britain were contacted in 1951 and the cohort of more than 40,000 respondents provided information at first contact and at six further time points, the last in 2001. As early as 1956, the study demonstrated the now well-known link between smoking and lung cancer [53]. The Framingham Heart Study [139], which began in 1948 with the enrolment and follow-up of approximately 5000 residents of the town of Framingham, Massachusetts, has led to numerous scientific publications, many of which report lifestyle and environmental factors related to cardiovascular disease that are commonly accepted today: smoking, blood pressure, cholesterol, diet, exercise. This study is not only the source of the cardiovascular risk score known as the 'Framingham risk score', but was the first study to use the term *risk factor*. Cardiovascular disease was also one of the outcomes of interest in the Nurses Health Study, which enrolled more than 120,000 nurses from around the US in 1976, with breast cancer as the primary outcome of interest. While this cohort study had many impacts on public health [38], it has also generated some controversy with an early publication reporting a protective effect of hormone therapy on cardiovascular disease risk [202] that was not supported by randomised clinical trials or other cohort studies. Similarly, the conclusion after 10 years follow-up of the cohort, that oral contraceptives conferred no increased risk of breast cancer, was also premature, with a recent publication reporting an association between exogenous hormones and breast cancer [13].

Since those early pioneering studies, cohort studies are widely used in epidemiological research and a recent initiative by the International Journal of Epidemiology encourages investigators to publish a 'Cohort Profile' as a means of stimulating better use of these valuable data resources. One recent cohort study that deserves special mention is the UK Biobank, which enrolled approximately half a million participants from 2006-2010, obtaining not only questionnaire data, but blood and urine specimens that were stored for later laboratory analysis, including genetic measurements. Health researchers can apply for access to the database, and this cohort has had an enormous impact on medical research, particularly in the field of genetics [206].

1.3.3 Case-control study

A common approach to investigating risk factors for a rare disease is to compare cases of the disease to 'control' individuals who do not have the disease. This design may be implemented in either a prevalence or incidence study, sampling some or all of the prevalent or incident cases and comparing them with a sample of the non-cases. Thus, the sampling strategy differs from that of the cross-sectional or cohort approach, where a random sample, perhaps stratified, is selected or followed over time, and cases in the sample identified. In the case-control study, the cases and controls are first selected, and then information is gathered on characteristics that may be associated with the disease. In contrast to the cohort design, the case-control design focuses on characteristics that are known at the time of sampling, such as prior exposures or medical history, and so is referred to as a *retrospective* design (see Figure 1.2). The idea of looking retrospectively for clues to current disease in a patient seems natural and logical, and even at the time of Hippocrates (300 - 400 BC) was common [190], but comparison of the patient's history with that of a control group appeared only in the last 100 - 200 years. As early as 1843, the association between occupation and pulmonary disease was investigated by comparing the occupations (i.e. the exposure) of men with pulmonary disease to men with other diseases [73], but the first publication of a case-control study is believed to be the paper by the remarkable physician-epidemiologist, Janet Lane-Claypon in 1926, where she compared 500 women with breast cancer to 500 controls who were free of breast cancer [112]. This ground-breaking study identified risk factors for breast cancer that are still considered in risk scores today, such as childlessness, older maternal age and breastfeeding. These and other historic studies were described by Breslow in his Fisher lecture in 1996 [21].

The efficiency of the case-control design has strong intuitive appeal. It seems wise to ensure that sufficient patients with the disease of interest are studied, and such 'cases' present themselves to the clinical researcher. In case-control studies of rare diseases, it is common for investigators to include all possible cases. Since the cases will almost always be a small proportion of the population, it is sufficient to compare them with a subset of the (many) non-cases. If a specific exposure or characteristic is found in a larger proportion of the cases than the controls, this would suggest that the exposure is a risk factor. However, these are not the proportions of real interest, since to compute the relative risk of disease in exposed compared to unexposed persons, we would need the proportions of diseased persons among the exposed and unexposed. We have seen earlier in this chapter that if we focus on odds rather than risk, then the odds ratio of disease in exposed versus unexposed persons can be obtained from case-control data as it is the same as the odds ratio of exposure in diseased versus non-diseased persons, i.e. in cases versus controls. Furthermore, if the disease is rare, as is often the case in case-control studies, the odds ratio will be close to the relative risk.

Selecting controls

The classic case-control design selects cases that accrue over a given time and subsequently identifies 'control' individuals who were not diagnosed with the disease of interest during the same time interval. As a simple example, a case-control study of SIDS (sudden infant death syndrome, also known as 'cot death') would compare infants who died of SIDS during their first year to a random sample of control infants chosen from all those who were alive on their first birthday. In a clinical case-control study of cancer recurrence, an investigator may define as cases all the patients whose cancer recurred within five years of their initial diagnosis, so that the comparison group would consist of individuals who were still free from a recurrence after five years. This way of choosing controls is called **exclusive sampling** (also known as cumulative incidence

Example 1.1. *Illustration of relative risk and odds ratio of disease during follow-up of a cohort of 10,000 exposed and 10,000 unexposed individuals.*

	Case: Yes	Case: No	
Exposed	4013	5987	10,000
Unexposed	956	9044	10,000
	4969	15,031	20,000

Compared to unexposed individuals, the relative risk of disease in the exposed group over the follow-up period is

$$\frac{4013}{10000} \div \frac{956}{10000} = 4.20$$

The odds ratio of disease in the exposed compared to unexposed individuals is, as expected, larger than the relative risk:

$$\frac{4013}{5987} \div \frac{956}{9044} = 6.34$$

This odds ratio is equivalent to the odds of exposure among cases relative to controls:

$$\frac{4013}{956} \div \frac{5987}{9044} = 6.34$$

sampling) since all those who become a case are excluded from being selected as a control. Example 1.1 provides an illustration of a cohort consisting of 10,000 exposed and 10,000 unexposed individuals, where during the follow-up, a total of 4013 cases were observed in the exposed group and 956 in the unexposed group.

Since the number of diseased individuals is typically (much) fewer than the number of non-diseased at the end of the study period, a classic case-control study does not compare the cases to all the non-cases, but to a random sample. In many research investigations, the controls are matched to the cases on some important characteristic(s), such as sex and age, but for now, we will assume the controls are a simple

TABLE 1.1: *Number of men with myocardial infarction (MI) among male physicians randomised to placebo or low-dose aspirin and followed up for five years. [170]*

	MI: Yes	MI: No	
Placebo	189	10,845	11,034
Aspirin	104	10,933	11,037

random sample with each individual having an equal probability of being selected. In Example 1.1, if all 4969 cases (exposed and unexposed) were to be compared to an equal number of controls sampled randomly from the 15,031 non-cases at the end of follow-up, then we would expect the proportion of exposure among these to be 5987/15031 and hence an odds of 5987/9044. Thus we would expect to get the same odds ratio for our comparison of 4969 cases and 4969 controls as that obtained from the whole cohort. While this is what we expect from conducting such a study within the cohort, the actual numbers that would be observed would vary from these values due to the random sampling of controls. This sampling variation will be smaller for larger sample sizes, so the ratio of controls to cases is often greater than the 1:1 in this example. However, it is rarely more than 5:1 as it has been shown that there is little gain in sampling more.

The simple example presented in the previous paragraph is sometimes referred to as a 'classic' case-control study, where cases are accrued over some time period and the controls are selected by exclusive sampling from those who are still non-cases at the end of follow-up. This design provides a 'clean' comparison that has the advantage of being intuitively appealing and easy to communicate; however, the only estimate of risk available from such data is an odds ratio. For rare diseases, the odds ratio will approximate the relative risk that would have been obtained by conducting a prospective cohort study instead of a case-control study, as can be verified for the Physicians' Health Study data in Table 1.1 where the odds ratio for placebo vs. aspirin is 1.832 and the relative risk is 1.818. But in Example 1.1 above, the disease is not rare (especially in the exposed), so the odds ratio was not a good approximation for the relative risk. However, there are alternative ways of sampling the controls that enable the computation of the relative risk, and even of the hazard ratio (instantaneous relative risk). If the 4969 cases in the example were compared to a random sample of 5000 individuals selected by **inclusive sampling**, then we would expect these controls to consist of 2500 exposed and 2500 unexposed individuals, i.e. to have an odds of 2500/2500=1 of exposure, so that the odds ratio would equal the relative risk:

$$\frac{4013}{956} \div 1 = 4.2$$

An alternative sampling design that is commonly used (for reasons that will become clear) is **concurrent sampling** (also known as incidence density sampling or risk set sampling), where the controls are selected from the population of non-cases at the same time (e.g. in the same year) as the case(s) occurred. We will see in later chapters that the odds ratio from this sampling design provides an estimate of the incidence rate ratio or hazard ratio without the need for the follow-up times of the individuals. This property underlies the importance of this sampling design in epidemiology, which is commonly referred to as the **nested case-control study** .

The extensions of the simple/classic case-control design that use inclusive or concurrent sampling are commonly known as the case-cohort design and nested case-control design. The odds ratio from each of the three designs provides a different measure of disease risk. These designs and the estimates available are summarised in Table 1.2.

1.3.4 Comparison of cohort and case-control design

The efficiency of the case-control design for studying rare diseases is well-recognised. Compared to a cohort study, it requires comparatively few subjects, and this advantage underlies its wide adoption in medical research where a single disease outcome (which defines a 'case') is of primary interest. The design allows the investigator to collect information on multiple exposures to determine their association with the disease. However, if there is a single exposure of primary interest, a cohort study that compares exposed and unexposed individuals is more efficient, especially if the exposure is rare. The cohort design has the advantage of enabling multiple outcomes to be studied, provided the necessary information is recorded during follow-up, but any exposures of interest need to be collected at baseline and/or subsequent time points. Other advantages and disadvantages of case-control studies and cohort studies commonly discussed in introductory textbooks are summarised below.

Differences in	Cohort Studies	Case-control Studies
Time and Cost	Follow participants over time, which not only delays the answer to the research question but can be very costly	Identify participants and gather data at a single time point; existing data resources can be used.
Temporal Order	Can establish a clear temporal order between exposure and outcome, one of criteria [18] supporting 'causal' exposure	May be difficult to establish time order: imperfect memory of subjects; sub-clinical disease contributing to the exposure
Loss to Follow-up	Cohort members may lose interest over time, move from study area, or die, resulting in reduced sample size and possible bias	Validity is assured at the time of enrolment if cases and non-cases are representative of the population and the data are unbiased
Exposure	Changes in habits over follow-up time may create difficulties in describing the effect of exposure on outcome	Investigators can define meaningful measures of prior exposure (level, duration, recency)
Incidence	Allow direct measurement of disease incidence, both overall and in the exposed and unexposed persons	Do not allow direct calculation of incidence; odds ratio can estimate relative risk (depends on sampling design)

1.4 Sources of Bias

Unlike randomised controlled trials which investigate an intervention in a carefully chosen group of volunteers, the purpose of an observational study is to observe some real-world population, with all its imperfections, and thus the potential for bias at every stage of the study from design to final reporting. A thorough presentation of sources of bias

TABLE 1.2: *Extended case-control designs with their corresponding sampling strategies, sampling time-frame and what the odds ratio estimates.*

Design	Sampling Strategy	When to Sample	Odds Ratio is an estimate of:
Classic case-control	**Exclusive sampling** Cumulative incidence sampling	End of follow-up	Incidence OR (≈ RR, IRR for 'rare diseases')
Case-cohort	**Inclusive sampling**	Beginning of follow-up	RR
Nested case-control	**Concurrent sampling** Incidence density sampling Risk-set sampling	Through-out follow-up	IRR

OR = Odds Ratio; RR = Relative Risk; IRR = Incident Rate Ratio

and suggested remedies is available in Chapter 6 of the methodological guide of the European Network of Centres for Pharmacoepidemiology and Pharmacovigilance [59].

1.4.1 Sampling bias

The individuals selected as the study participants may not be representative of the target population, which is referred to as **sampling bias** or **observation bias**. This may be due to incomplete knowledge of the population from which the sample is drawn (i.e. the primary study base). Where a list or register of the population of interest is available, then it should be checked for its completeness and validity before using it as a sampling frame. Even where the data are of high quality, it will only be available from the time when recording began, so that earlier events will not be captured: the resulting bias from such incompleteness is known as truncation bias, often called left truncation bias. A well-recognised example in cancer epidemiology is pancreatic cancer, which is difficult to diagnose and has poor survival. As a result, cohort studies using national cancer registers of incident cases will underestimate the actual incidence in the population if the cause of death information is not included [134], and case-control studies that require contact with patients will also miss those who are too ill to participate.

In situations where the registration of the disease outcome is essentially complete for the years covered by the register, such as breast cancer diagnosis in Sweden [132], truncation bias can be avoided be restricting the study cohort to ages that are covered by the register. However, where the exposure under investigation is a health condition in the same individual or a family member, there is potential for truncation bias. For example, an investigation of the relative risk of breast cancer in women in Sweden with/without an affected mother will identify both the outcome (cancer diagnosis) and exposure (mother's cancer) using the national cancer register. The outcome will be essentially complete for the cohort of women who can be linked to their mothers using the Multi-Generation Register [56], as these were all born since 1932, and were at most 26 years old in 1958. However, the exposure (mother's cancer) is subject to truncation as diagnoses in mothers prior to the start-up of the cancer register in 1958 will have no record: the amount of such bias will depend on the extent of truncation, the pattern of disease risk with age, and the underlying relative risk [124, 123].

Perinatal epidemiology is particularly susceptible to truncation bias: the risks of adverse pregnancy outcomes estimated from national registers may be biased due to miscarriages that go unrecorded. In addition to failing to capture (very) early miscarriages, national birth registers typically do not register pregnancies/deliveries prior to a specified cut-off gestational age. For example, in Sweden, only pregnancies that proceed to at least week 22 of gestation are currently registered, with a 28 week cut-off used prior to July 2008 [60]. A recent article and commentary in *Epidemiology* proposed that such truncation bias may underlie the long-debated counter-intuitive protective effect of smoking on preeclampsia, suggesting bias from a higher risk of miscarriage in smoking mothers [130].

Another source of sampling bias that can arise, even where the sampling frame is accurate, is the lack of care in selecting a truly random sample. Hospital-based case-control studies that select a subsample of all cases are particularly vulnerable to sampling bias from the choice of cases to be included. For example, an investigator may trust their judgement that selecting an easy, haphazard sample of cases in their practice is no worse than undertaking the careful steps that yield a random sample where all individuals in the study base have an equal chance of being selected. A more serious situation arises with **convenience sampling**, where an investigator simply makes use of easily-accessible cases or records. The appropriate choice of controls for a case-control study can be challenging, especially for case-referent studies where it can be difficult, or even impossible, to define and enumerate the secondary study base from which the controls should be selected. This has been widely discussed since the 1980s by eminent epidemiologists and biostatisticians [20, 148, 223, 224].

Studies conducted on individuals presenting for clinical care are prone to a specific type of sampling/selection bias, known as **Berkson bias** [229], if both the exposure and the outcome (and thus the association between them) influence an individual's attendance at the clinic or other facility where the study is being carried out. This bias was first recognised by the physician Joseph Berkson in 1946 [12], when he described how the choice of controls in a hospital-based study of a prevalent disease could lead to a spurious association, if the exposure being studies is another disease or condition associated with hospitalisation. Known as *Berkson's fallacy*, this is subject to ongoing debate [198], but is unlikely to have contributed to many reports of biased findings, since most case-control studies are of incident cases and it is rare for the primary exposure of interest to be another disease.

1.4.2 Response bias

The potential for bias in the study sample does not end once a representative sample of the population has been successfully identified: some of the individuals invited to participate in the study may decline, and those who are willing and ultimately enrolled may no longer be representative of the intended target population. The term **response bias** is used to refer to this contribution to the lack of representativeness of the study sample, as it is a consequence of the response of those contacted. Such bias has been well-recognised in survey sampling, with a dramatic example in 1936 when a poll of more than two million individuals conducted by the Literary Digest in the US predicted that Alf Landon would win the presidential election: 57% of the approximately two million respondents stated that they would vote for Landon, but he received only 36.5% of the popular vote. This famously bad prediction was based on data that was subject to both sampling bias and response bias [201]: the individuals contacted for the survey were readers of Literary Digest, registered car owners or listed telephone users, a sampling frame that did not represent the majority of voters in 1936; ten million participants were contacted, so the 2.4 million responses represent the minority who cared enough to participate and there was a clear danger of response bias. While we may be tempted to ridicule the obvious statistical blunders of this historic survey, current scientific methods failed to predict the results of the Brexit referendum in the UK and the presidency of Donald Trump in the US, and there is widespread publication today of unscientific results from internet surveys and 'satisfaction' buttons such as when passing through airport security!

1.4.3 Measurement bias (information bias)

Given that the investigators have succeeded in enrolling a representative sample of exposed and unexposed persons in a cohort study, or cases and controls in a case-control study, the subsequent collection of information through interviews, questionnaires, or direct measurement of participant characteristics may be subject to bias from several sources. For example, the differing perceptions of patients with a disease compared to healthy controls when asked to respond to questions about their physical and mental well-being, and the different level of alertness in a study clinician conducting a clinical examination of an individuals known to be a case. Randomised trials are often designed to eliminate, or at least minimise, some or all of this **measurement bias**: in placebo-controlled trials, the participants are randomly assigned to an active intervention or a placebo (an inactive/harmless substance) that are prepared to be indistinguishable, and where there is thought to be a risk of measurement bias due to the clinical investigators, they too are 'blinded' and so do not know which treatment an individual has been assigned. This type of trial is known as 'double-blind' and there is also a 'triple-blind' variation, where the data analyst does not know the treatment assignment but works with an uninformative group label (e.g. 'A' and 'B'), lest they be biased in their approach to the analysis or interpretation of results.

In contrast to randomised clinical trials, participants in observational studies will know their status with respect to exposure (in cohort studies) or disease (in case-control studies) so that the potential for measurement bias in their responses can be a serious concern. Blinding the clinical or research staff when assessing or interviewing the participants could reduce measurement bias, especially in a case-control study, but this would present major practical and logistical challenges. A particular form of measurement bias to which the case-control design is susceptible is **recall bias**. This is the term used to describe the tendency for those affected by disease to remember adverse events or exposures in their past in their attempt to explain their misfortune.

The examples discussed in the preceding paragraph are all of *systematic* measurement error, where there is a tendency for the error to be in a specific direction: for example, for a case to recall more adverse exposures or be aware of more disease in their family, or for a study clinician to note fewer side-effects in a patient whom they know is taking a placebo. However, a measured exposure or outcome can also vary randomly (spuriously) with no overall tendency in either direction from the 'true value'. Where continuous variables with this **random measurement error** are used to define categorical variables, such as binary exposures and outcomes, this can result in **misclassification error** since it can result in an individual being classified in the wrong category.

The consequences of misclassification error in measures of association depends on whether it is the exposure or the outcome that is subject to misclassification, and on whether the misclassification has a different effect in different groups of individuals: where the misclassification of outcome is the same for exposed and unexposed individuals in a cohort study, or for the cases and controls in a case-control study, the error is described as **non-differential misclassification error**. Simple non-differential misclassification of the exposure in a cohort study where the outcome is not subject to measurement error, or the outcome in a case-control study where the exposure is not subject to measurement error, will result in the comparison of two groups that are more similar than the correctly classified groups and thus a dilution of the association: the relative risk or odds ratio will be biased towards 1.0 (no association). In a cohort study with no misclassification of the exposure status but non-differential misclassification of the outcome, the relative risk will have little or no bias but will have greater variability, so that a larger sample may be needed to see an effect. A similar situation arises in a case-control study with non-differential misclassification of the case status. A simple introduction to measurement error is provided in Chapter 4 of the BMJ online book 'Resources for Readers: Epidemiology for the Uninitiated' [35].

A discussion of random measurement error in continuous variables using illustrative graphics [91] provides a useful summary and intuitive interpretation that applies to any variables. Random measurement error in continuous variables is widely recognised and understood by medical researchers: for example, the blood pressure of an individual varies throughout the day, and even from one moment to another, so that a single measurement cannot be considered the 'true' value. Such *biological variation* is also manifest in the measurement of haemoglobin, cholesterol, or indeed any biomarker: the random variation in the biological material results in differences in two samples taken at different times, or at the same time, or even when the same sample is split in two. Where the exact same biological material is measured twice, and there is no reason to believe that the specimen can have altered, then there can still be random fluctuations due to the imperfection of the measuring instrument (or the operator!). The (small) random fluctuations due to the sensitivity of an instrument are referred to as *technical errors.* The fluctuations due to measurement error can be reduced by averaging several replications: for example, blood pressure monitors are designed to average three readings and many laboratory assays are conducted in duplicate, or more replicates if the result is to be used a reference. Another common example is the measurement of 'dietary intake', which is conducted using average amounts from a '24-hour recall' or from a food frequency questionnaire (FFQ) that the respondent completes over the course of a week. Given that the 'true' intake of foodstuffs, or food components, is notoriously hard to measure, it is no surprise that nutritional epidemiology is the focus of much of the published work on measurement error bias in epidemiology. Where repeated measurements of an exposure are available, there are statistical methods available for correcting for measurement error [100].

An appreciation of measurement error bias, even for the simple situations presented here, can encourage better design of epidemiological studies and more careful data analysis. In real applications, the nature and consequences of measurement error can be complex. For example, the measurement error in the outcome of a cohort study may be different for exposed and non-exposed individuals, or in a case-control study, the measurement error in the exposure may be different in cases and controls: these situations are referred to as *differential measurement errors* or in the case of categorical outcomes and exposures, *differential misclassification.* In such settings, the bias resulting from the measurement error is more complex, depending on a number of factors including the magnitude of the error and the extent by which it differs in the different groups. Even where measurement error is non-differential, the simple effect on bias for a single binary exposure (or outcome) does not generalise to an exposure variable with more than two categories: this can be understood intuitively when we consider that the misclassification will influence the reference category, resulting in a change in odds ratios for other categories, which could lead to a true trend becoming undetectable or a false trend being observed. Effects of measurement error on bias also becomes much more complex if more than one measurement in the study is affected.

1.4.4 Time-related bias

Time-related biases receive much less attention than the biases discussed above, but with the widespread use of analysis methods involving time, the potential for such biases needs to be considered carefully. These types of bias arise due to incorrect definition and/or analysis methods for an exposure or outcome with respect to time [59]. A simple example is the **time-window bias** that arises in case-control studies if cases and controls have their exposure ascertained from different time windows [209]: for example, if cases have their exposure assessed over a longer time-window than controls, the odds ratio for the effect of exposure on the disease outcome will be exaggerated. Another type of time-related bias is **truncation bias**, which results from ignoring left truncation. Returning to the familial breast cancer example from section 1.4.1 and assuming all mothers who have no recorded breast cancer to be cancer-free, then the relative risk for their respective daughters would be underestimated. Truncation bias due to the start-up date of registration should always be considered in register-based studies, and the study population chosen to minimise the potential for such bias.

In cohort studies, where time is an integral part of the design, there are several types of time-dependent bias. Bias due to incorrect definition of the exposure period arises where subjects who become cases during the study period are assumed to have been exposed from the beginning of follow-up. An amusing pedagogic example provided by Sylvestre, Huszti and Hanley [212] is the erroneous claim that Oscar winners live 4 years longer than non-winners, a result that arises from an analysis that assumes that actors or actresses are born winners! On a more serious note, this kind of bias can lead to flawed conclusions in studying the benefit of an intervention, especially if there is a relatively long waiting time and the patients in need of the intervention have an increased mortality. The bias arises if the follow-up for an exposed individual includes time during which it is impossible for them to experience the outcome, and is referred to as **immortal time bias**. Kidney transplantation was used to provide a detailed illustrative example of this bias in a cohort study [78] and the bias in a case-control design has been illustrated in the re-analysis of data on the benefit of statins in treating lung cancer [209].

Other common terms for time-related biases that arise in cohort studies are **lead-time bias** and **length-time bias**. The 'lead-time' is the time between an early diagnosis (for example due to screening) and the time when the disease would have been diagnosed by routine clinical procedures. In the evaluation of the benefits of cancer screening, if individuals are followed from the time of diagnosis, there will be an apparent survival advantage for those screened, and correction of this lead-time bias is an important component of screening studies. Length-time bias, which is also a concern in screening studies, arises due to the slower-growing and/or less lethal tumours being more likely to be detected by screening, while a fast-growing or lethal tumour is more likely to result in symptoms, clinical diagnosis, and perhaps death, before the patient's screening appointment came due. A recent field in breast cancer epidemiology that is focused on understanding this issue is the study of 'interval breast cancer' [87], i.e. cancers arising between two screening appointments.

1.4.5 Confounding bias

Finally, if the study has managed to circumvent all the biases discussed so far, and a careful and correct data analysis has been conducted and an estimate of risk computed, this may be biased due to the presence of a **confounding** factor that went unrecognised by the investigators. A confounder is a variable that influences both the exposure and the disease, generating a misleading relationship between them so that the apparent effect of the exposure on the risk of disease is exaggerated or diluted (i.e. biased). As a simple example, an observational study of infants of HIV-positive mothers that finds a lower risk of diarrhoea in formula-fed infants than in breast-fed infants may conclude that formula protects infants from diarrhoea, but the educational level of the mother may be a confounder if better educated mothers tend to choose formula feeding and can also provide their infant with a more hygienic living environment. Examples of confounding abound in the medical and epidemiological literature and this important issue will be dealt with in detail in the following chapters, as the control of confounding is central to the design and analysis of *controlled* epidemiological studies.

1.5 Which Design?

Faced with a real question concerning prevalence, incidence or risk of a health outcome, the choice of study design will be dictated, not only by the primary measure of interest, but by issues such as feasibility, expediency, cost and other concerns. Thus, even where risk factors for a 'rare outcome' are to be identified, a case-control study may not provide the first clues (or the final evidence). Likewise, although the effect of a rare exposure on disease incidence can be quantified in a cohort study, the speed or feasibility of a cross-sectional or case-control study might be critical in the choice of an informative cohort. The different designs have contributed to many important discoveries that we take for granted today, with several fascinating examples presented in a special issue of the *Annals of Epidemiology* dedicated to the 'triumphs of epidemiology' [162].

Before there was any understanding of the role of folate in protecting against spina bifida, there had been several decades of simple descriptive epidemiological studies showing that this condition varied not only with maternal factors but also over time and place, suggesting that the maternal and physical environment were both important. This pointed the finger at nutritional factors, and although initial efforts to conduct a randomised trial of a multivitamin were thwarted, a large (non-randomised) trial showed a dramatic reduction in the risk of neural tube defects in infants born to mothers who took the multivitamin. Around the same time, a case-control study was conducted of Vietnam veterans, to investigate exposures that might help to explain their higher risk of having a child with birth defects, and vitamin intake was found to be associated with a halving of the risk. Finally, a cohort study was conducted where vitamin consumption was recorded early in pregnancy, thereby eliminating recall bias as the mother would not yet know whether or not she was carrying an affected child. All of these efforts, from descriptive to case-control to cohort, have together resulted in folic acid being added to staple foods in many countries, thereby preventing most cases of spina bifida and anencephaly and their tragic handicaps, deserving to be hailed as 'a modern miracle from epidemiology' [166].

The term 'sudden infant death syndrome' (SIDS) was first used in 1969 to describe the sudden death of an infant where no specific cause of death could be identified. Although there was an increase in the incidence in the following decades, clinical and laboratory investigations made no progress in identifying the cause. There had been very little epidemiological work, and none at all that followed up a cohort of infants from birth, which was not surprising as a very large cohort would be required to study such a rare condition. If a cohort of infants at higher risk could be identified, then a modest sample size could be used, which together with the short follow-up (12 months maximum or even 2-4 months, the peak event time) would result in cost- and time-efficient answers to the questions concerning risk factors. Using a scoring system, researchers in Tasmania conducted a cohort study in the late 1980s of infants considered to be at high risk, focusing on environmental factors, such a room temperature, prompted by the known higher incidence in winter and in cooler climates. Concurrent with this cohort study, a case-control study was also conducted in Tasmania, to obtain more detailed retrospective information for infants who died of SIDS, and case-control studies were also conducted in the UK and New Zealand. In the 20 years prior to this work, there had been reports of prone sleeping position being associated with the risk of SIDS, one of these from a case-control study in Northern Ireland, but these received little interest in the field, which was focused on finding more clinical explanations. Again, it was a clue from a simple descriptive study that changed the attitudes: ethnic Chinese babies in Hong Kong (who were normally placed supine to sleep) had much lower risk than infants of European immigrants to Hong Kong. This prompted intervention studies of sleeping position that demonstrated a protective effect of supine sleeping position. By the late 1980s, there were nine case-control studies all reporting the prone position to be a risk factor, but there was much concern about recall bias of the mothers who had lost their infant, especially as there was so much debate about sleeping position at that time. National interventions promoting supine position were launched in several countries, demonstrating dramatic reductions in SIDS: prone sleeping position was considered to be the causal factor in at least half of the deaths. The simple advice about sleeping position that emanated from all of this research effort has resulted in saving the lives of many infants around the world, and stands as a tribute to the power of epidemiological methods [54].

Current awareness of the toxic effect of lead is often focused on pollution from traffic and industry, but knowledge about the dangers of lead exposure for the human brain has been known for more than two thousand years: the Greek physician who treated Nero is reputed to have said 'lead makes the mind give way'. Initially considered a serious risk factor in exposed adults, such as miners, the harm of lead in children came under serious epidemiological investigation in the last 50 years. The evidence from earlier studies of children with cognitive problems was weak due to '1) small sample size; 2) inadequate attention to confounders; 3) possible selection bias; 4) insensitive outcome measures' [161]. All of these are issues that can be appreciated from the discussion in the previous sections, with the exception of 'confounders' which can be loosely defined as alternative explanations, and will be dealt with in detail in the next chapter.

Using the lead level in teeth as a proxy for the level in bone, investigators in Boston identified a small cross-sectional study of schoolchildren with high and low exposure to lead (54 and 100 children respectively) and found significantly poorer cognition levels of the highly-exposed children. Prompted by the knowledge that lead can cross the placenta, the same research group conducted a cohort study of more than 11,000 newborn children, gathering information on lead levels in the umbilical cord and in the child's blood at six follow-up times, from 6 months to 10 years age, finding significant adverse effects of lead levels on neurodevelopmental outcomes. Today, it is well accepted that lead is a silent danger to the developing brain, increasing risks of cognitive, memory and behavioural problems in children. Lead exposure has also been associated with deficits in IQ and verbal ability in adults. The epidemiological work in this field has 'triumphed' in the elimination of lead from petrol and paints, and should serve as an inspiration for researchers to scrutinise other potential toxins with the same fervour.

1.6 Electronic Data Resources

Much of the discussion above assumes traditional epidemiological studies conducted in real time that involve enrolling individuals 'now' and following them for many years into the future (in a cohort study) or determining their prior exposures (in a case-control study) as depicted in

Figure 1.2. The time saving of such a case-control study compared to a cohort study would be accompanied by considerable cost savings, since the data collection in the case-control study would typically involve a single contact with the study subjects, while the follow-up of individuals in a cohort study, and 'tracing' those lost, could involve significant efforts and costs over a long time period. However, with the electronic recording of populations and their health events in recent decades, the experience of a cohort may already be available in a database. The availability of population data for many years into the past, enables us to identify individuals 'back then' and 'follow' them over time until the latest time point for which the electronic data has been recorded. Hence we can study events and trends over time in a cohort without waiting for data to accumulate, so that time efficiency is no longer an issue in the choice of study design. The concerns about bias can also be much reduced if the quality of the electronic data is high. Given population data of high quality, the traditional 'pyramid of evidence', ranking the main study designs for the strength of their scientific evidence, is no longer appropriate [217, 157]: the strength of evidence depends on the validity of the design and analysis in addressing the research question, and not on the choice of design.

A cohort study that uses previously-recorded data is called a **retrospective cohort** study or **retrospective longitudinal** study. For case-control studies, electronic registers are a convenient way of identifying cases of a disease and perhaps also appropriate controls (depending on the population registers available). Where all the relevant to the research question is available in the electronic database, a cohort/incidence study is often considered to be the gold standard, although it can sometimes be easier to define the research question from a case-control perspective. If after identifying the study participants, the research question requires additional collection of material (such as biological specimens) or data, then the efficiency of the case-control design may have a dramatic impact on the total study cost. In the past, computational efficiency was an important advantage of the case-control design (especially for rare outcomes) but this is rarely an important consideration with the computing power that is now routinely available.

For health research, the value of any electronic register is greatly enhanced if it is possible to link it to other registers in the same population. This requires not only that data are gathered electronically, but that the records of any individual can be 'connected' by a unique identifier. The personal number assigned to all citizens and residents in the

Scandinavian countries [133] enables such 'data linkage' and is a major factor in the contribution of those countries to register-based epidemiology. For example, to study how a woman's long-term health depends on her reproductive history would require information about her pregnancies/deliveries from the birth register and her subsequent health events from hospital or other health-care registers.

The availability of the study population in an electronic database also overcomes many of the sources of bias outlined above, provided the database itself has a high level of completeness and quality. Electronic population registers also open up the possibility of sampling strategies other than the simple cross-sectional, cohort and case-control designs, that allow more flexible and efficient use of the data resources. Such designs will be introduced and compared in later chapters, and illustrations provided of their application to study disease occurrence or risk in a well-defined cohort or population.

1.7 Exercises

1. Describe the properties (both strengths and limitations) of each of the classic epidemiological designs when they are implemented using data from electronic registers.
2. Present the arguments for which of the classic designs (cohort, cross-sectional and case-control) would be most practical and efficient for the study of benign prostate hyperplasia. Explain why.(Note: this condition presents with unspecific symptoms, can by asymptomatic for a long time and may be discovered at screening).
3. Use the ideas in *Effects of errors in classification and diagnosis in various types of epidemiological studies* by Diamond and Lilienfeld in Am Jour Pub Health 1962 (VOL. 52. NO. 7) to plan a validation step for a study that you have worked with or are familiar with, where there was concern about misclassification bias.
4. For the paper on the association of childhood-onset IBD with psychiatric disorders and suicide in JAMA Paediatrics 2019 (PMC6704748), is the bias an example of "immortal time bias"? Explain. Do you think the authors efforts to control for bias is "reasonable"?

2

From Tables to Logistic Regression Models

This chapter will begin by presenting exposure-outcome information from the classic epidemiological designs (cohort, cross-sectional, case-control) on simple tables, from which one can estimate the association between the exposure and outcome. From the simplest 2-by-2 tables describing a binary exposure and binary outcome, a RR or OR can be estimated along with its confidence interval. Where it is reasonable to assume a common association across several strata (e.g. age groups), an estimate of the common underlying OR or RR can be computed from the stratified tables. These same estimates can be obtained from the logistic regression model, which offers a more general and flexible tool for studying the association between a binary outcome and explanatory variables.

2.1 Estimating RR or OR from 2-by-2 Tables

Assuming a sample of individuals for whom a binary exposure and binary outcome are known, this information can be represented on a 2-by-2 table. For example, in Chapter 1 we presented such a table for the approximately 22,000 physicians who participated in the investigation of aspirin and myocardial infarction, and this information is presented again in Table 2.1. Readers may note a change in how the information is presented compared to previously: the individuals exposed to aspirin are now on the first row and the reference group (placebo) is on the second row. The numbers of individuals with the outcome (MI) are presented in the first column and the numbers without the outcome in the second column, as before. We will adopt this convention throughout this text. i.e. exposed in the first row and outcomes/cases in the first column. While any arrangement of a 2-by-2 table is valid, this convention, which is widely used, will simplify the presentation of some general formulae.

TABLE 2.1: *2-by-2 table of aspirin use and myocardial infarction (MI).*

	MI		
	Yes	No	
Aspirin	104	10,933	11,037
Placebo	189	10,845	11,034

If we denote the counts in the four cells of a 2-by-2 table by a, b, c, d:

	Outcome	
	Yes	No
Exposed	a	b
Unexposed	c	d

then for the Aspirin and MI data in Table 2.1,

$$a = 104 \qquad b = 10,933 \qquad c = 189 \qquad d = 10,845$$

and we can write the RR and OR for aspirin users compared to placebo as:

$$RR = \frac{a}{(a+b)} \div \frac{c}{(c+d)} \tag{2.1}$$

$$OR = \frac{a}{b} \div \frac{c}{d} = \frac{ad}{bc} \tag{2.2}$$

Note that the OR does not change if we switch the rows and columns, i.e. the OR of disease in exposed compared to unexposed is the same as the OR of exposure in diseased compared to non-diseased. This important property of the OR, which we already saw in Chapter 1, underlies the major contribution of the case-control design to epidemiological research.

The RR or OR calculated from a sample provides an estimate of the quantity we are interested in, i.e. the 'true' RR or OR in the whole study population, which is referred to as the **parameter** of interest. Another sample from the same population would likely yield a different value for the RR or OR, which is also a valid estimate of the true parameter. This variation of a quantity from sample to sample is called **sampling variation**. To quantify our confidence in an estimate we obtain from a (single) research study sample, we need to understand the sampling variation. If the sample size is large, the estimates from different samples would be similar, and any one sample provides a reasonable estimate of the true parameter. However, for a small sample size, there can be large variation from one sample to another, so that the result from a single sample might not be close to the true parameter. A description of all the possible estimates that could arise is called the **sampling distribution**. While there are ways of deriving the sampling distribution theoretically, it will be illustrated below by mimicking the random sampling in an electronic 'cohort'.

2.2 Sampling Distribution of a RR or OR

The sampling distribution of a RR or OR will be illustrated here using a cohort similar to that used in [181] based on data from [77]. There are 50,000 cohort members, the outcome of interest is coronary heart disease (CHD), and the variables recorded include binary variables for sex (male/female), smoking status (smoker/non-smoker) and anti-hypertensive treatment (yes/no). The cohort has approximately equal numbers of males and females (25,660 and 24,340 respectively), with 1,251 male cases and 669 female cases. Thus, the true RR of CHD in males compared to females in this large cohort is:

$$\frac{1251}{25,660} \div \frac{669}{24,340} = .0488 \div .0275 = 1.77$$

Taking random samples of 2500 individuals and computing the RR for each sample, the distribution of the RR obtained in different samples can be examined graphically. The distribution of values obtained over 500 samples is shown in Figure 2.1a. A feature of the sampling distribution of a RR is that it is not symmetric. However, if we use the (natural) log scale, and instead of the RR from each sample, plot the ln(RR),

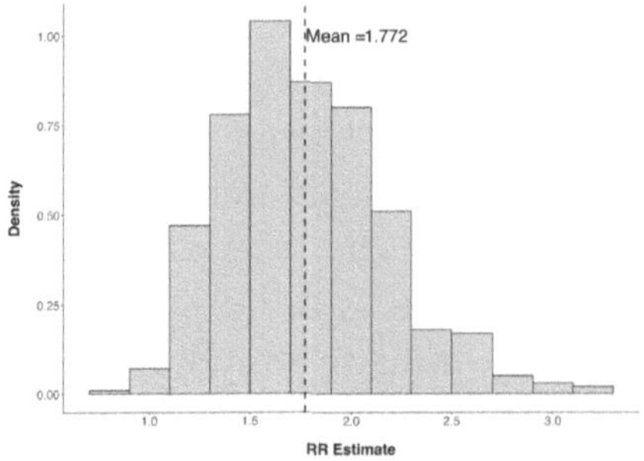

(a) *Distribution of RR estimates*

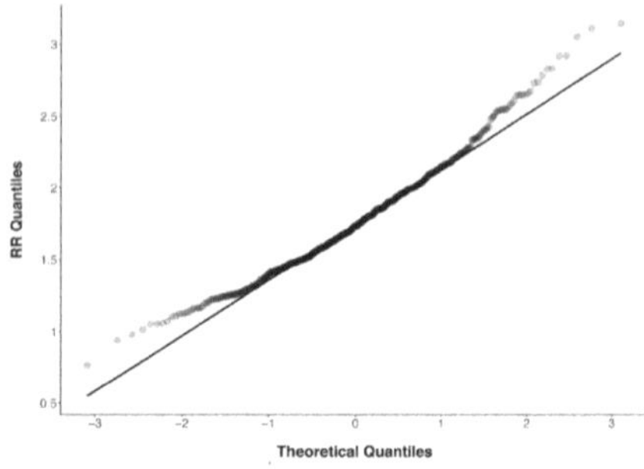

(b) *Q-Q plot of RR estimates*

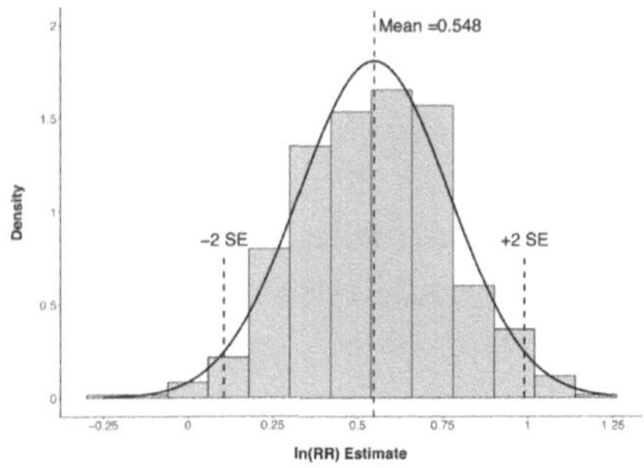

(c) *Distribution of ln(RR) estimates*

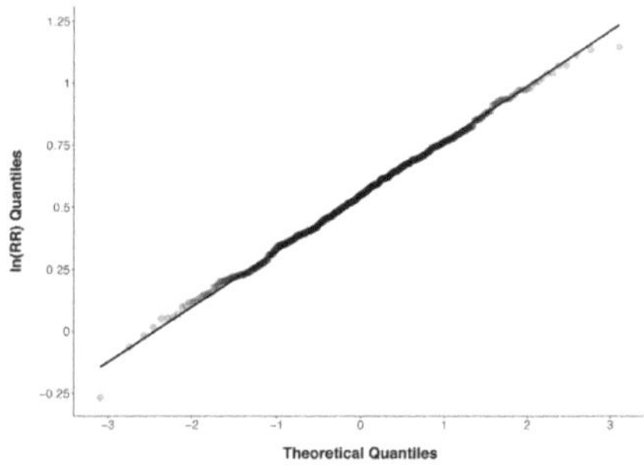

(d) *Q-Q plot of ln(RR) estimates*

FIGURE 2.1: *Distribution and Q-Q plots of RR and ln(RR) estimates for 2500 individuals over 500 samples. Data from simulated Singapore Chinese Health Study Cohort [77].*

we obtain a symmetric distribution, as illustrated in Figure 2.1c. From statistical theory, it can be shown that the distribution of the ln(RR) is not only symmetric, but is (approximately) normal, as we see from the QQ-plot in Figure 2.1d compared to the QQ-plot of the RR estimate in Figure 2.1b: the QQ-plot compares the observed quantiles to their expected values if the data were normally distributed. This normal distribution is centered at the true parameter, and will have a smaller variation for larger sample sizes. Thus, provided we know the standard deviation of the sampling distribution (more correctly called the **standard error**, we can say that 95% of samples will yield estimates that lie within 1.96 standard errors of the true parameter, or equivalently, that a single sample's estimate $\pm$ 1.96 standard errors provides a 95% confidence interval for the true parameter (on the natural log scale). In a real research study, only one study sample is available, so the standard error is unknown as this is the standard deviation of the distribution of all possible ln(RR) values that one might have obtained. However, the standard error can be estimated from the study sample using simple formulae that have been derived from statistical theory. For large sample sizes, the counts in a 2-by-2 table (denoted by a,b,c,d as before) can be used in Equations 2.3 and 2.4 to obtain good estimates of the standard error of the ln(RR) and ln(OR), as well as the 95% confidence intervals. The step-by-step calculations are provided in Examples 2.1 and 2.2.

	Outcome Yes	No
Exposed	a	b
Unexposed	c	d

$$\text{SE of } \ln(\text{RR}) = \sqrt{\frac{\frac{b}{a}}{b+a} + \frac{\frac{d}{c}}{d+c}} \tag{2.3}$$

$$\text{SE of } \ln(\text{OR}) = \sqrt{\frac{1}{a} + \frac{1}{b} + \frac{1}{c} + \frac{1}{d}} \tag{2.4}$$

While it is instructive to see how the confidence interval is calculated, such calculations are commonly done by online calculators or statistical software packages by simply providing the four numbers from the 2-by-2 table or by opening the sample dataset and requesting the required analysis. It is left as an exercise to reproduce the confidence interval above using the **Openepi** calculator (www.openepi.com), or any statistical software.

Example 2.1. *Confidence interval for a RR*

A single random sample of 10,000 from the cohort of 50,000 described above, produced the following 2-by-2 table:

	Outcome	
	Yes	No
Exposed	230	4885
Unexposed	106	4779

From these data, we can calculate:

$$RR = 2.072$$
$$ln(RR) = 0.7285$$

$$\text{SE of } ln(RR) = \sqrt{\frac{\frac{4885}{230}}{4885+230} + \frac{\frac{4779}{106}}{4779+106}} = .1157$$

so that the 95% confidence interval for the population $ln(RR)$ is

$$0.7285 \pm 1.96(.1157) = (.5017, .9533)$$

and by taking the anti-log (i.e. exponentiating), we get the 95% confidence interval for the RR:

$$= (e^{.5017}, e^{.9533})$$
$$= (1.652, 2.599)$$

Note that this interval contains the true population RR of 1.77 that was calculated at the beginning of Section 2.2.

Example 2.2. *Confidence interval for an OR*

The OR, with 95% confidence interval can be computed for the sample of 10,000 in a similar way as for the RR:

$$OR = 2.123$$
$$ln(OR) = 0.7528$$

$$\text{SE of } ln(OR) = \sqrt{\frac{1}{230} + \frac{1}{4885} + \frac{1}{106} + \frac{1}{4779}} = .1191$$

and the 95% confidence interval for the population ln(OR) is

$$0.7528 \pm 1.96(.1191) = (.5194, .9862)$$

and by taking anti-log, the 95% confidence interval for the OR:

$$= (e^{.5194}, e^{.9862})$$
$$= (1.681, 2.681)$$

2.3 Stratification and Confounding

Although much of this book will be concerned with binary outcomes and categorical exposures, this section will be introduced with an example of a continuous exposure and continuous outcome that allows the ideas to be communicated graphically. In an article in CHANCE in 2008 [225], the authors described an online dating service that collected information from respondents on a number of characteristics, including index finger length, height and ideal partner's height. Why the index finger length might be useful information becomes clear when we view the data. In the scatter plot in Figure 2.2a, representing 100 individuals similar to those in the original survey, it is clear that there is a positive correlation (r=0.72) between finger length and height, as we might expect. The best-fitting straight line to the points in the plot has a slope of 5.9, which means that for every additional centimetre in finger length, the average height of an individual is 5.9 centimetres taller. Thus, by requesting the finger length, the dating service obtains an estimate of the applicant's

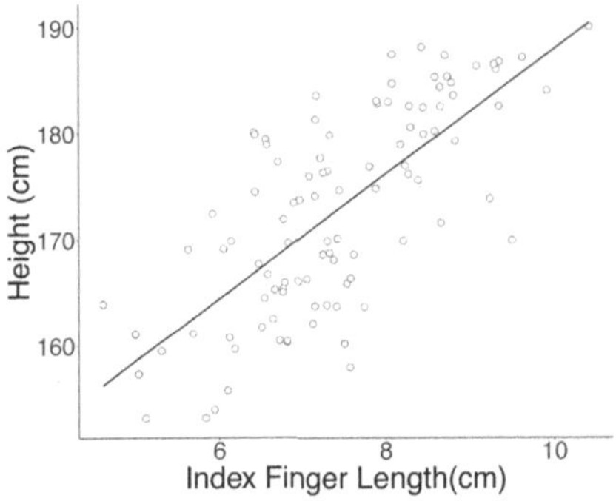

(a) *Association between index finger length and height of 100 individuals.*

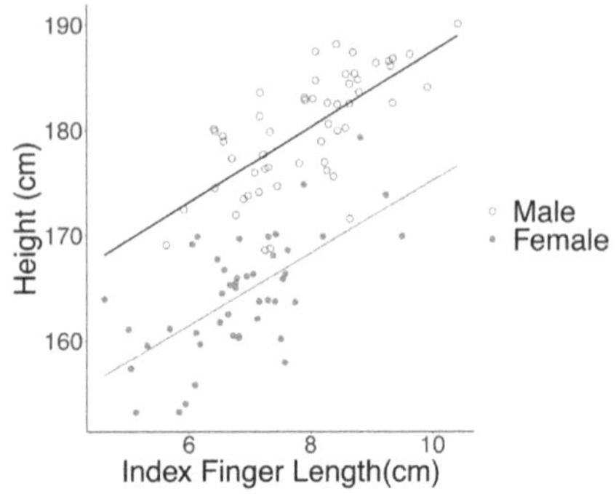

(b) *Association between index finger length and height of 54 males and 46 females.*

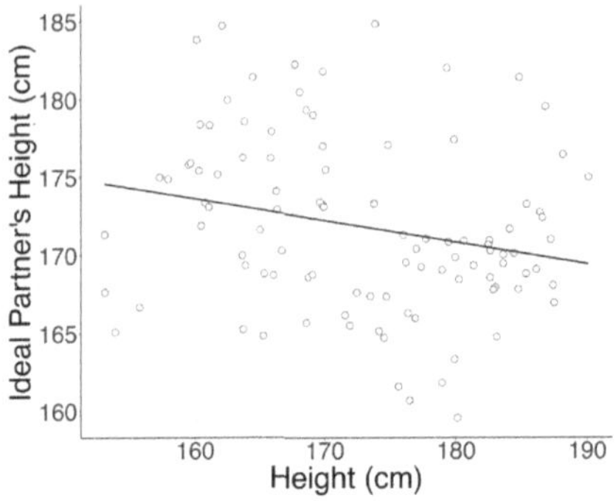

(c) *Association between height and ideal partner height of 100 individuals.*

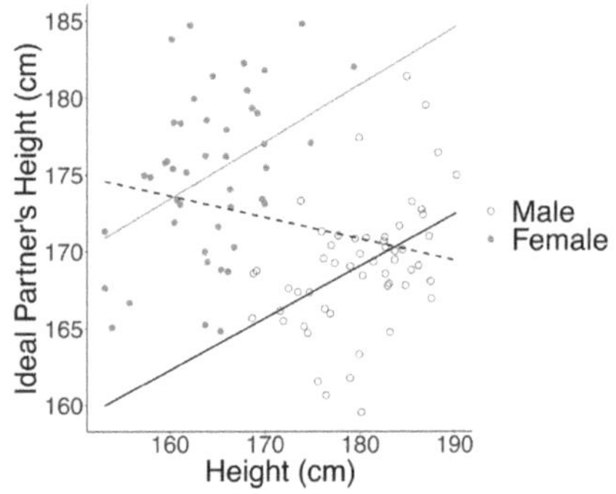

(d) *Association between own and ideal partner height of 54 males and 46 females.*

FIGURE 2.2: *Crude and stratified associations between index finger length and height, and height and ideal partner's height.*

height, where a direct request for height might have been considered a more sensitive question and elicited less truthful answers!

The correlation and slope just mentioned represent the **crude** relationship between finger length and height when we examine all the data. But if we look at males and females separately, we see that the crude slope gives a false impression, as the association between finger length and height is not as strong as the crude model suggests: the increase in average height with each centimetre increase in finger length is approximately 3.5 cm (3.6 cm for males and 3.45 cm for females, Figure 2.2b). We say that the association between finger length and height is **confounded** by sex, as the true relationship that exists between these measures in both men and women respondents has been masked due to sex differences: males are much taller and tend to have longer index fingers (approximately half are longer than 8cm, while most females have index fingers shorter than 8cm). When there is a potential confounding factor (such as sex in this example), the separate analysis of the relationship in the different groups/strata defined by the factor is called a **stratified analysis**. If this analysis reveals that there is a common relationship in all the strata that was masked by the crude analysis, then this common value is reported and referred to as the **adjusted** estimate.

Assuming the small difference in males and females in our example is due to spurious sampling variation, then it is reasonable to report a common value of the slope relating finger length to height for males and females. From the stratified analysis, we see that this is approximately 3.5cm, but the exact value can be obtained by fitting a simple linear regression model, that expresses height as a function of finger length and sex, from which the estimate of the coefficient of finger length is found to be 3.53cm (see Table 2.2). Thus, we can report that the average increase in height per additional centimetre of finger length is 3.53cm, *adjusted for sex*. For this example, it seemed obvious that there was indeed a common value in the two groups, but linear regression analysis also allows a formal test of this assumption (by including an interaction term in the model), and unsurprisingly, this test was not significant (p=0.85) for the data presented here (last column of Table 2.2).

A simple graphical tool, known as a DAG (directed acyclic graph) is often used to display the potential confounding of the relationship between variables. For our example, the DAG in Figure 2.3 illustrates that being male is associated with both being *taller* (denoted by the plus sign) and having a *longer* index finger.

In the example above, the crude effect was an exaggerated estimate: adjusting for the confounding due to sex removed this positive bias and

TABLE 2.2: *Estimates of the slope (with p-value) from linear regression of height on index finger length, using crude, adjusted and interaction analyses.*

	Crude	Adjusted	Interaction
Index finger length	5.90 (<.001)	**3.53** (<.001)	3.45 (<.001)
Male	–	11.89 (<.001)	10.79 (0.0732)
Index finger length (within males)	–	–	0.151 (**0.85**)

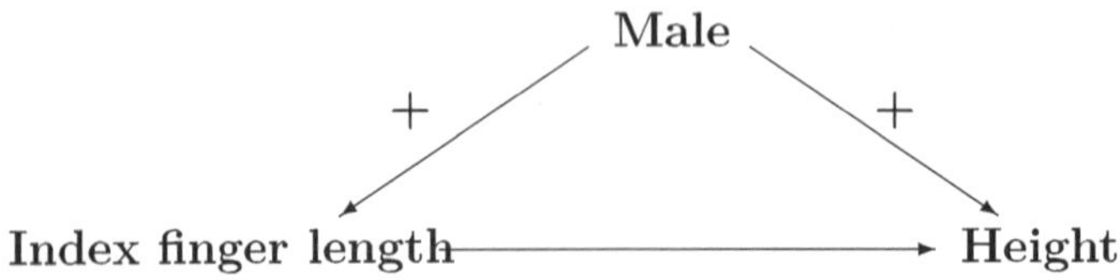

FIGURE 2.3: *Relationship between index finger length and height confounded by sex.*

revealed that the estimate of the common slope for males and females was smaller than the crude slope. However, depending on how the confounding factor is associated with the two variables whose (linear) relationship is being studied, the effect of confounding can also result in negative bias, where the crude effect is 'diluted' rather than exaggerated, or even in a change in the direction of the relationship, as illustrated in the next example.

Figure 2.2c uses similar data to those in the paper by Wainer et al [225] to plot the heights of 100 individuals against their ideal partner's height in . If one preferred their partner to have a height the same as their own, then the points would be expected to fall on a diagonal line (slope = 1), indicating that for every one centimetre taller a respondent is, their ideal partner is also one centimetre taller. However, it is clear that the plot has a *negative* slope, and from a simple linear regression analysis, the best fitting line to the points has a slope of -0.144, which means that for every one centimetre taller the respondent, their ideal partner is *shorter* by approximately 0.144 cm. This is the *crude* relationship between height and ideal partner's height when we examine all the data, but a stratified analysis reveals a *positive* slope in both males and females (Figure 2.2d: taller individuals prefer taller partners, with a similar trend/slope in the two groups). The common slope describing the average increase in the ideal partner's height per 1 centimetre increase in an individual's own height, *adjusted for sex*, is estimated from a linear regression model of ideal partner's height as a function of both the individual's own height and their sex. The difference between this adjusted estimate (0.35 cm) and the crude estimate (-0.144) is due to confounding by sex: females tend to be shorter and to prefer taller partners, as illustrated by the clustering of their data points in the top left corner of Figure 2.2d and by the DAG in Figure 2.4.

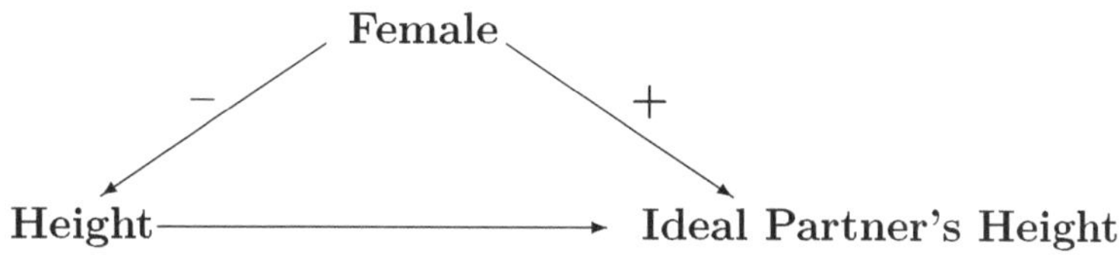

FIGURE 2.4: *DAG of sex as confounder of height and ideal partner's height.*

In the simple examples above, it was clear that there was confounding, as the adjusted slope was quite different from the crude value, and in one case even of the opposite sign. If the adjusted value had been close to the crude value, we might have concluded that there was no confounding and reported the crude/overall estimate – but how close is close? If the adjusted estimate differs by more than 10% from the crude value, it is standard practice to report the adjusted estimate. This simple rule-of thumb, also called the 'change-in-estimate' criterion, was first proposed by Miettinen [146] in the context of risk estimates, and has been widely adopted due to its simplicity and good performance [140], although it can be somewhat conservative in some settings[121].

2.3.1 Interaction (effect modification)

The previous examples had rather elegant results: the change in height for each centimetre increase in finger length was similar for males and females, the change in preferred partner height for each centimetre change in one's own height was also similar for males and females, and these (common) relationships were apparent from the data. However, in many applications, a stratified analysis will reveal not only that the crude estimate is inappropriate, but that there is a *different* relationship in the two strata. When this occurs, we say the effect of the predictor variable on the outcome is *modified* by the stratum variable, or that there is an *interaction* between the predictor and the stratum variable. This is illustrated in Figure 2.5, which presents a scatter plot (and fitted linear regression models) for 250 individuals (110 males, 140 females) in the Framingham teaching dataset available from *https://biolincc.nhlbi.nih.gov/teaching/*, which is a subset of the data from the Framingham Heart Study [139] [125].

The crude increase in the average systolic blood pressure for each additional year of age is approximately 1mmHg (slope = 0.85), but a

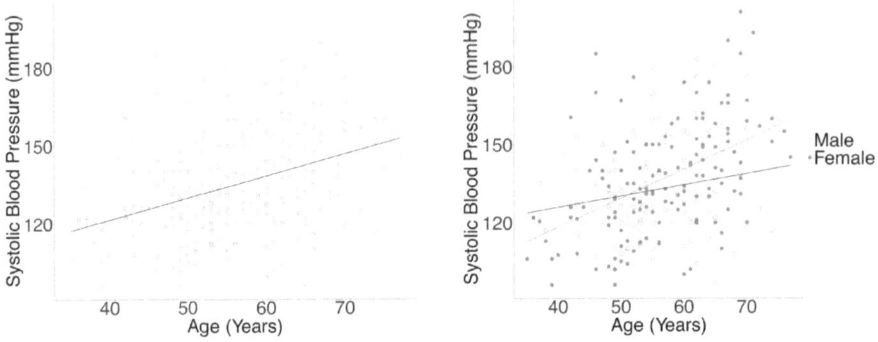

(a) *Association between age and systolic blood pressure of 250 individuals.*

(b) *Association between age and systolic blood pressure (110 males, 140 females).*

FIGURE 2.5: *Crude and sex-stratified associations of age and systolic blood pressure in the Framingham Teaching dataset.*

stratified analysis reveals that the blood pressure rises more gradually with age for men (slope = 0.43 compared to 1.12 for women). A formal statistical test using an interaction term indicates that this difference is significant (p=.01).

2.3.2 Confounding of a risk estimate

Depending on the study design, the effect of an exposure on an outcome can be quantified by a RR, OR, or IRR. In Chapter 1, the examples of risk were all simple *crude* (i.e. overall) effects, obtained by comparing the exposed and unexposed individuals. However, the relationship between an exposure and an outcome can be distorted if there is a variable that is associated with both the exposure and the outcome, i.e. a *confounding factor*. A classic example that was reported as early as 1982 [82], and has been described in numerous papers [242], is the crude association between lung cancer and alcohol consumption that can arise due to confounding by smoking. From the information provided in the paper by Zang and Wynder [242], the cross-tabulation of lung cancer and alcohol consumption in males (Table 2.3) can be constructed.

Combining the two lowest and two highest alcohol categories, the OR for the association between high alcohol intake and lung cancer is 1.78. However, this crude OR may be confounded by other factors, most notably smoking, which is a well-known risk factor for lung cancer and is also associated with drinking alcohol. For example, in Table 2.4, a crude

TABLE 2.3: *Association of lung cancer in males with levels of alcohol intake (measured as 'whiskey-equivalent' ounces per day).*

		Lung Cancer	
		Yes	No
Alcohol Intake	<1	1090	3976
	1–3.9	806	2244
	4–6.9	378	783
	≥ 7	679	1166
		2953	8169

association of the same magnitude as above (OR=1.78) is apparent, even though there is no association in either of the smoking strata.

The confounding effect of smoking in this example has resulted in a spurious association between alcohol consumption and lung cancer. This is referred to as *positive confounding* as the crude OR is exaggerated: not only does it suggest a larger effect, it suggests an association for which there is no evidence in the stratified analysis. When a stratified analysis reveals an association with common OR not equal to 1.0, then positive confounding results in the crude OR being further from 1.0, while a crude OR closer to 1.0 is referred to *negative confounding.* Thus, while positive confounding results in exaggeration of the true association, negative confounding results in a dilution, or masking, of the true relationship. In the extreme case of negative confounding, a real association may be missed because the OR for the crude association is close to 1.0.

To illustrate this type of distortion of the relationship between an exposure and an outcome, we use a simple example from the textbook by Kirkwood and Sterne [104]. The data is presented in Table 2.5 and

TABLE 2.4: *2-by-2 tables of association between alcohol consumption and lung cancer, overall and stratified by smoking status.*

	Overall			Smoker			Non-smoker		
	Lung Cancer			**Lung Cancer**			**Lung Cancer**		
	Yes	No		Yes	No		Yes	No	
Heavy Drinker	1057	1949	3006	786	665	1451	271	1284	1555
Light Drinker	1896	6220	8116	702	591	1293	1194	5629	6823
	2953	8169	11122	1488	1256	2744	1465	6913	8378
	OR = 1.78			**OR = 1.0**			**OR = 1.0**		

TABLE 2.5: *2-by-2 table of association between type of residence and presence of leptospirosis antibodies.*

	Antibodies Yes	Antibodies No	
Rural Residence	60	140	200
Urban Residence	60	140	200
	120	280	400

OR = 1.0

describes the presence of antibodies to leptospirosis in 400 people, 200 from each of a rural and urban area of residence.

The odds of testing positive for antibodies is 60/140=0.429 for both rural and urban residence, yielding an OR of 1.0, from which we might conclude that area of residence is not associated with antibody status. However, an analysis stratified by sex gives the results in Table 2.6: an OR of 2.57 in males and 1.71 in females.

Thus, there is an association between area of residence and antibodies in both groups, although we cannot yet say if it is higher in males than females or the difference is just spurious sampling variation (we will return to this later). The association was not apparent in the crude analysis due to confounding by sex, which is related to the exposure and the outcome: females are more likely to live in a rural area and less likely to have antibodies, as represented in the DAG in Figure 2.6.

The extent of confounding, which depends on the direction and magnitude of the relationships between the confounder and exposure, and between the confounder and outcome, can even result in the crude OR

TABLE 2.6: *2-by-2 tables of association between type of residence and presence of leptospirosis antibodies, stratified by sex.*

Male

	Antibodies Yes	Antibodies No	
Rural	36	14	50
Urban	50	50	100
	86	64	150

OR = 2.57

Female

	Antibodies Yes	Antibodies No	
Rural	24	126	150
Urban	10	90	100
	34	216	250

OR = 1.71

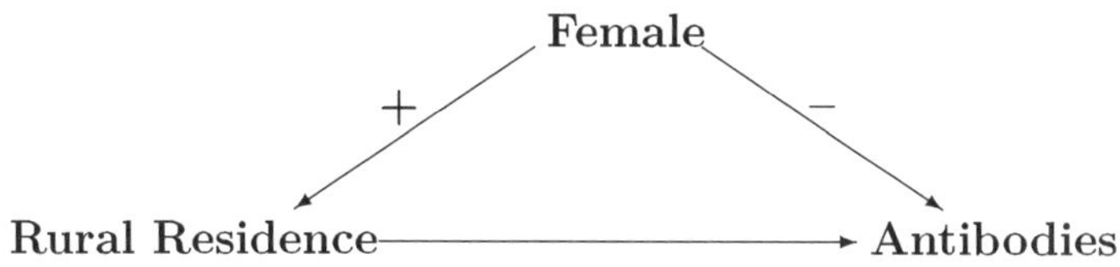

FIGURE 2.6: *DAG illustrating female sex as a confounder of the association between rural residence and antibodies.*

indicating an association in the opposite direction to the relationship in the strata, which is known as **Simpson's paradox**. In popular science, this paradox is usually described as the reversal of a relationship when data is considered in aggregate form, due to a 'lurking' variable having been overlooked. Numerous examples are presented in the popular and scientific literature. An interesting recent example [31] is the apparent discrimination against women applicants to Graduate School at the University of California, Berkeley: when analysis considered the academic departments and their admission rates (the lurking variables!), women tended to do better. In a presentation of Simpson's paradox from an epidemiological perspective in the International Journal of Epidemiology in 2011 [83], the authors 'unravel' the paradox with the aid of DAGs, and emphasise the importance of knowledge of the research area for meaningful statistical analysis of epidemiological data.

It will by now be clear that the crude association between an exposure and disease in a population is of limited interest without some further knowledge of whether/how the association varies across the strata defined by some characteristic of interest (e.g. male and female, age groups, socioeconomic status). A characteristic that is associated with both the exposure and the outcome may confound the relationship between the two and it is standard practice to consider any such variable as a potential confounder. If a stratified analysis indicates that there is a common association that differs from the crude association due to confounding, then the *adjusted* value, which estimates the common underlying association, is reported. To define a confounder as 'a variable that is associated with both the exposure and the outcome' is rather loose, and for some such variables, the stratified analysis will result in an adjusted/common OR that is not (much) different from the crude OR. In situations where there is a common OR in the population, a more complete definition of a confounder is a factor that is associated with the exposure *in the control group* (and therefore also in those with the outcome) and is associated with the outcome in both the exposed and unexposed (Chapter 3 of [24]). The strength of these associations will determine the extent of the confounding, and a change of more than 10% is considered meaningful confounding and deserving of an adjusted risk estimate to be reported.

2.3.3 Mantel-Haenszel odds ratio

In the example in Table 2.4 above of a common disease-exposure relationship across strata, the numerical values have been idealised to provide the *exact* same OR in each of the strata. However, in a real application, random selection of the study sample will result in some differences in the ORs across strata, even if there is indeed a common OR in these strata in the population. The questions then arise as to how to decide if it is reasonable to assume a common OR in the population, and, if such assumption is reasonable, how to estimate this common OR from the available sample data. These two issues will be addressed in reverse order, by first presenting how one estimates the common (adjusted) OR when it is clear from an informal inspection of the stratified tables that it is reasonable to do so. The decision regarding whether it is reasonable to assume a common OR will be addressed formally in Section 2.4.3. For now, assume a confounding factor with only two levels, where the stratified 2-by-2 tables relating exposure to disease suggest a common odds ratio. Denoting the two tables as in Table 2.7, the **Mantel-Haenszel estimator** of the common OR is given by Equation 2.5:

TABLE 2.7: *Stratified 2-by-2 tables of exposure and disease status.*

Stratum 1

	Outcome: Yes	Outcome: No
Exposed	a_1	b_1
Unexposed	c_1	d_1
		n_1

Stratum 2

	Outcome: Yes	Outcome: No
Exposed	a_2	b_2
Unexposed	c_2	d_2
		n_2

$$\widehat{OR}_{MH} = \frac{\frac{a_1 d_1}{n_1} + \frac{a_2 d_2}{n_2}}{\frac{b_1 c_1}{n_1} + \frac{b_2 c_2}{n_2}} \tag{2.5}$$

This is similar to the simple OR ($\frac{ad}{bc}$) in that the products of the main diagonal elements (a and d) appear in the numerator and the products of the off-diagonal elements (b and c) appear in the denominator, but now these products are scaled by the number of observations in the stratum and then summed. Returning to the data in Table 2.4 for alcohol consumption and lung cancer stratified by smoking status, the Mantel-Haenszel OR is:

$$\begin{aligned}\widehat{OR}_{MH} &= \frac{\frac{786\times591}{2744}+\frac{271\times5629}{8378}}{\frac{665\times702}{2744}+\frac{1248\times1194}{8378}} \\ &= 351.367/347.988 \\ &= 1.0097\end{aligned}$$

As we would expect from inspection of the data, the common OR is very close to 1.0, indicating no association between alcohol and lung cancer, *when adjusted for smoking.*

If there are more than two strata, the Mantel-Haenszel estimator sums the main diagonal terms and off-diagonal terms over all strata, in the same way, to obtain the numerator and denominator. For K strata:

$$\widehat{OR}_{MH} = \frac{\frac{a_1d_1}{n_1}+\frac{a_2d_2}{n_2}+\cdots+\frac{a_Kd_K}{n_K}}{\frac{b_1c_1}{n_1}+\frac{b_2c_2}{n_2}+\cdots++\frac{b_Kc_K}{n_K}} \tag{2.6}$$

or indexing the strata by i, this is usually abbreviated as

$$\widehat{OR}_{MH} = \frac{\sum\frac{a_id_i}{n_i}}{\sum\frac{b_ic_i}{n_i}} \tag{2.7}$$

An illustration using the Framingham teaching dataset is presented in Example 2.3. The crude OR for the association between coronary heart disease (CHD) and diabetes is 2.12, which differs from the ORs in the three age strata: 1.73, 1.40 and 1.54. Assuming for now that there is a common OR in each stratum (and that the differences between these three is due to random variation), the Mantel-Haenszel estimate of that common OR from Equation 2.7 is 1.50.

Example 2.3. *Mantel-Haenszel OR for association between prevalent coronary heart disease (CHD) and diabetes in Framingham subjects aged 42–71.*

Overall

	Diabetes Yes	Diabetes No	
CHD	12	175	187
No CHD	104	3214	3318
	116	3389	3505

OR = 2.12

Age 42–51

	Diabetes Yes	Diabetes No	
Yes CHD	1	32	33
No CHD	28	1553	1581
	29	1585	1614

OR = 1.73

Age 52–61

	Diabetes Yes	Diabetes No	
Yes CHD	4	74	78
No CHD	47	1221	1268
	51	1295	1346

OR = 1.40

Age 62–71

	Diabetes Yes	Diabetes No	
Yes CHD	7	69	76
No CHD	29	440	469
	36	509	545

OR = 1.54

$$\widehat{OR}_{MH} = \frac{\dfrac{1(1553)}{1614} + \dfrac{4(1221)}{1346} + \dfrac{7(440)}{545}}{\dfrac{28(32)}{1614} + \dfrac{47(74)}{1346} + \dfrac{29(69)}{545}} = \mathbf{1.50}$$

Mantel-Haenszel (adjusted) relative risk

In the discussion of confounding above, the OR was the measure of association between exposure and disease. However, the same principles apply to other measures of risk. Denoting the overall and stratified (two strata) tables as in Table 2.8, the RR describing the association in the population is estimated as

$$\widehat{RR} = \frac{a/(a+b)}{c/(c+d)}$$

and where the assumption of a common RR is reasonable, the Mantel-Haenszel estimate of the adjusted RR is given by:

TABLE 2.8: *Overall and stratified 2-by-2 tables.*

	Overall Disease: Yes	Overall Disease: No	Stratum 1 Disease: Yes	Stratum 1 Disease: No	Stratum 2 Disease: Yes	Stratum 2 Disease: No
Exposed	a	b	a_1	b_1	a_2	b_2
Unexposed	c	d	c_1	d_1	c_2	d_2
		n		n_1		n_2

$$\widehat{RR}_{MH} = \frac{\frac{a_1(c_1+d_1)}{n_1} + \frac{a_2(c_2+d_2)}{n_2}}{\frac{c_1(a_1+b_1)}{n_1} + \frac{c_2(a_2+b_2)}{n_2}} \tag{2.8}$$

which for K strata generalises to:

$$\widehat{RR}_{MH} = \frac{\sum \frac{a_i(c_i+d_i)}{n_i}}{\sum \frac{c_i(a_i+b_i)}{n_i}} \tag{2.9}$$

where the summation is taken over $i = 1, \ldots K$.

For the alcohol and lung cancer example from Table 2.4, the estimate of the crude RR is:

$$\widehat{RR} = \frac{a/(a+b)}{c/(c+d)} = \frac{1057/(1057+1949)}{1896/(1896+6220)} = \frac{.3516}{.2336} = 1.505$$

and the Mantel-Haenszel estimate of the adjusted RR is:

$$\begin{aligned}\widehat{RR}_{MH} &= \frac{\frac{786(702+591)}{2744} + \frac{271(1194+5629)}{8378}}{\frac{702(786+665)}{2744} + \frac{1194(271+1248)}{8378}} \\ &= \frac{591.072}{587.693} \\ &= 1.0057\end{aligned}$$

Thus, we would report that the RR of lung cancer in heavy drinkers compared to light drinkers, *adjusted for smoking*, is 1.0057, almost the same as the adjusted OR. As seen previously, the RR tends to be closer to 1.0 than the OR (here RR= 1.505 vs. OR= 1.73) and this is also true for the adjusted estimates, although in this example the difference is very small ($OR_{MH} = 1.0097$ vs. $RR_{MH} = 1.0057$).

2.4 Association, Homogeneity and Trend

In the examples so far in this chapter, we have focused on RR and OR as the measures of association between an exposure and an outcome. Constructing a confidence interval for the RR or OR enables a formal test of association: if the 95% confidence interval excludes 1.0, the hypothesis of no association can be rejected at significance level .05. Thus, in the simple worked examples at the beginning this chapter (Examples 2.1 and 2.2), the RR and OR both lead to the conclusion that there *is* an association between aspirin and MI.

2.4.1 Chi-squared test of association

There are other ways to view the question regarding association. Instead of a ratio measure such as RR or OR, a difference in proportions can also be assessed: the difference in the prevalence of the outcome in exposed and unexposed individuals in a cohort study, or the difference in the prevalence of exposure in cases and controls in a case-control study. These tests can be conducted using the **Pearson Chi-squared test**, which compares the counts observed in the table to the expected counts *if there was no association.* In the absence of an association, these counts will be similar, and conversely, a large difference would suggest an association – but how similar, and how large?

The row totals in Table 2.9(a), n_e and $n_{\bar{e}}$, denote the overall numbers of exposed and unexposed individuals, and the column totals, n_c and $n_{\bar{c}}$, denote the numbers of cases and non-cases. The total sample size is denoted by the grand total, n. The overall proportion of individuals with disease is n_c/n, so if there is no association between exposure and disease, we would expect this same proportion among the n_e exposed and among the $n_{\bar{e}}$ unexposed individuals, so that the 'expected' numbers of observations would be as in Table 2.9(b). Similarly, the overall proportion without the disease, $n_{\bar{c}}$, can be used to fill in the expected counts in the other two cells, and it can be seen that for any cell:

$$\text{Expected count} = \frac{(\text{row total}) \times (\text{column total})}{\text{grand total}} \qquad (2.10)$$

Note that it is actually only necessary to calculate one of the expected

TABLE 2.9: *(a) Observed counts in a 2-by-2 table and (b) the corresponding expected counts under the assumption of no association between exposure and outcome.*

(a)

	Outcome: Yes	Outcome: No	
Exposed	a	b	n_e
Unexposed	c	d	$n_{\bar{e}}$
	n_c	$n_{\bar{c}}$	n

(b)

	Outcome: Yes	Outcome: No	
Exposed	$\frac{n_c . n_e}{n}$		n_e
Unexposed	$\frac{n_c . n_{\bar{e}}}{n}$		$n_{\bar{e}}$
	n_c	$n_{\bar{c}}$	n

counts, as all the others can be obtained by subtraction from the row or column totals! The discrepancy between the observed and expected tables is calculated by summing, for each cell, the squared difference between the observed and expected counts, scaled by the expected count. The scaling allows the differences in any cell to be 'normalised' to represent a meaningful contribution to discrepancy, since a small difference in a cell with a larger count is less important, and vice versa.

$$\text{Total discrepancy} = \sum \frac{(\text{Observed-Expected})^2}{\text{Expected}} \qquad (2.11)$$

If there is no association in the table, it can be shown that in repeated samplings of n individuals where there are n_c cases, $n_{\bar{c}}$ non-cases, n_e exposed and $n_{\bar{e}}$ unexposed, the discrepancy which will arise due to randomness alone (if there is no difference in the proportion of disease in the exposed and unexposed groups in the population) has a skewed distribution known as a Chi-Squared distribution with 1 degree of freedom and denoted by $\chi^2_{(1)}$. Because of this, the discrepancy calculated from the sample is called the 'Chi-Squared statistic'. The $\chi^2_{(1)}$ distribution is actually the square of a standard normal, so that 95% of the values are less than $(1.96)^2$. Thus, a discrepancy larger than 3.84 is evidence of an association at the 5% significance level. The cut-offs for significance levels of 5%, 1 % and 0.1% are provided in the first row of Table 2.10 for convenience.

The total numbers of heavy and light drinkers among lung cancer cases and non-cases from the overall counts in Table 2.4 are presented again in Table 2.11, with the expected counts in parentheses in each

TABLE 2.10: *Cut-off values for the $\chi^2_{(1)}$, $\chi^2_{(2)}$ and $\chi^2_{(3)}$ distributions corresponding to 5%, 1% and 0.1% of values in the upper tail.*

Tail	0.05	0.01	0.001	.0001
$\chi^2(1)$	3.84	6.63	10.83	15.14
$\chi^2(2)$	5.99	9.21	13.82	18.42
$\chi^2(3)$	7.81	11.34	16.27	21.11

cell. At first glance, it can be seen that the observed counts differ from what would be expected from just random variation (in the absence of any association): the top left cell has a larger count than expected (i.e. there are more cases among the heavy drinkers) and there are also some differences in the other cells. The total discrepancy is:

$$\frac{(1057-798)^2}{798}+\frac{(1949-2208)^2}{2208}+\frac{(1896-2155)^2}{2155}+\frac{(6220-5961)^2}{5961}=156.82$$

Comparing this to the values from the $\chi^2(1)$ distribution in Table 2.10, the probability of such a large value is very unlikely (<.0001) so the discrepancy between the observed and expected table is unlikely to be due to random variation. Thus there is strong evidence of an association between alcohol intake and lung cancer.

If more than two proportions are compared, then the discrepancy has a χ^2 distribution with $K-1$ degrees of freedom, $\chi^2_{(K-1)}$ where K is the number of categories: for example, a value ≥ 5.99 would indicate a significant difference (at the 5% significance level) between three proportions (Table 2.10). For a table with R rows and C columns, the

TABLE 2.11: *2-by-2 table of observed (and expected) counts from alcohol and lung cancer data example.*

	Lung Cancer		
	Yes	No	
Heavy drinker	1057 (798)	1949 (2208)	3006
Light drinker	1896 (2155)	6220 (5961)	8116
	2953	8169	11122

Chi-squared test is conducted in the same way by computing the total discrepancy between the observed and expected table. However, the distribution of the values that this discrepancy can take in repeated random samples when there is no association, depends on the number of rows and columns of the table: it is a χ^2 distribution with $(R-1) \times (C-1)$ degrees of freedom.

2.4.2 Test of association in paired data: McNemar's Test

When the available data compares paired observations for their exposure and outcome, the information can be represented on a 2-by-2 table, where the counts no longer represent independent individuals, but pairs. Such data arise naturally in twin studies, where the comparison of the exposure status of a diseased twin and the exposure status of their disease-free co-twin provides valuable insight: if the twins are identical, then all genetic differences are automatically adjusted in the comparison. Similarly, in studies of paired organs, one of which is diseased, non-genetic exposures can be investigated from the paired data. Matched case-control studies attempt to adjust for nuisance confounders by selecting one or more controls for each case that 'match' the case with respect to the potential confounders that are not of interest. Where there is just one control per case, this gives rise to paired data. To present paired data on a 2-by-2 table (see Table 2.12), we record the numbers of pairs where:

- the case and control are both exposed
- the case and control are both unexposed
- the case is exposed and the control is unexposed
- the case is unexposed and the control is exposed

If there is an association between the exposure and disease, there will be more pairs where the case is exposed and the control is unexposed (n_{10}). It should be intuitively clear that the concordant pairs, where both case and control are exposed (n_{11}) or unexposed (n_{00}), do not contribute information about the relationship between disease and exposure. The information is contained in the discordant pairs, and if there is no association between exposure and disease, we would expect these $n_{11} + n_{00}$ to be equally split. The 'discrepancy' between the expected equal split and the observed values of n_{10} and n_{01} is known as **McNemar's Chi-squared** and is simply:

TABLE 2.12: *2-by-2 table of paired data.*

	Control Exposed Yes	Control Exposed No
Case Exposed	n_{11}	n_{10}
Case Unexposed	n_{01}	n_{00}

$$\chi^2 = \frac{(n_{10} - n_{01})^2}{(n_{10} + n_{01})} \tag{2.12}$$

If there is no association between exposure and outcome, this quantity has a $\chi^2(1)$ distribution, so large values enable the null hypothesis (of no association) to be rejected.

As an illustration, we use data from a paper that investigated the association between radiation for breast cancer and the risk of a subsequent lung cancer [174]. For all women who were diagnosed with a lung cancer, a comparison of the laterality of the lung cancer with respect to whether that side of the body was irradiated (when the breast cancer was treated) is a paired design, where the pairs consist of the breasts of the same woman. Each lung cancer can be classified as to whether it was diagnosed on the same side as the breast cancer, and if that breast cancer was radiated. The paired data offers a means of testing whether the occurrence of lung cancer on the same side as the breast cancer is associated with exposure to radiation. From the published data, the following counts are available: 61 women who received radiotherapy for their breast cancer and developed a lung cancer on the same side; 45 who developed lung cancer on the contralateral side; 53 women who did not receive radiotherapy, 25 of whom developed lung cancer on the same side. Example 2.4 presents this paired data and conducts a McNemar χ^2 test of the association between radiation and lung cancer, using the information in the discordant lung-breast pairs.

Example 2.4. *McNemar test of association between radiotherapy for breast cancer and subsequent lung cancer on the same side (from [174])*

	Breast Exposed: Yes	Breast Exposed: No
Lung Ca on same side: Yes	61	25
Lung Ca on same side: No	45	28

$$\chi^2 = \frac{(25-45)^2}{(25+45)}$$
$$= 5.714$$
$$\text{p} = .017$$

2.4.3 Test of homogeneity

In Section 2.3.3, we calculated the common Mantel-Hanszel OR estimator after an informal inspection suggested a similar association in each stratum. However, before computing a Mantel-Haenszel estimator, the homogeneity of the OR across the strata can be tested formally. The statistical methods for assessing if the data are consistent with a common underlying association are referred to as tests of 'homogeneity'. There are a number of such tests, including the earliest test proposed by Woolf in 1955 [236] and the Breslow-Day-Tarone test [24] that is commonly provided by statistical software packages. All the tests of homogeneity are very similar in spirit to the simple Chi-squared test of association in Section 2.4.1, as they are based on comparing the observed data in each stratum to what would be expected if there was a common OR, and assessing the magnitude of the total discrepancy. For example, if the 2-by-2 table for each stratum i is represented as in Table 2.7, then the discrepancy first proposed by Breslow and Day was:

$$\text{Discrepancy} = \frac{(a_c i - a_i^{est})^2}{\text{Var}(n_i)} \tag{2.13}$$

where the a_i are the numbers of exposed cases observed in each stratum, the superscript *est* denotes the estimates of these numbers under the hypothesis that there is a common OR (the Mantel-Haenszel estimator of Equation 2.7) and *Var* denotes the variance.

As with the simple Chi-squared test of association, the discrepancies between the observed and expected numbers are each squared, scaled by the variance, and then summed to give an overall discrepancy. Scaling by the variance allows the difference for each stratum to make a meaningful contribution to the discrepancy, since strata with high variability will have less influence on the total. Under the null hypothesis of a common OR across the strata, this discrepancy tends to be somewhat larger than a $\chi^2_{(K-1)}$ distribution, where K is the number of strata. With a correction proposed by Tarone [213], the discrepancy has an approximate $\chi^2_{(K-1)}$ distribution where the sample size is large compared to the number of strata [131] and is known as the Breslow-Day-Tarone test statistic.

Other tests of homogeneity differ with respect to the aspect of the observed data that is used for the comparison (Equation 2.13 above used the exposed cases), how the expected value of this quantity is estimated, and what is used as the scaling factor. For example, the Woolf test focuses on the ln(OR), and compares the ln(OR) in each of the strata to the weighted average over all strata (i.e. the estimate of a common ln(OR)), summing all the differences to obtain an overall discrepancy. Other tests of homogeneity use a similar approach to the Breslow-Day test above, but instead of using the Mantel-Haenszel OR as the estimate of the common OR, make other choices. Although worked numerical examples of tests of homogeneity can be found (e.g. Table 4.3 of the book by Breslow and Day [24] which is available online from IARC) such calculations are now commonly done using statistical software or a statistical calculator such as **openepi.com**.

Returning to the Framingham data on the prevalence of CHD and diabetes that was presented in Example 2.3, we can now test formally whether it was reasonable to assume a common OR in the three age strata.

Example 2.3 (continued). *Framingham Heart Study: prevalent coronary heart disease (CHD) and diabetes in three age groups.*

	Age 42–51 Diabetes			Age 52–61 Diabetes			Age 62–71 Diabetes		
	Yes	No		Yes	No		Yes	No	
Yes CHD	1	32	33	4	74	78	7	69	76
No CHD	28	1553	1581	47	1221	1268	29	440	469
	29	1585	1614	51	1295	1346	36	509	545
	OR = 1.73			**OR = 1.40**			**OR = 1.54**		

Test of homogeneity: $\chi^2 = 0.04$ p=0.98

The total discrepancy is very small, just 0.04. Comparing this to a $\chi^2_{(2)}$ distribution , the data is consistent with the hypothesis of a common OR in the three strata (p-value = 0.98) and so we conclude that it was reasonable to compute the Mantel-Haenszel estimate and present it as an estimate of this common OR, as done earlier in Example 2.3.

A less obvious example is provided by the data in Table 2.5 describing the prevalence of antibodies to leptospirosis in urban and rural populations. Although the sample data suggests that males and females have different risk, the Breslow-Day-Tarone test of homogeneity has a p-value of 0.46, suggesting that the difference may be due to randomness (and not an underlying systematic difference between the two groups in the population), so that the adjusted OR of 2.13 might be reported. It is worth noting here that the Breslow-Day-Tarone test of homogeneity is lacking in statistical power, so a real difference in groups might be missed if relying solely on this test.

2.4.4 Effect modification of an exposure-disease relationship

If a stratified analysis or test of homogeneity indicates that the relationship between exposure and disease differs across the groups, then it is not reasonable to assume a common OR or RR. Instead, we would suppose that the effect of the exposure on disease differs in the various strata in the population, with larger effects in some group(s) and smaller effect(s) in others. In the epidemiological literature, this is referred to as *effect modification* (the effect of the exposure is *modified* by the stratum variable) and in the statistical literature this is commonly called *interaction.*

When there is evidence of effect modification, it is clearly not meaningful to estimate a *common* risk estimate! If there are only a small number of strata and there is no obvious pattern in the relationship, the separate RRs or ORs can be reported. Example 2.5 presents the association between prevalent hypertension and diabetes in the Framingham data, overall and stratified by sex. Comparing the total discrepancy of 7.13 to a $\chi^2_{(1)}$ distribution, the test of homogeneity is significant (p= 0.0076) so we would not assume a common OR in males and females, and instead would report an estimated OR of 1.43 for males and 4.14 for females.

Example 2.5. *Framingham Heart Study: prevalent hypertension (HTN) and diabetes*

	Overall			Males			Females		
	Diabetes			**Diabetes**			**Diabetes**		
	Yes	No		Yes	No		Yes	No	
Yes HTN	67	1237	1304	25	520	545	42	717	759
No HTN	49	2152	2201	32	951	983	17	1201	1218
	116	3389	3505	57	1471	1528	59	1918	1977
	OR = 2.38			**OR = 1.43**			**OR = 4.14**		

Test of homogeneity: $\chi^2 = 7.13$ p=0.0076

2.4.5 Dose-response, test for trend

Until now, we have been addressing the following simple questions concerning the association of a binary exposure with a binary outcome:

- is there evidence of an association? (Chi-squared test) and how strong is it? (crude OR)
- is it reasonable to assume the association is common across strata? (inspection of OR across strata, test of homogeneity)
- what is the strength of the common association? (Mantel-Haenszel OR)
- is there evidence of confounding? (compare Mantel Haenszel OR to crude OR)

In many applications, the exposure will not be a simple binary variable, but may consist of a number of ordered categories, for example age groups. In such settings, an examination of the data may reveal a steady increase or decrease in the risk with the 'dose' of exposure. Such dose-response effect may provide important insight and is one of the Bradford-Hill [18] criteria for causation. For an exposure that is a risk factor, an increasing dose-response would be expected (i.e., more exposure associated with higher risk), while for a protective factor, it would be decreasing (i.e., more exposure, less risk).

An example which was presented in Table 2.3 earlier in this chapter, concerned alcohol consumption among lung cancer cases and healthy controls, where alcohol intake was classified into four (ordinal) levels. The numbers of lung cancer cases and controls in each group are presented again here in Table 2.13, where the odds of lung cancer (i.e. the ratio of cases to controls) and ln(odds) for each of the four exposure levels appear to be increasing with alcohol intake.

A simple Pearson Chi-squared test examines whether there is evidence of an association between alcohol intake and lung cancer. The discrepancy between the observed an expected counts is 186.8. Comparing this to the $\chi^2_{(3)}$ distribution (see Table 2.10) the p-value is <0.0001, indicating very strong evidence of an association. Consistent with the very low p-value, a plot of the ln(odds) values (Figure 2.7) demonstrates a very clear relationship and the strong linear pattern suggests that the effect of alcohol on the lung cancer risk could be described by the increase in risk (on the ln(odds) scale) per unit increase in daily intake. We will return to this idea again in the section on logistic regression below. For now, a simple crude test of the linearity of the relationship could be conducted by estimating the slope of the four ln(odds) values by simple

TABLE 2.13: *Odds of lung cancer in males for different levels of alcohol intake (measured as 'whiskey-equivalent' ounces per day).*

		Lung Cancer			
		Yes	No	odds	ln(odds)
Alcohol Intake	<1	1090	3976	.274	-1.295
	1–3.9	806	2244	.359	-1.024
	4–6.9	378	783	.482	-0.730
	≥7	679	1166	.582	-0.541
		2953	8169		

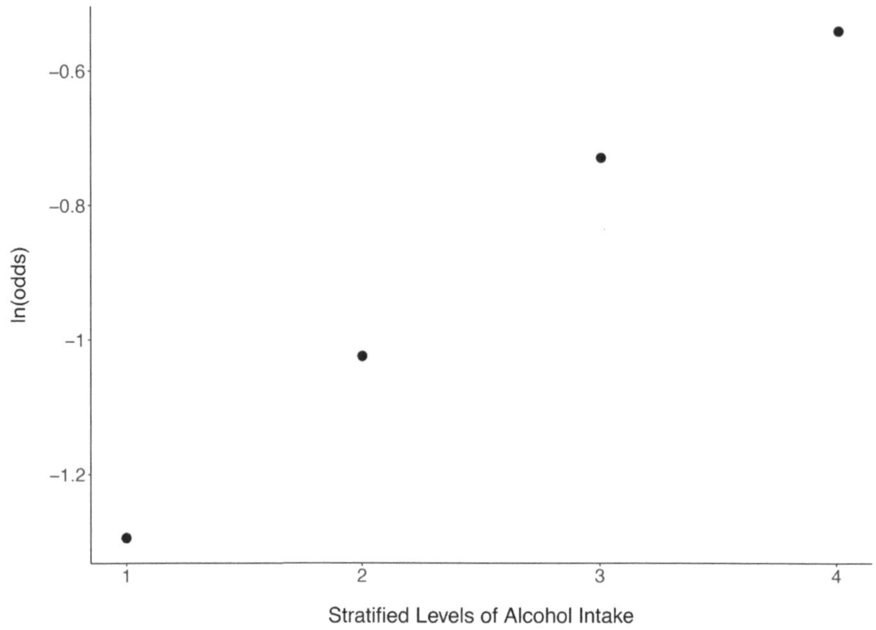

FIGURE 2.7: *Scatter plot of ln(odds) of lung cancer for different levels of alcohol intake, illustrating a clear trend.*

least squares regression and testing whether this slope is significantly different than zero.

The Breslow-Day method [24] uses the tabulated data to test for a *linear* trend in the ln(odds) across the levels of exposure. The method first assigns an exposure 'score' x_i, to each stratum i and then compares the total exposure score for the cases in each of the strata to what would be expected if there was no trend (i.e. if the exposure scores in all strata were the same for all individuals, the average value). Where the exposure levels are categories of a continuous variable, it is common to use the midpoints as the scores'. This would be straightforward in the diabetes example above, with age scores of 46.5, 56.5 and 66.5, but it may be unclear how to assign a score to the highest or lowest category in examples like the alcohol and lung cancer example. Without further knowledge of the range of exposure values, integer scores can be used. For equally spaced strata, such as in the diabetes example, simply using scores 1,2,3 will give the same result as the midpoints, but where strata are not equally spaced, the trend being examined by using integer scores is the change in ln(odds) between neighbouring strata and not the trend per unit change in the actual exposure value.

Similar to the χ^2 tests already encountered, the appropriately scaled discrepancy has a Chi-squared distribution ($\chi^2_{(1)}$). Such tests are rarely computed by hand, since they can be implemented by statistical calculators and packages by simply providing the counts in the table. However it is helpful to understand that the χ^2 test statistic in Equation 2.14 is again a discrepancy, scaled by a variance term. With x_i, n_i and n_{1i} denoting the exposure score, number of observations and number of cases for the ith stratum, the numerator compares the total score observed for the cases to the total score expected if there was no trend (all N_1 cases had the average score in the sample, $\bar{x}$). With p denoting the overall proportion of cases and N the total sample size, the terms in the denominator represent the variance in the total number of cases and their scores.

$$\frac{[\sum_{i=1}^{K} n_{1i}x_i - N_1\bar{x}]^2}{p(1-p)N[\sum_{i=1}^{K} \frac{n_i x_i^2}{N} - \bar{x}^2]} \tag{2.14}$$

Trend in OR across strata

When a stratified analysis of an exposure-disease relationship suggests an increasing or decreasing pattern in the strength of the relationship across strata, but the test of homogeneity fails to reject the hypothesis of a common OR, this could be due to a lack of power. Thus, it is of interest to have a more sensitive test of whether the data provide evidence of a trend in the ORs across the strata in the underlying population. By assigning scores for the (ordinal) strata, the Breslow-Day test for trend offers a test that is sensitive to a linear trend in the ln(OR) across the strata. The test statistic is similar in form to Equation 2.14 and again has a $\chi^2(1)$ distribution under the null hypothesis of no association. Example 2.6 provides an illustration using the Framingham data. The crude OR for the association between diabetes and cardiovascular disease is 4.06. A stratified analysis suggests that there is heterogeneity in the OR across age groups, but the $\chi^2(1)$ test of homogeneity is not significant. However, the stratified analysis indicates a decrease in the OR with increasing age, and the more sensitive test for trend finds evidence of such a trend.

Example 2.6. *Framingham Heart Study: association between diabetes and cardiovascular disease (CVD).*

Total

	CVD Yes	CVD No	
Diabetes	72	44	116
No Diabetes	974	2415	3389
	1046	2459	3505

OR = 4.06

Stratified by Age Category

	Ages 42–51 CVD Yes	Ages 42–51 CVD No		Ages 52–61 CVD Yes	Ages 52–61 CVD No		Ages 62–71 CVD Yes	Ages 62–71 CVD No	
Diabetes	17	12	29	31	20	51	24	12	36
No Diabetes	334	1251	1585	416	879	1295	224	285	509
	351	1263	1614	447	899	1346	248	297	545
	OR = 5.31			**OR = 3.28**			**OR = 2.54**		

χ^2 **Test of Homogeneity** $\chi^2 = 2.01$ p=0.3659

χ^2 **Test of trend:** χ^2=43.50 p<0.001

2.5 Logistic Regression

Regression analysis is used to model the relationship between variables, or more specifically, to model the impact of various factors (X) on an outcome of interest (Y), in order to answer the questions:

- Is there a relationship between variables X and Y?
- How does Y change if X changes?
- What is the best guess for Y for given value(s) of X?

- How good is that guess?
- How much of the variation in Y is explained by the X variables (together or alone)?
- ... and finally: does X cause Y?

Different models are useful depending on the type of outcome variable. If the outcome variable Y is continuous and there is a single predictor variable X (also continuous), **simple linear regression** (also known as 'least squares') fits the best straight line to the data. The model assumes that in the population, the expected (or average) Y is related to X by the simple straight-line formula in Equation 2.15.

$$E(Y|X) = \alpha + \beta X \tag{2.15}$$

where $E(Y|X)$ should be read as 'the expected value of Y, given the value of X'. The slope of the line, β, is the change in the expected value of Y when X changes by one unit, and α is the intercept, so that the underlying (linear) relationship is completely described by these two parameters. The relationship can also be written:

$$Y = \alpha + \beta X + \epsilon \tag{2.16}$$

which states that for a *specific* X value, the corresponding Y is the expected or average Y at that X, plus a random error component, ϵ. The 'least squares' line is that which minimises the total squared error, i.e. the discrepancy between the line and the actual data. Several examples of such relationships were presented earlier in this chapter using data on finger length, height and ideal partner's height (Figure 2.2). A glance at those plots will make it clear that the error term, ϵ, represents the random variation of the *individual* Y values around the expected level for any X: the linear model fitted to the data assumes this random variation to have a normal distribution.

For a dichotomous outcome variable, such as disease (Yes, No), a linear relationship is not meaningful, and in this setting, the **logistic regression model** is widely used to model the underlying (unobserved) probability of disease as a function of various independent variables, such as exposure(s) and confounders. In the simple case of a single continuous exposure variable X, and assuming disease Y is coded as (1=Yes, 0=No), the logistic model for the probability that Y=1 for a given X is:

$$P(Y = 1|X) = \frac{e^{\alpha+\beta X}}{1 + e^{\alpha+\beta X}} \tag{2.17}$$

The probability of disease among the unexposed is

$$P(Y = 1|X = 0) = \frac{e^{\alpha}}{1 + e^{\alpha}} \tag{2.18}$$

so that α contains the information about the prevalence (in the unexposed). While at first glance this may seem like a very awkward model, if we instead describe how the *Odds* of Y, and from that, the ln(odds), which is also called the **logit**, depends on X

,

$$\text{Odds}(Y = 1|X) = \frac{P(Y = 1|X)}{1 - P(Y = 1|X)} \tag{2.19}$$

$$= e^{\alpha+\beta X} \tag{2.20}$$

$$\text{logit}(Y = 1|X) = \alpha + \beta X \tag{2.21}$$

we see that the logistic model for the probability is actually a simple linear model for the ln(odds). Unlike simple linear regression, where the errors are assumed to have a normal distribution, the errors in the logistic model have a binomial distribution, as it is modelling probabilities (proportions) and not continuous outcomes. The α and β that 'best fit' the data are found by a method called 'maximum likelihood', not 'least squares' as in linear regression. However, many of the ideas for linear regression apply to logistic regression and it will often be helpful to return to the linear regression examples earlier in this chapter to help visualise some of the ideas that are not so 'visible' in a logistic regression analysis.

Readers may still think it rather awkward to decide to model the ln(odds), but there are many surprises in store! We will soon see that this model provides a simple and flexible method for estimating ORs, adjusting for confounding and assessing effect modification, from much more complex data than can be handled by the tables in the previous sections. In the following sections, we revisit a range of settings, from the simplest 2-by-2 table, to confounding and effect modification, and consider the estimation of ORs using the logistic regression model.

For the simple case of a single dichotomous exposure X, taking the values 1=exposed, 0=unexposed, the logistic model for disease Y (1=disease, 0= no disease) assumes that:

$$\text{If X=1: Odds}(Y=1) = e^{\alpha+\beta(1)} = e^{\alpha+\beta} \quad (2.22)$$

$$\text{If X=0: Odds}(Y=1) = e^{\alpha+\beta(0)} = e^{\alpha} \quad (2.23)$$

$$\text{OR} = e^{\beta} \quad (2.24)$$

The parameter α is the ln(odds) of disease in the unexposed individuals, so e^{α} represents the odds and thus the prevalence. The coefficient β of exposure in the equation is the ln(OR) for exposed vs. unexposed individuals. Equivalently, the exponent of the exposure coefficient (i.e. e^{β}) is the OR for exposure. If instead of a 2-by-2 table with counts a, b, c, d, we have a dataset with a record for each of the individual n observations, with their binary exposure status X and binary outcome Y recorded as 0/1 variables, then a simple logistic regression analysis that specifies Y as the outcome and X as the exposure, finds the estimates of α and β that provide the 'best fit' to the data (using the maximum likelihood method). Unsurprisingly, the estimate of β, which we denote as $\hat{\beta}$ will be exactly the same as the ln(OR) that we could calculate from the simple 2-by-2 table of the counts obtained by cross-tabulating the exposure and outcome variables in the dataset.

For example, a logistic regression of the Framingham data with diabetes as outcome and CHD as exposure gives the following, which is exactly what was obtained earlier from the 2-by-2 table in Example 2.3.

Example 2.3 (continued). *Framingham Heart Study: prevalent coronary heart disease (CHD) and diabetes*

	Exposure	**Odds Ratio**	**95% CI**
Unadjusted	Prevalent CHD	2.12	1.14 – 3.93

If an exposure has more than two levels, for example levels $0, 1, 2 \ldots K$, with 0 denoting the reference level, then the logistic model for the ln(odds)(Y=1) at each level, without assuming any pattern (such as a trend) is given by the equations in Table 2.14 (a), i.e. a different β in each stratum.

TABLE 2.14: *(a) Model for a different ln(odds) at each level of a stratum variable, with level 0 as reference; (b) the corresponding odds in each stratum.*

$$
\begin{array}{llcll}
\textbf{(a)} & \ln(\text{odds})(\text{Y=1}) & = & \alpha & \text{for level 0} \\
 & & = & \alpha+\beta_1 & \text{for level 1} \\
 & & = & \alpha+\beta_2 & \text{for level 2} \\
 & & = & \alpha+\beta_3 & \text{for level 3} \\
 & & \dots & & \\
 & & = & \alpha+\beta_K & \text{for level K}
\end{array}
$$

$$
\begin{array}{llcll}
\textbf{(b)} & \text{Odds(Y=1)} & = & e^{\alpha} & \text{for level 0} \\
 & & = & e^{\alpha+\beta_1} & \text{for level 1} \\
 & & = & e^{\alpha+\beta_2} & \text{for level 2} \\
 & & = & \dots & \\
 & & = & e^{\alpha+\beta_K} & \text{for level K}
\end{array}
$$

Thus the OR for level 1 versus level 0 =

$$\frac{e^{\alpha+\beta_1}}{e^{\alpha}} = e^{\beta_1}$$

and the OR for any level i (relative to the reference level) is e^{β_i} (Table 2.14 (b)). For a dataset with n individual observations, each recording a binary outcome and an exposure level from 0 to K, a logistic regression analysis will report the ln(OR) for each level of the exposure versus a reference: these will be exactly the same as the ln(OR) that would be computed from a $K \times 2$ table (such as Table 2.13) that uses the same reference. It is not uncommon, if a categorical variable has a small number of levels, to replace the variable by several 'dummy' (binary) variables, one for each level except the one considered as reference. A typical example would be a four-level BMI variable, with categories normal, underweight, overweight, obese: by creating a binary (yes/no) variable for the underweight, overweight and obese categories, the OR for each of these (relative to the normal BMI) will be estimated by logistic regression.

If, instead of comparisons with the reference level, it was of interest to compare two (other) levels of the exposure, the relevant OR can be easily found from the difference in the β coefficients of the two levels being compared (j and i), as follows:

$$\begin{aligned}\text{ln(odds) for level j} &= \alpha + \beta_j \\ \text{ln(odds) for for level i} &= \alpha + \beta_i \\ \text{Change in ln(odds)} &= \beta_i - \beta_j \\ \text{OR (i vs. j)} &= e^{\beta_i - \beta_j}\end{aligned}$$

2.5.1 Adjusted OR from logistic regression

If there is a common value of OR relating response (Y) to a binary exposure (X=0,1) in each of several strata (e.g. age strata), then this can be modelled as:

$$\begin{aligned}\text{ln(odds) for stratum 1} &= \alpha_1 + \beta X \\ \text{ln(odds) for stratum 2} &= \alpha_2 + \beta X \\ &\cdots \\ \text{ln(odds) for stratum K} &= \alpha_K + \beta X\end{aligned}$$

The different α values model the fact that the actual odds (or risk) may be different from stratum to stratum, but the *same* β value in each stratum implies that the OR for $X = 1$ (exposed) compared to $X = 0$, *regardless of stratum*, is e^{β}. Defining a categorical variable Z with K levels, the equations above can be written

$$\text{ln(odds)}(Y = 1) = \alpha + \beta X + \gamma Z$$

where α now represents the ln(odds) in unexposed ($X = 0$) individuals in the reference stratum: if stratum 1 is chosen as the reference, then $\alpha = \alpha_1$ and the coefficients γ represent the difference between α_1 and the ln(odds) in the other strata defined by Z. For example, for the common OR for the association between prevalent CHD and diabetes in the different age groups in the Framingham Heart Study in Example 2.3, we would fit a logistic regression model with diabetes specified as the outcome and two predictor variables (the binary variable CHD and the three-level age category). The coefficient of CHD from the regression provides the estimate $\hat{\beta}$ of the common ln(OR), β, and on exponentiating, $e^{\hat{\beta}}$ gives an adjusted OR (see Example 2.3 continued) that is essentially the same as the Mantel-Haenszel OR we computed earlier!

Example 2.3 (continued). *Framingham Heart Study: association between prevalent coronary heart disease (CHD) and diabetes*

	Exposure	Odds Ratio	95% CI
Adjusted	Prevalent CHD	1.50	0.799 – 2.83

2.5.2 Logistic regression model with interaction term

When there is evidence of heterogeneity, it is not appropriate to assume a common β describing the association of interest. In this case, the risk of disease depends not only on the exposure status of an individual, but on which stratum they belong to. Thus, the ln(odds) is no longer just a function of the exposure as in the simple examples above, but needs to model a different association between exposure and disease for the different strata. As a simple illustration, we return to Example 2.5 where the association between prevalent hypertension and diabetes differed for males and females. Denoting diabetes (the outcome) as Y, the indicator for hypertension (the exposure) as X, and a binary variable Z denoting the sex (with Z=0 for males, and Z=1 for females), then the ln(odds) can be written as:

$$\text{logit } (\text{Y=1}|\text{X, Z}) = \alpha + \beta_1 X + \beta_2 Z + \gamma X * Z \qquad (2.25)$$

where β_1 describes the exposure effect, β_2 the sex effect and γ the additional effect of exposure in stratum Z=1 (females) since the product X*Z will be zero except for records with X=1 and Z=1. For the different values of X and Z, we examine the values taken by the logit (and hence the odds) in columns 3 and 4 of Table 2.15. The final column presents the OR of exposure in each of the groups compared to (X=0, Z=0) as reference. Thus, β_1 provides an estimate of the effect of exposure in the stratum with Z=0, β_2 provides the effect of being female (Z=1) among the unexposed individuals (X=0). If $\gamma = 0$, the OR for exposure (X=1 vs. X=0) is e^{β_1} for both Z=0 and Z=1, but when γ is non-zero it represents the additional contribution to the odds for individuals who are both exposed and female, i.e. the magnitude of the effect modification.

TABLE 2.15: *Logit, odds and OR (with first group as reference) for the different values of X and Z.*

X	Z	logit	Odds	OR
0	0	α	e^{α}	$\frac{e^{\alpha}}{e^{\alpha}} = 1$
1	0	$\alpha + \beta_1$	$e^{(\alpha+\beta_1)}$	e^{β_1}
0	1	$\alpha + \beta_2$	$e^{(\alpha+\beta_2)}$	e^{β_2}
1	1	$\alpha + \beta_1 + \beta_2 + \gamma$	$e^{(\alpha+\beta_1+\beta_2+\gamma)}$	$e^{(\beta_1+\beta_2+\gamma)}$

The first row in Example 2.5(continued) presents the crude OR from a logistic regression analysis of the Framingham data with diabetes as outcome and hypertension as exposure. As before, this is identical to what is obtained from the 2-by-2 table. To model the effect of sex, and its potential modification of the exposure effect, two additional terms are added to the logistic model: the binary sex variable (Z), and the interaction term, which we will denote by X*Z. If X and Z are numeric, the interaction variable can be constructed by multiplying X (exposure) and Z (sex) as this will create a variable that takes the value 1 when both X and Z are =1. However, it is rarely necessary to do this, as most software packages allow the user to specify any categorical variables whose interaction is of interest and present the output in terms of the levels of those variables.

Example 2.5 (continued). *Framingham Heart Study: prevalent hypertension (X) and diabetes (Y): modification by sex (Z)*

	Exposure	Odds Ratio	95% C.I.
Unadjusted	Hypertension	2.38	1.63 – 3.46
Interaction Model	Hypertension	1.43	0.84 – 2.44
	Sex (Female)	0.42	0.23 – 0.76
	Sex* Hypertension	2.90	1.33 – 6.33

The OR of 1.43 is the effect of the exposure in males (the reference group) which agrees with what we obtained from the stratified analysis in

Example 2.5. The interaction term is significant (the confidence interval excludes 1.0), indicating that there is heterogeneity between males and females, consistent with our significant test of homogeneity earlier. The logged values of the ORs 1.43 and 2.90 correspond to β and γ in the equations above, so that the ln(OR) for the effect of the exposure in females is ln(1.43)+ln(2.90) = 1.42, an OR of $e^{1.42} = 4.14$ in agreement with the stratified analysis.

2.5.3 Modelling a linear effect of a continuous variable

When there is a continuous exposure of interest or a continuous confounder requiring adjustment, data analysts will often categorise the continuous variable and use techniques similar to those in the previous sections to estimate the effect in the different categories of the exposure or to adjust for differences across the different categories of the confounder. However, it may be more appropriate to model the effect of the continuous variable: the risk of disease may rise/fall steadily with the value of the continuous exposure or the effect of the exposure may change for every small change in the (continuous) confounder. The logistic function encountered earlier in Equation 2.17 and which is presented again below in Equation 2.26 provides a very flexible model for the effect of a continuous variable on the probability of a binary outcome. For example, Figure 2.8 illustrates the probabilities computed from logistic functions with different α and β parameters for a continuous covariate X. A larger value of β reflects a steeper increase in risk with increasing X, and the value of α reflects the level of X at which risk begins to rise, i.e. the level that discriminates between the low and high risk individuals.

As seen previously in the discussion of a binary exposure, if the probability follows a logistic regression model, the ln(odds) is a *linear* function of X.

$$P(Y = 1|X) = \frac{e^{\alpha+\beta X}}{1 + e^{\alpha+\beta X}} \tag{2.26}$$

$$\ln\{(\text{Odds}(Y = 1|X)\} = \alpha + \beta X \tag{2.27}$$

Figure 2.9 provides an example of a logistic curve and corresponding ln(odds) for a continuous X ranging from 0 to 50 units. The parameter β now represents the change in ln(odds) *per unit change in* X so that the interpretation is:

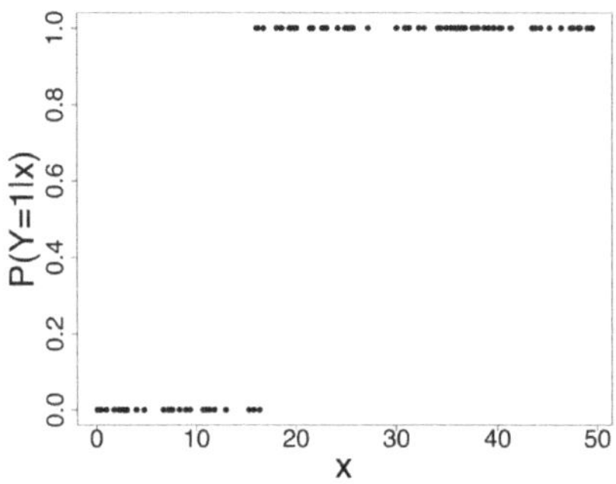

(a) *Points for logistic function with* $\alpha = -6$ *and* $\beta = 0.4$

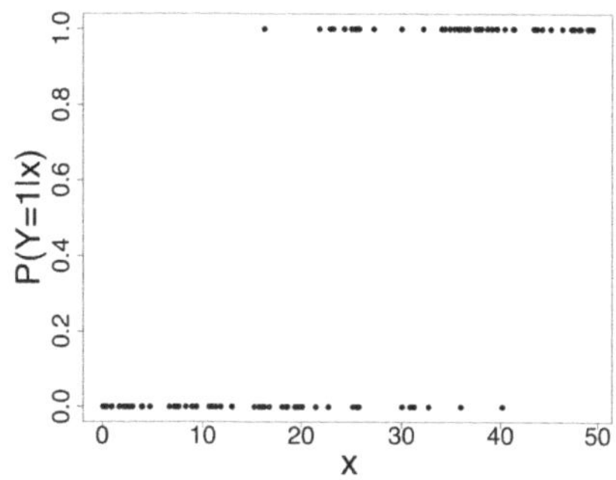

(b) *Points for logistic function with* $\alpha = -6$ *and* $\beta = 0.2$

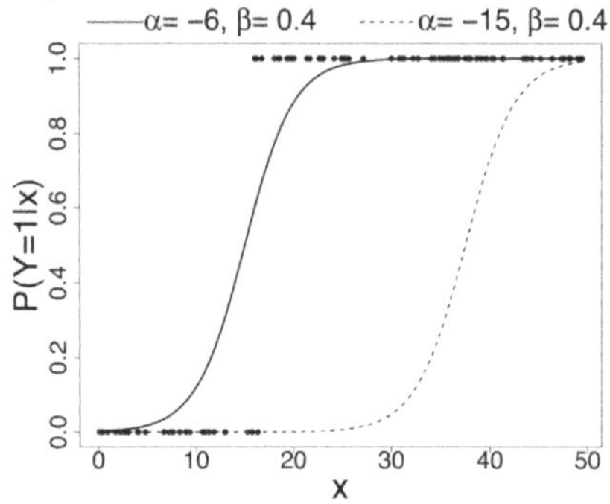

(c) *Two logistic functions with* $\beta = 0.4$

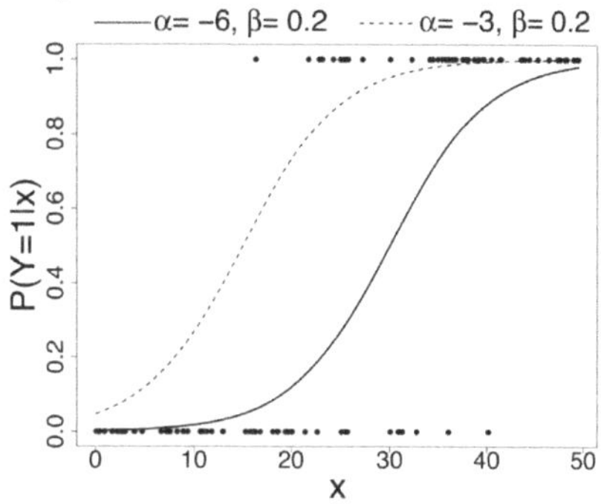

(d) *Two logistic functions with* $\beta = 0.2$

FIGURE 2.8: *Points and curves of logistic functions with varying* α *and* β *values.*

$$e^{\beta} = OR \text{ for unit change in X} \tag{2.28}$$

$$e^{2\beta} = OR \text{ for a change of 2 units} \tag{2.29}$$

$$e^{k\beta} = OR \text{ for a change of k units} \tag{2.30}$$

A first assessment of whether it is reasonable to fit a linear effect for a continuous variable is to examine the trend across categories generated from the variable, by plotting the ln(odds) versus the midpoints of the catergories. Such a plot for the ln(odds) of CHD versus categorised SBP in the Framingham data has a clear linear pattern, so a simple logistic regression model for the risk of CHD as a function of an individual's SBP is $logit(CHD = 1|SBP) = \alpha + \beta * SBP$. This results in an estimate $\hat{\beta} = 0.0198$ per unit change in SBP, i.e., 0.198 per 10 units, a crude OR of

1.22 (Example 2.7, first row). A model that includes a binary variable for sex (with females as the reference group) and a categorical age variable (with the youngest individuals, aged <40, as the reference) gives the estimates in the middle panel of Example 2.7, from which the OR per 10 units change in SBP, adjusted for sex and age group, is 1.19. Note that there is an apparent trend in the effect of age, and a model that adjusts for a linear effect of age rather than for age categories, gives very similar results for the ORs for SBP and male sex (Example 2.7, lower panel). The OR per one year increase in age is 1.04, which is equivalent to an OR of 1.48 per 10 units increase, consistent with the estimates for the age groups, which differ from each other by approximately this factor.

In the example above, the effect of SBP on CHD is not confounded by age and sex, as the crude and adjusted estimates of the OR are similar. It made little or no difference whether age was included as a categorical variable or as a linear term: in such situation, the model with linear trend has greater statistical power, especially if some categories have a small number of individuals. Sometimes adjustment for a categorised version of a continuous variable results in a smaller adjustment to the crude OR, especially if only a few categories are used. This suggests some residual confounding due to differences that are not adjusted adequately, for example a trend in the risk with age within the (wide) categories.

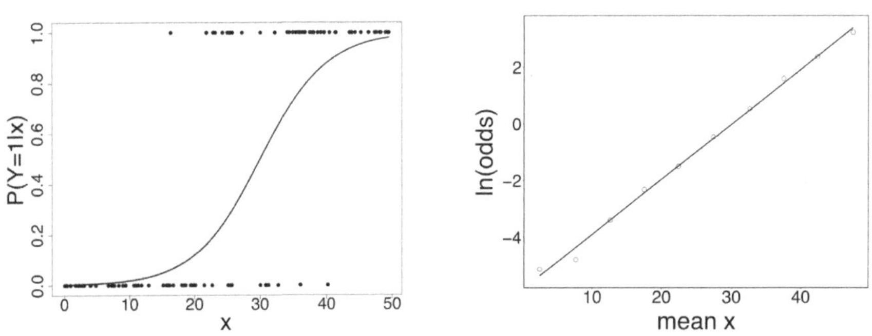

(a) *Points and curve for logistic function with* $\alpha = -6$ *and* $\beta = 0.2$

(b) *Ln(odds) plot for the logistic function and points in (a)*

FIGURE 2.9: *Points and curve of logistic function with* $\alpha = -6$ *and* $\beta = 0.2$ *(a) and corresponding ln(odds) plot (b).*

2.5.4 Multivariable logistic regression

In real applications, the logistic regression models will often be more complex than the examples presented above, as there may be more than one exposure of interest, and several potential confounders, some of which modify the exposure effect(s), and some of which may be continuous and perhaps exhibit a dose-response. In addition, the relationship between an exposure and outcome may have a trend across categories of an ordinal stratum variable. While it is technically straightforward to fit a complex model to data, care must be taken that coefficients are interpreted correctly with respect to the chosen reference categories, particularly in the presence of effect modification. If the final model has no

Example 2.7. *Framingham Heart Study: linear effect of systolic blood pressure (SBP) on coronary heart disease (CHD).*

	Covariates	Odds Ratio	95% C.I.
Unadjusted	SBP*	1.22	1.18 – 1.26
Adjusted by:			
Sex and age group	SBP*	1.19	1.15 – 1.23
	Male	2.40	2.09 – 2.76
	Age <40	1.0	–
	Age 40–49	1.34	1.04 – 1.74
	Age 50-59	1.92	1.48 – 2.50
	Age ≥60	2.64	1.99 – 3.50
Sex and linear age	SBP*	1.18	1.14 – 1.22
	Male	2.41	2.09 – 2.77
	Age	1.04	1.03 – 1.05

* *per 10 mm change in systolic blood pressure (SBP)*

interaction terms, then the coefficient for any covariate is the estimate of the common effect of that factor in individuals who have the same values for all other variables.

For example, a model with K explanatory variables (exposure(s) and confounders) denoted by $X_1, X_2, \ldots X_K$ is written:

$$\ln(\text{odds}) = \alpha + \beta_1 X_1 + \beta_2 X_2 \ldots \beta_K X_K \tag{2.31}$$

$$\text{odds} = e^{\alpha}(e^{\beta_1 X_1})(e^{\beta_2 X_2}) \ldots (e^{\beta_K X_K}) \tag{2.32}$$

$$= (\text{base odds}) OR_1 OR_2 \ldots OR_K \tag{2.33}$$

so that the logistic model for how the risk of disease depends on the explanatory factors is *multiplicative* on the odds scale. In the simplest case where all the X variables are binary, the odds for an individual with a given covariate profile is the base odds' (i.e. the odds when all X values are zero) multiplied by the OR values for all X variables with value 1). In the general case where the X variables may be binary, categorical or continuous, the base odds, e^{α}, is the odds of disease in the chosen reference group, which can be defined using a specific category for binary/categorical variables and the average values for continuous variable, although other choices may be preferred depending on the application.

In the simple model in Equation 2.31 above, there were no interactions included between the explanatory factors. Thus, the e^{β_i} values are the ORs describing the (common) effect of the explanatory variables X_i in individuals in each of the strata defined by the other X variables, i.e., the OR for the effect of X_i in those with the same values for all other X variables. Where there is an interaction term in the model, and thus no common effect for the 'interacting' variables, the reporting of results depends on the primary research question. If the interaction involves only confounders (and not the main exposure of interest), then it is meaningful to report the OR for the exposure effect as an adjusted OR. If the interaction term represents a non-homogenous effect of the main exposure at different levels of another covariate, then it is not meaningful to report the single OR of the main exposure, but instead the ORs should be reported for specific sub-groups of interest. Some simple guidelines for reporting interactions are provided in the paper by Knol et al. [108].

2.5.5 From prospective to retrospective models

For cohort or cross-sectional data, the logistic model is a *regression model* in the usual sense, in that the covariate(s) X can be fixed or chosen and the random outcome Y is then modelled as a function of X. As seen earlier, the α parameter in the model represents the prevalence in the population from which the sample was drawn. However, for case-control data, we cannot model the probability of disease, as the sampling of the study subjects is dependent on disease status. For example, in a study where an equal number of cases and controls are selected, the 'prevalence' in the sample (50%) is completely determined by the design (equal numbers of cases and controls) and carries no information about the actual prevalence in the underlying population. For case-control data, we can however model the probability of disease *conditional on being sampled* and from this we can estimate effects of interest.

Assume that in the underlying population, the probability of disease is described by the logistic function as before:

$$\text{Prob}(Y = 1|X, Z) = \frac{e^{\alpha+\beta X}}{1 + e^{\alpha+\beta X}} \tag{2.34}$$

We cannot model this from case-control data, but we *can* model the probability conditional on being sampled, which is written as $P[Y = 1|X, Sampled]$ or $P[Y = 1|X, S = 1]$ where S is an indicator variable for being sampled. If the probability of an individual in the population being sampled for the study is π_1 for cases and π_0 for controls, then using Bayes theorem, $P[Y = 1|X, S = 1]$ can be rewritten as in Equations 2.35 to 2.38.

$$P[Y = 1|X, S = 1]$$

$$= \frac{P[Y = 1, X, S = 1]}{P[X, S = 1]} \tag{2.35}$$

$$= \frac{P[X]P[Y = 1|X]P[S = 1|X, Y = 1]}{P[X, S = 1]} \tag{2.36}$$

$$= \frac{P[X]P[Y = 1|X]P[S = 1|X, Y = 1]}{P[X]P[Y = 1|X]P[S = 1|X, Y = 1] + P[X]P[Y = 0|X]P[S = 1|X, Y = 0]} \tag{2.37}$$

Cancelling P[X] and using the sampling probabilities, π_1 and π_0, for cases and controls:

$$= \frac{\frac{e^{\alpha}}{e^{\alpha+\beta X}}\pi_1}{\frac{e^{\alpha}}{e^{\alpha+\beta X}}\pi_1 + (1 - \frac{e^{\alpha}}{e^{\alpha+\beta X}})\pi_0}$$

$$= \frac{e^{\alpha^*}}{e^{\alpha^*+\beta X}} \tag{2.38}$$

$$\text{where } \alpha^* = \alpha + ln(\frac{\pi_1}{\pi_0}) \tag{2.39}$$

In Chapter 1, the OR describing the association between an exposure and outcome in a population was estimated from the 2-by-2 table constructed from either a cohort or case-control sample. Equivalently, if a logistic model describes how the risk of disease in the underlying population depends on an exposure X, then the OR can be estimated either from cohort or case-control data. The risk in the sampled case-control data is described by the same logistic model as the risk in the population (or a cohort sample) with the same exposure effect β but different α (i.e. a different base odds as we would expect. In summary:

$$\text{logit } P[Y = 1|X] = \alpha + \beta X \tag{2.40}$$

$$\Longrightarrow \text{logit } P[Y = 1|X, S = 1] = \alpha^* + \beta X \tag{2.41}$$

$$\text{where } \alpha^* = \alpha + ln(\frac{\pi_1}{\pi_0}) \tag{2.42}$$

and π_1 and π_0 are the sampling fractions of cases and controls from the study population. If all cases and all controls are sampled (i.e. $\pi_1 = \pi_0 = 1$) so that the whole cohort is available, then α^* is the same as α and we are fitting the population model. Regardless of the sampling strategy for cases and controls, the exposure effect β that is estimated from a logistic model is the same exposure effect as in the prospective data from a cohort study. The only difference in the case-control analysis is that the population prevalence is no longer represented by the intercept term. However, if the sampling fractions for cases and controls are known, the prevalence can be recovered from the α^* estimate using the relationship between α^* and α in Equation 2.42 above. This idea of recovering population estimates from biased data using sampling weights is an important theme in much of the later chapters of this book.

The validity of the logistic regression model applied to retrospective data, for which Prentice and Pyke presented formal proof in 1979 [173], has led to its wide adoption for the analysis of exposure effects from epidemiological data in the last few decades. In addition, there have been numerous methodological developments to enable case-control data to yield estimates of other quantities that were initially thought to be accessible only from cohort data. These methods will constitute a significant portion of the remaining sections of this book, which will explore the various ways of 'controlling' epidemiological studies of different designs to obtain the desired estimates.

2.5.6 Matched data

An alternative to adjusting for confounders at the analysis stage, as in the previous sections, is to use a **matched design** for sampling the study subjects. This is most commonly used in case-control studies, where the controls are chosen to match' the cases on one or more confounders. Where the confounders define large strata, within which the number of controls is randomly chosen to be a constant times the number of cases, the design is called a **frequency matched**. Where the matching variables define more individual characteristics and a specific number of controls is selected to match each individual case, the design is **individually matched**: one-to-one matching results in the paired data that was presented earlier. In matched case-control studies, it is common to have up to 5 controls per case. When the control data is readily available (for example from a database or register), investigators may select more than 5 controls per case, but additional controls will only result in modest gains in efficiency if there are no more cases. For studies that incur a cost for every individual enrolled, such as the early examples of clinic-based case-control studies, the balance between cost and information led to the widespread use of between 3 and 5 controls per case. For a binary exposure, a case-control study that selects all cases and M times as many controls captures a fraction M/(M+1) of the information in the whole cohort [24], so that approximately 80% of the total cohort information is available from a 1:4 case-control study. While this simple rule of thumb is useful, in any specific application the power of the study depends not only on the ratio of controls to cases, but also on the magnitude of the RR to be estimated and the prevalence of the exposure in the non-cases. The expression developed and used in early work on sample size and efficiency of case-control designs ([29, 20]) was used to generate Figure 2.10 which displays the number of cases required in a 1:1 case-control study as a function of the RR and the prevalence of exposure among the controls.

Such sample size calculation can be readily done today using software tools: for example, the on-line calculator, **Openepi.com**, provides sample size and power calculations for a simple (non-matched) case-control study, and Stata's **power mcc** command offers automated or customised tables and graphs (https://www.stata.com/features/power-and-sample-size/).

Matching on confounders is also employed in cohort studies, although the term matched cohort' is more rarely used to describe such studies than their case-control counterparts. For frequency-matched cohort stud-

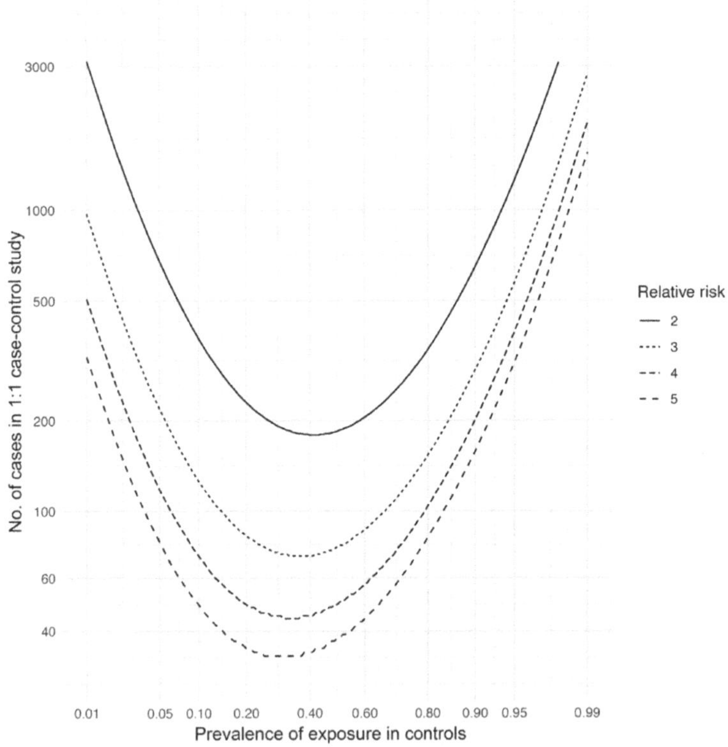

FIGURE 2.10: *Plot of number of cases required in a 1:1 case-control sample for a power of 95% and significance level 5%, as a function of prevalence and RR.*

ies, this is unsurprising when we consider that the analysis of disease risk in a cohort, even where the explanatory variables have been used to select subjects, fits in the usual regression paradigm where sampling can depend on explanatory variables. In case-control studies, matching is not only dependent on the explanatory variables used in the matching, but also on the outcome, as the matching forces the selected controls to be similar to the cases on some characteristics. Thus the relationship between the matching factors and the outcome is disturbed in the study sample. In either the cohort or case-control design, there is an appropriate method of analysing matched data, which is introduced for the case-control design in the following paragraphs.

Frequency matched case-control data

Consider a frequency matched case-control study where cases and controls are matched in a ratio of 1:K on a single stratum variable with levels 1,2, ... S. The stratum variable may be a single variable (e.g. age-group) that is known for each member of the population, or it may be a combination of two or more variables (e.g. sex and age-group). If the disease is rare, all cases may be included in the study (i.e. a sampling fraction of 1.0), but each stratum will have a different sampling fraction for controls in order to select just K from those available. In the more general design, where a fixed number of cases (not all) are also selected from each stratum, then the sampling fraction of cases will also vary across strata. Denoting the sampling fraction of cases and controls in a specific stratum s as π_{1s} and π_{0s}, and assuming a common exposure effect, β, in all strata, then if the relationship between the exposure X and outcome in the population is described by the logistic function, the model describing the sampled data in stratum s is:

$$\text{logit } P[Y = 1|X, Sampled] = \alpha^{*s} + \beta X \text{ in stratum } s \quad (2.43)$$

$$\text{where } \alpha^{*s} = \alpha^{s} + ln(\frac{\pi_{1s}}{\pi_{0s}}) \quad (2.44)$$

so that the common β can be estimated by fitting a logistic model including a term for each stratum.

If a frequency-matched case-control study uses fine matching, the logistic model in 2.43 will involve a large number of stratum effects, α^{*s}. These effects are not of intrinsic interest, so it is not efficient to use the information in the data to estimate them. If instead, each case is individually matched to one or more controls, then the matching factors do not enter into the analysis, as will be explained in detail in the following section.

2.6 Individually Matched Data

Although power calculations will rarely suggest just one control per case, there are numerous settings where case-control pairs are the natural (and only) data available. For example, in sibling studies it is common to compare an affected and unaffected sibling in an effort to adjust for genetic and shared family environment. Studies of twins are particularly valuable, as monozygous twins share 100% of their genetic material and dizygous twins share 50%. Thus comparisons of case-control monozygotic twin pairs offer full adjustment for genetic factors, comparisons of the strength of an association in monozygotic and dizygotic twins enables the separation of genetic and shared family factors, and finally a comparison of twins reared together to those reared apart provides estimates of the contribution of a non-shared environment. Studies of spouses are also valuable where risk estimates are to be adjusted for the adult environment.

2.6.1 OR from paired data

As with the McNemar test, the OR for paired data uses only the discordant pairs, since only these contribute information about the relationship between the exposure and outcome. The paired OR, which measures the association between exposure and outcome *adjusted for the common factors of the pair* is simply the ratio of the numbers of the two types of discordant pairs, i.e. the ratio of the odds of exposure in those with the outcome compared to controls. It can be easily seen that this simple ratio is actually the Mantel-Haenszel estimate of the OR, where each pair is a stratum! For a binary exposure, the pairs are of four different types, depending on the exposure status of the case and control in the pair. Thus, each pair can be represented on a 2-by-2 table (see Table 2.16), where Y=1 denotes the case in the pair and Y=0 their corresponding control, and the counts are defined as before: n_{11} concordant exposed, n_{00} concordant unexposed, n_{10} discordant with the case exposed and n_{01} discordant with the control exposed. Assuming a common OR in the different strata/pairs, the Mantel-Haenszel estimator of this common

OR can be easily computed as the two individuals in each matched pair can be described by one of just four tables, two concordant and two discordant. Denoting the case and control by Y=1 and Y=0:

$$\text{Numerator} = 0(n_{11}) + 0(n_{00}) + \frac{1}{2}(n_{10}) + 0(n_{01}) \tag{2.45}$$

$$\text{Denominator} = 0(n_{11}) + 0(n_{00}) + 0(n_{10}) + \frac{1}{2}(n_{01}) \tag{2.46}$$

$$OR_{MH} = \frac{n_{10}}{n_{01}} \tag{2.47}$$

The standard error of the paired OR (on the natural log scale) also depends only on the two discordant counts and is similar in form to the standard error presented earlier for independent observations.

	Control Exposed	
	Yes	No
Case Exposed	n_{11}	n_{10}
Case Unexposed	n_{01}	n_{00}

$$\text{paired } OR = \frac{n_{10}}{n_{01}} \tag{2.48}$$

$$\text{SE of } ln(OR) = \sqrt{\frac{1}{n_{10}} + \frac{1}{n_{01}}} \tag{2.49}$$

Applying this to the radiation and lung cancer data from Example 2.4 provides the paired OR with 95% confidence interval for the association as in Example 2.4 (continued).

TABLE 2.16: *Summary of the pairs from a matched-pair case-control design.*

	Concordant pairs				**Discordant pairs**			
	Y=1	Y=0	Y=1	Y=0	Y=1	Y=0	Y=1	Y=0
Exposed	1	1	0	0	1	0	0	1
Unexposed	0	0	1	1	0	1	1	0
No. pairs	n_{11}		n_{00}		n_{10}		n_{01}	

Example 2.4 (continued). *Confidence interval for paired OR from Example 2.4.*

$$\text{Paired } OR = 45/25 = 1.8$$
$$\ln(\text{OR}) = 0.5878$$
$$\text{SE of } \ln(\text{OR}) = \sqrt{\frac{1}{45} + \frac{1}{25}}$$
$$= .249$$

The 95% confidence interval for the ln(OR) is

$$0.5878 \pm 1.96(.249) = (.09976, 1.0758)$$

Taking anti-log, the 95% confidence interval for the OR:

$$= (e^{.09976}, e^{1.0758})$$
$$= (1.10, 2.93)$$

2.6.2 Conditional logistic regression

When cases are individually matched to one or more controls, then analysis of the matched sets can be based on the *conditional* probability that it was the case (and not any of the controls) in the set, that had the outcome. For paired data, denoting X_1 as the case exposure value and X_0 as the control value, this is the probability that the event should have happened to the individual with X_1 (i.e. the case), conditional on one of the pair having had the event. This is not an absolute probability but expresses the risk to the case as a proportion of the risk to any one of the set (Equations 2.52 and 2.53).

$$P(Y=1|X_1) = \frac{e^{\alpha+\beta X_1}}{1+e^{\alpha+\beta X_1}} \tag{2.50}$$

$$P(Y=1|X_0) = \frac{e^{\alpha+\beta X_0}}{1+e^{\alpha+\beta X_0}} \tag{2.51}$$

$$\frac{P(Y=1|X_1)}{P(Y=1|X_1)+P(Y=1|X_0)} = \frac{\frac{e^{\alpha+\beta X_1}}{1+e^{\alpha+\beta X_1}}}{\frac{e^{\alpha+\beta X_1}}{1+e^{\alpha+\beta X_1}} + \frac{e^{\alpha+\beta X_0}}{1+e^{\alpha+\beta X_0}}} \tag{2.52}$$

$$= \frac{e^{\beta X_1}}{e^{\beta X_1} + exp^{\beta X_0}} \tag{2.53}$$

The likelihood to be maximised is this product over all N pairs

$$\Pi_{i=1}^{N} \frac{e^{\beta X_{i1}}}{e^{\beta X_{i1}} + e^{\beta X_{i0}}} \tag{2.54}$$

or equivalently

$$\prod_{i=1}^{N} \frac{e^{\beta(X_{i1}-X_{i0})}}{1 + e^{\beta(X_{i1}-X_{i0})}} \tag{2.55}$$

which is known as the **conditional logistic regression** model. Note that any pair i with concordant exposure for case and control ($X_{i1} = X_{i0}$) will not contribute to the likelihood, as the β cancels out, and so the estimate that maximises the likelihood depends only on the discordant pairs. In fact, for the simple case of a binary exposure, the estimate of the crude OR is simply the ratio of discordant pairs with an exposed case to discordant pairs with an exposed control, as already seen in Table 2.16 using Mantel Haenszel arguments.

The conditional likelihood for paired data is a special case of the likelihood for K:1 individually matched data. For 3 controls per case, and labelling their exposure values as X_{01}, X_{02} and X_{03}, the likelihood from Equation 2.54 becomes:

$$\prod_{i=1}^{N} \frac{e^{\beta X_{i1}}}{e^{\beta X_{i1}} + e^{\beta X_{i01}} + e^{\beta X_{i02}} + e^{\beta X_{i03}}} \tag{2.56}$$

Again, sets where the case and their controls are all concordant for exposure make no contribution to the likelihood. This is also true for 1:K individually matched case-control data, although as the number of controls is increased, it is less likely that the whole set will have the same exposure value. The exception is when one is studying a very rare exposure, and we will return in later chapters to sampling designs that are useful and efficient in such settings.

For a 1:K matched study, the general form of the conditional likelihood from Equation 2.56 is:

$$\prod_{i=1}^{N} \frac{e^{\beta X_1}}{e^{\beta X_1} + \sum_{j=1}^{K} e^{\beta X_{0j}}} \tag{2.57}$$

2.7 Exercises

1. Reproduce the RR and OR for the following 2-by-2 table using an online calculator (such as **openepi.com**) and a statistical software program (such as the *immediate* commands in **Stata**).

	Outcome Yes	No
Exposed	230	4885
Unexposed	106	4779

2. The following three tables from Example 2.3 in Chapter 2 provide a summary of prevalent CHD and diabetes in three age groups in the Framingham teaching dataset.

	Age 42–51 **Diabetes** Yes	No		Age 52–61 **Diabetes** Yes	No		Age 62–71 **Diabetes** Yes	No	
Yes CHD	1	32	33	4	74	78	7	69	76
No CHD	28	1553	1581	47	1221	1268	29	440	469
	29	1585	1614	51	1295	1346	36	509	545

(i) Use an online calculator (such as **openepi.com**), to find the crude OR, the three separate ORs, and the Mantel-Haenszel OR.

(ii) Is there evidence of heterogeneity in the ORs in the three age categories? In other words, is it reasonable to assume the ORs are homogeneous and report the adjusted OR? Justify your response.

3. Example 2.6 in Chapter 2 presents the relationship between diabetes and CVD for individuals aged 42 and older in the Framingham teaching dataset.

(i) Reproduce the stratum-specific ORs using levels 1-3 of the categorised age variable **agecat1** (four categories: $0 = 32 - 41, 1 = 42 - 51, 2 = 52 - 61, 3 = 62 - 71$) in the dataset `Chap2_framingham_exercises.dta`.

(ii) On pages 142-146 of Breslow and Day [24], the authors provide the usual test of homogeneity and an alternative test of the null hypothesis (homogeneity) against the alternative hypothesis of a linear trend in the ORs across strata. Verify that the usual test of homogeneity is not significant for the ORs from (i) but the Breslow and Day test is significant. How is this possible?

4. The following table is taken from Table 4 of *Chlordecone exposure, length of gestation and risk of preterm birth* by Kadhel et al, in American Journal of Epidemiology, 2014 (PMID: 24401561).

Chlordecone level μg/L	Total births	Preterm births
< 0.14	163	16
0.14-0.28	165	21
0.29-0.51	162	23
0.52-0.97	165	30
≥ 0.98	163	25

(i) Enter these data in an online calculator (such as **openepi.com** or a statistical software package (where you should 'expand' the data to create a record for each individual) and conduct a Chi-squared test of the association between chlordecone level and preterm birth.

(ii) Using an appropriate command for dose-response, test for evidence of a trend for increasing risk with increasing exposure, using scores 1 to 5 for the categories.

Looking at the separate ORs in the categories, you will note that all except one are non-significant, yet the trend you found is borderline significant. Comment.

(iii) Plot the ln(odds) of preterm birth against the categories of chlordecon, coded simply as levels 1 (< 0.14 μg/L), 2 (0.14-0.28 μg/L), 3 (0.29-0.51 μg/L), 4 (0.52-0.97 μg/L), 5 (≥ 0.98 μg/L).

(iv) Repeat the test in (ii) using the midpoints of the categories as the scores, except for the highest category which may contain outliers (use a value of 1 or other value that is motivated by the data presented in the paper). Compare to your result in (ii).

(v) Explain and compare your conclusions in part (i) and (ii).

5. Table 2.3 in Chapter 2 presents the following data on alcohol intake and lung cancer:

		Lung Cancer	
		Yes	No
Alcohol Intake	<1	1090	3976
	1-3.9	806	2244
	4-6.9	378	783
	≥ 7	679	1166

(i) Test for a trend in risk with alcohol level using a statistical calculator or software package, assigning "scores" to the alcohol intake categories or simply using the values 1,2,3.

(ii) Table 2.4 in Chapter 2 includes the following tables of heavy/light drinking and lung cancer:

	Smoker			Non-smoker		
	Lung Cancer			**Lung Cancer**		
	Yes	No		Yes	No	
Heavy	786	665	1451	271	1284	1555
Light	702	591	1293	1194	5629	6823
	1488	1256	2744	1465	6913	8378

Use the appropriate four numbers from this information to calculate the OR for the association between smoking and lung cancer. Would you expect this association to be confounded by drinking? Why/why not?

(iii) These data are available as Stata and R datasets named `alcohol_lungcancer_smoking`. Open the dataset, display the table in (i) above and request a test of trend.

(iv) For the same data, find the OR for the association between smoking and lung cancer. Check if it is confounded by alcohol and compare to your expectation in (ii).

6. The data in Exercise 2 above represents baseline visit information for individuals aged 42 or older in the Framingham teaching dataset (`Chap2_framingham_exercises`), including the following variables:

   diabetes (0=no diabetes, 1=diabetes)

   prevchd (0=no prevalent CHD, 1=prevalent CHD)

   agecat1 (4 age categories: 32-41, 42-51, 52-61, 62-71)

   (i) Reproduce the counts shown in Exercise 2.

   (ii) Run a logistic regression command to get the crude OR and check it against your answer from Exercise 2.

   (iii) Test for heterogeneity of the OR across the three age groups and compare to your results from using an online calculator in Exercise 2.

   (iv) Estimate the OR adjusted for age group and compare to your answer in Exercise 2.

7. The following tables are from Example 2.5 in Chapter 2 describing the 3505 individuals aged 42 or older:

	Overall		Males		Females	
	Diabetes		**Diabetes**		**Diabetes**	
	Yes	No	Yes	No	Yes	No
Yes HTN	67	1237	25	520	42	717
No HTN	49	2152	32	951	17	1201
	116	3389	57	1471	59	1918

   (i) Compute the three ORs (overall, males, females).

   (ii) Using the dataset `Chap2_framingham_exercises`, run a logistic regression model with interaction term to reproduce the results presented in **Example 2.5 (continued)** in Chapter 2.

   (iii) How can the OR for females found in (i) be obtained from the output in (ii)?

8. This and the following four exercises are based on the same dataset as Exercise 6 above (`Chap2_framingham_exercises.dta`) which contains baseline data for individuals in the Framingham

teaching dataset that was used in the Examples in Chapter 2. The variables include:

randid (individual identification number)

sex (1=male, 2=female)

age (age, in years)

agecat1 (4 age categories in 10-year intervals: 32-41, 42-51, 52-61, 62-71)

agecat2 (age categories in decades: < 40, 40-49, 50-59, 60-70)

diabetes (0=no diabetes, 1=diabetes)

prevchd (0=no prevalent CHD, 1=prevalent CHD)

anychd (0=any CHD during follow-up, 1=no CHD during follow-up)

prevhyp (0=no prevalent hypertension, 1=prevalent hypertension)

sysbp (systolic blood pressure in mmHg)

sbpcat (8 systolic blood pressure categories: 110-119, 120-129, 130-139, 140-149, 150-159, 160-169, 170-179, 180-189)

(i) Fit a simple logistic model to estimate the ln(odds) of CHD (variable name **anychd**) as a linear function of systolic blood pressure (variable name **sysbp**) for individuals with systolic blood pressure between 110 and 189 (i.e. 110 $\leq$ **sysbp** $\leq$ 189). Obtain the coefficient of systolic blood pressure and the corresponding OR.

(ii) The coefficient in (i) is the change in the ln-odds per unit change (i.e. 1mm Hg) in systolic blood pressure, which is not clinically meaningful. Multiply the coefficient by 10 to get the change in ln-odds per 10mm change in systolic blood pressure, and exponentiate this to give the OR associated with a 10mm increase in systolic blood pressure.

(iii) Create a new variable **sbp10** by dividing **sysbp** by 10 and refit the logistic model from (i). Compare the OR to your result from (ii).

(iv) Fit the logistic model with the categorical blood pressure **sbpcat** using the lowest as reference, and record the ORs for the other seven categories. Are the results consistent with (iii)?

9. (i) In the previous exercise, we assumed a linear relationship between the ln(odds) of CHD (variable name **anychd**) and systolic blood pressure (variable name **sysbp**). To check if this is reasonable, plot the ln(odds) of CHD versus the median systolic blood pressure for each of the categories in **sbpcat** (representing the systolic blood pressure levels $110 \leq$ **sysbp** ≤ 189). From the graph, does it seem reasonable to assume a linear effect of blood pressure in a logistic model?

   (ii) Repeat (i) stratified by male and female and plot the two sets of ln-odds on the same graph. Is it reasonable to assume a linear effect in both groups? Is it reasonable to assume a common linear effect in the two groups?

10. (i) Reproduce Example 2.7 from Chapter 2 (CHD outcome, SBP exposure) for individuals with systolic blood pressure between 110 and 189 (i.e. $110 \leq$ **sysbp** ≤ 189) in the dataset `Chap2_framingham_exercises.dta`.

    (ii) Compare the fit of the models with categorical and continuous age using the likelihood ratio test in your software.

11. For the 3505 subjects aged 42 and older in the Framingham dataset described in Exercise 8 above (i.e. excluding the youngest age category in the variable **agecat1**), this exercise examines the association between CVD (variable name **cvd**) as outcome and any CHD (variable **anychd**) as exposure.

    (i) Find the odds ratios, overall and within the three age strata.

    (ii) Examine the tests of homogeneity and trend? Is it reasonable to report a Mantel-Haenszel OR? Is it reasonable to assume a linear effect of age?

    (iii) Fit a logistic model with age as a categorical variable. Comparing the adjusted OR to the overall OR in (i), is there evidence of confounding?

    (iv) Fit another model with age as a continuous (linear) effect. Compare the adjusted odds ratios from this model and the model in (iii) and comment.

12. (i)Using the data `Chap2_framingham_exercises.dta`, run a logistic regression analysis of diabetes in the cohort of

individuals aged 40 and older. Record the crude OR for the effect of prevalent CHD (variable name **prevchd**) on diabetes (variable name **diabetes**), also the ln(OR) and the intercept of the logistic model.

(ii) Select a case-control sample consisting of all cases and an equal number of controls (chosen randomly: use a "seed" so that you can reproduce your results if needed).

(iii) Re-run the logistic regression using the case-control sample, again recording the crude OR, and also the ln(OR) and intercept. Compare to your estimates in (i): the OR or ln(OR) should agree to within sampling variation, but the intercept will likely be very different.

(iv) Verify that equation 2.39 in Chapter 2 describes the relationship between the intercept from your case-control dataset and the intercept for the cohort.

13. For the 2-by-2 table describing paired data below (or using a small numerical example), show that by regarding each pair as a stratum, the Mantel-Haenszel OR is the concordant OR.

	Control Exposed	
	Yes	No
Case Exposed	n_{11}	n_{10}
Case Unexposed	n_{01}	n_{00}

14. Using the data in `Chap2_framingham_exercises.dta`, create a matched case-control sample of diabetes cases and one control per case, matched on the age category variable **agecat2**. Save as a temporary dataset to use for the following tasks examining the association of prevalent diabetes with prevalent CHD.

(i) Create the paired 2-by-2 table of the association between CHD and Diabetes for individuals aged 40 years and older.

(ii) Use the counts in the table to conduct the McNemar test of association.

(iii) Calculate the paired OR from your table, and provide the 95% confidence interval.

(iv) Repeat the test and OR estimation using the temporary dataset that you stored.

15. The dataset `RSV_data_exercise.dta` contains data from a 1:2 matched case-control study of severe RSV disease in infants in Kenya, reported in *Absence of Association between Cord Specific Antibody Levels and Severe Respiratory Syncytial Virus (RSV) Disease in Early Infants: A Case Control Study from Coastal Kenya* by Nyiro JU, Sande CJ, et al. in PLoS One 2016 (e0166706). The variables of interest for this exercise are:

    matchset: a unique number identifying a case and their controls

    controlno: control number (1,2)

    case: indicator for case (1) or control (0)

    ntitre0: antibody titre

    bwt: birth weight (Kg)

    underwt: indicator for low birth weight

    `gest_agew`: gestational age (weeks)

    premature: indicator for prematurity

    (i) Open this dataset and create an indicator for a high titre ($\geq$ the median rounded to 2 decimal places).

    (ii) Drop one control from each set and examine the table of the remaining case-control pairs for an association between high titre and RSV.

    (iii) Compute the paired OR and 95% confidence interval for the crude association between high titre and RSV.

    (iv) Reproduce the published results for Model 1.

    (v) Reproduce the published results for Model 2.

16. (i) Using the RSV data with just one control per case as in the previous exercise, use an appropriate command to obtain the Mantel-Haenszel OR where the pairs define the strata. Verify that this is the same as the paired OR computed from the discordant pairs.

(ii) For the same data as in (i), run a conditional logistic regression, conditioning on pair, and verify that you get the same OR for the high antibody titre.

(iii) Repeat the Mantel-Haenszel calculation and conditional logistic regression, but adjusting for prematurity. These results will not be the same, as these two methods make different assumptions about the underlying true "common" OR. State what is being assumed common in the two analyses.

(iv) Describe how the assumptions in (iii) could be checked if there were sufficient data (the RSV dataset is too small).

3

Extensions to Classic Epidemiological Studies

3.1 Missing/Incomplete Data

In the previous chapter, the relationship between an exposure X and a binary outcome Y was represented by a logistic regression model. In all the illustrative examples, it was assumed that all exposure and confounder information was available for all study subjects. However, in real applications, it is common to have missing values (also called **incomplete data**) for one or more variables. When only a few study subjects have incomplete data, then it is reasonable, and standard practice, to exclude them from the analysis, which is referred to as a **complete case** analysis. If the proportion of subjects with incomplete data is not negligible, a complete case analysis will also be valid, provided the exclusion of incomplete cases does not result in any bias. The simplest situation is when the missing values in the dataset are **missing completely at random (MCAR)**, so that the individuals with complete data, who are available for analysis, are a random sample and thus representative of the larger dataset. Although the random sample will provide unbiased estimates of the OR, there will be a loss in precision (i.e. wider confidence intervals) due to the smaller sample size.

There are other patterns of incomplete data for which a complete case analysis is also unbiased. If missingness depends *only* on the binary outcome, with a different proportion of cases and non-cases having incomplete data, then a logistic regression is also valid, since the available (complete) data is essentially a case-control study! Perhaps less obvious is the fact that if missingness depends *only* on the exposure or confounders (i.e., is random with respect to outcome), a logistic regression analysis will also provide unbiased estimates of the OR: this is because the logistic regression model (Equation 3.1) models the probability of a binary outcome Y, *conditional on* the values of exposure X and confounders Z, that may be continuous variables.

$$\text{Prob}(Y = 1|X, Z) = \frac{e^{\alpha+\beta_1 X+\beta_2 Z}}{1 + e^{\alpha+\beta_1 X+\beta_2 Z}} \tag{3.1}$$

As with all regression models, observations with specific values of the independent variables (in this case X and Z) can be chosen by the investigator for the study of their association with the *dependent* outcome variable (here Y). However, if missingness depends on the outcome *and* exposure, then a standard logistic regression analysis of the complete cases will not provide a valid estimate of the odds ratio, as the relationship between Y and X in the available data may be biased. If the missingness depends on Y and Z (but not on X), then a logistic regression model that includes Z as a confounder will provide a valid adjusted OR, exp^{β}, for the exposure, but the confounder's own effect may be biased. This will be of no concern to the investigator if the purpose of measuring and including the confounder(s) was simply to get an adjusted OR for the exposure. In fact, it is common in case-control studies for investigators to sample cases and controls within strata defined by important confounders (for example males and females, or age groups), and to analyse the resulting data using logistic regression with adjustment for the stratification factors. One such variation of the simple case-control design, which samples equal numbers of cases and controls within pre-defined strata in the population, is referred to as a 'balanced' design [24].

3.1.1 Intentionally missing data

Incomplete data may be due to values that are 'missing' in the usual sense: errors in recording, questions not asked/answered in a questionnaire, loss of laboratory measurements due to insufficient biological samples or contamination, and other problems. However, data can be missing due to the investigators intentionally measuring some variable(s) only for a subsample of the study subjects. Such **missing-by-design** data might be due to a smaller sample being sufficient to answer the current research question, with the larger sample of subjects being intended for future investigations. Where exposures are expensive or difficult to measure (e.g. dietary factors, biochemical or genetic markers), investigators may decide to obtain these measurements only for a subsample of study subjects, due to cost or time constraints.

There are numerous examples of such intentionally missing exposure data. Here we will present two studies, whose data will be used as illustration. First, a case-control study of the association between sexually transmitted diseases and ectopic pregnancy [194] provides an interesting example where the incomplete exposure data was due to both kinds of missingness: an overlooked/forgotten variable in planning the study and the decision later in the study to measure it only for a subsample. The total sample size was 979 (264 cases and 715 controls), and the variables collected from the beginning of the study included contraceptive use, number of sex partners and history of gonorrhoea. From one year after the study was initiated, serum samples were collected in one of the study counties (for logistical reasons) and a chlamydia antibody test conducted in all cases and a 50% subsample of controls. In addition, all black study subjects not included in this sampling were recontacted to provide a blood sample. Thus, the subsample of controls is clearly not a simple random sample, but depends on the outcome and other factors. As a result of this sampling strategy, only 327 out of the 979 patients had measurements for chlamydia antibody.

A second example is a cross-sectional survey of Helicobacter pylori (H. Pylori) infection in 679 school children aged 10–12 years from 11 Stockholm schools, to determine the risk to children from infected family members [105]. For all study children, information was gathered on household socioeconomic factors, and for immigrant children, whether the family's country of origin had a high or low H. pylori prevalence. To investigate the additional contribution of H. Pylori infection in family members, the investigators wished to ensure that they included schools where the known risk factors (immigrant background and low socioeconomic status) were represented. As a result of these considerations, the H. Pylori infection status was determined for the family members of all children from the four schools with highest prevalence, and for infected children from the other seven schools.

3.2 Two-stage Studies

The two examples of intentionally missing data introduced above are examples of two-stage studies ([243]) where data on some covariates is ascertained only for a subsample of study subjects. The first stage of a typical two-stage study consists of the response variable and some covariates for all study subjects, while the second-stage data consist of any other covariates of interest for a subsample of subjects. The covariates recorded for all subjects at the first stage will usually be easy-to-get or cheap exposure variables and confounders, with the more expensive or hard-to-get covariates ascertained only for the subsample of subjects at the second stage. The first-stage data may include a crude measure (called a 'proxy' or 'surrogate') of the 'true' exposure that will be measured at the second stage. Such designs are intuitively appealing to researchers with limited resources who need to gather expensive specialised data, and indeed these designs are often implemented, although appropriate analysis requires non-standard methods. In designing a two-stage study, the investigators will plan to select the second-stage sample using stratified random sampling within the strata defined by some of the variables available at the first stage. A simple illustration is provided in Figure 3.1 for a study with binary outcome and a single binary confounder Z, so that there are four strata defined by the outcome and confounder. The total study sample in each of these strata is denoted by N_{ij} using the same notation for subscripts as in Chapter 2: i denotes the values of the binary (0,1) confounder and j the values of the binary outcome. The small n_{ij} denote the (smaller) numbers of subjects that are selected from each of the strata in the second stage. The ratio $\frac{n_{ij}}{N_{ij}}$ is called the second stage **sampling fraction**. Provided the second-stage

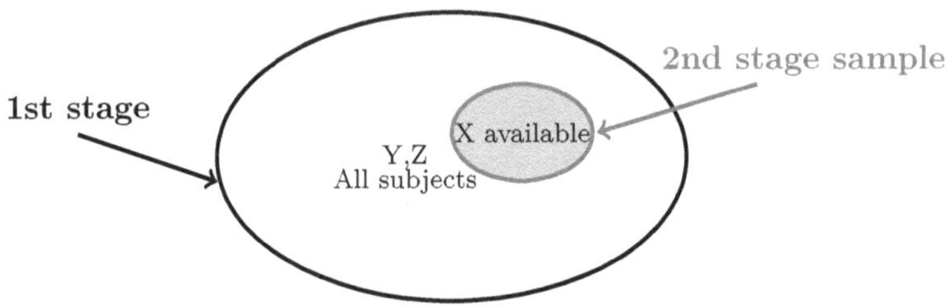

	Y=1	Y=0
Z=1	N_{11}	N_{10}
Z=0	N_{01}	N_{00}

1st Stage

Y=1	Y=0
n_{11}	n_{10}
n_{01}	n_{00}

2nd Stage

FIGURE 3.1: *Illustration of two-stage sample for a study with binary outcome Y and a single binary confounder Z available for all subjects, but exposure X only measured on a subsample of subjects in each of the (Z, Y) strata.*

data is randomly sampled within the strata, the n_{ij} subjects in each stratum can be 'upweighted' to represent all N_{ij}, so that we can conduct a **weighted logistic regression** of the complete data, with weights equal to N_{ij}/n_{ij} (i.e. the reciprocal of the sampling fractions).

The next section provides a brief presentation of the statistical properties of the weighted estimator for interested readers, but this is not essential reading as it can be understood intuitively. However, all readers do need to be aware that when a weighted analysis is conducted, an adjustment needs to be made to the naive standard error to recognise that the data analysed do not consist of N independent observations: analysis is based on only the n observations in the second-stage sample, which are 'upweighted' to represent the larger total number N. Software packages routinely offer a correction for this dependence using a conservative **robust standard error**.

3.2.1 Statistical explanation

The use of weighted regression for analysing two-stage data has been motivated above by an intuitive argument. Some readers may prefer to see a more statistical explanation, but this section is not essential for understanding what follows.

Using the same notation as in Chapter 2 and in Equation 3.1 above, Y denotes a binary outcome, X the exposure of primary interest and Z the other covariates. In the two-stage designs described above, X is the incomplete (exposure) variable, available only for a subsample of individuals, called the second-stage sample. The outcome Y and other covariates Z are available for all individuals at the first stage. For simplicity, assume that Z is a single categorical confounder, and that the second-stage subjects have been randomly sampled within the strata defined by Y and Z. Let us assume that the objective is to estimate the OR describing the effect of X on the outcome.

If we had complete data (X and Y for all individuals), the ln(OR) would be obtained from a simple logistic regression, which finds the value of β that maximises the likelihood of the observed data,

$$L(\beta) = \Pi P_{\beta}(Y_i|X_i)$$

or equivalently, maximises the log-likelihood

$$ln(L_{\beta}) = \sum ln(P_{\beta}(Y_i|X_i)$$

by setting the derivative to zero and solving for β. Thus, the required estimate is the solution to

$$\sum S_\beta(Y_i|X_i) = 0$$

where S denotes a 'score' component, i.e. the derivative of the log-likelihood. However, in the two-stage dataset, X and Y are only known for the second-stage sample, while for all other observations, we have only Z and Y and so cannot compute the score. If the relationship between X and Z, $P(X|Z)$, was known, then the maximum likelihood solution can be found using the Expectation Maximisation (EM) algorithm [50], which is an iterative method for maximising the sum of the log-likelihood components for the complete observations and the 'expected' components for the incomplete observations.

However, the functional relationship between an exposure and confounder is rarely known, or of interest, in epidemiological models, so an alternative is to adopt the idea of the EM algorithm and replace the score components of the incomplete observations by the average score of similar observations that are complete. If the second-stage data has been obtained by randomly sampling from the strata defined by Y and Z, then for an incomplete observation in stratum (Y, Z), the average of the scores of the complete observations in the stratum can be used as the 'expected' or 'estimated' score [179]. Replacing the unknown scores of the incomplete observations by these estimates, the equation to be solved for β is thus the sum of all the score components for the complete observations in the dataset, and the estimated scores for the incomplete observations. When these terms are gathered, the equation can be simplified to be written in terms of only the complete (second-stage) observations:

$$\sum_{i \in 2^{nd} stage} \frac{N_{Z_i Y_i}}{n_{Z_i Y_i}} S_\beta(Y_i|X_i) \qquad (3.2)$$

This is exactly the weighted likelihood that was introduced in the previous section, where the complete observations in each stratum are upweighted by the inverse of the sampling fraction in their stratum.

3.2.2 Two-stage illustration: Framingham data

In the Framingham teaching dataset, there are 3,026 cohort members who had their cholesterol (both HDL and LDL) measured at their third visit. This cross-sectional sample consisted of 777 subjects with a diagnosis of coronary heart disease (CHD) and 2249 non-cases. The sampling and analysis of two-stage data will be illustrated using these data to estimate the effect of HDL and LDL on CHD, adjusted for sex and hypertension. The HDL and LDL levels, which were recorded as integer values, have been categorised as follows:

LDL		**HDL**	
≤100 mg/dL	Desirable	≥60 mg/dL	Desirable
101–159 mg/dL	Moderate	41–59 mg/dL	Borderline
160–189 mg/dL	High	≤40 mg/dL	Low
≥190 mg/dL	Very high		

To mimic a two-stage study where HDL and LDL were only measured for the 777 cases and a random selection of 777 non-cases, the values are set to missing for a random selection of 1472 controls. Thus the data available for analysis consist of the 3026 cohort members, with exposure information available only for the cases and an equal number of randomly-selected non-cases. To mimic another two-stage study of approximately the same size (n=1554) but with a balanced sample from the eight strata defined by CHD, sex and hypertension, 1554/8 = 194 subjects should be randomly chosen from each stratum. However, some strata have fewer that 194 subjects (see Table 3.1) so all these records (120+81) would be selected, leaving 1353 subjects to be sampled ran-

TABLE 3.1: *Number of observations in each of the strata defined by CHD, sex and hypertension for the Framingham illustration of a two-stage study.*

Stratum	CHD	Sex	Hypertension	N
1	0	M	No	390
2	0	M	Yes	479
3	0	F	No	631
4	0	F	Yes	749
5	1	M	No	120
6	1	M	Yes	315
7	1	F	No	81
8	1	F	Yes	261

domly from each of the other six strata (225 from each), resulting in an approximately balanced second-stage sample of size 1551. By setting the HDL and LDL to missing for all except the 1551 selected individuals, the data consists of all details for the 1551 second-stage sample but missing exposure for the remainder of the subjects. The full dataset of 3026 individuals is analysed using standard logistic regression (all weights = 1) to provide a comparison with the two-stage analyses. For the two-stage data that includes all 777 cases and 777 randomly selected controls, cases are assigned a weight of 1 and controls a weight of 2249/777 (i.e. total number of controls divided by the number of randomly selected controls). For the balanced sample, a weight of 1 is assigned to the individuals in the two fully sampled strata, and a weight of s/225 (where s is the stratum size) to all others.

The results from logistic regression of the full sample and the two-stage samples are presented in Example 3.1, where it can be seen that the reweighted analysis of the two-stage samples provides estimates very similar to those from the whole cohort. This is what would be expected when sample sizes are reasonable in all the strata. The confidence intervals (not shown) were almost identical to those from the full cohort, indicating that the stratified samples captured most of the information in the cohort.

In this illustrative example, the prevalence of CHD was high (26%) and the second-stage sample size was large (approximately 50% of the total sample), but for lower prevalence and/or smaller second-stage sample, a balanced design can protect against sparse data and result in better estimates. This is illustrated in Example 3.1 (continued) which presents the results from taking half the sample size, i.e. a two-stage sample with half the cases (388) and the same number of random controls, and a two-stage design of the same size (777) but balanced across the eight strata as before. The estimates from the balanced design are closer to the values from the full data and the LDL effect is estimated with better precision (narrower confidence intervals).

Only two simple designs have been used here for the purpose of illustration of the validity of weighted regression for the analysis of two-stage data. However, the choice of design in a research study will depend on a number of factors. For example, researchers may plan to include all cases at the second stage, with controls (perhaps several times as many as cases) selected as a balanced sample. The issue of how to choose the most efficient two-stage design for a given study will be dealt with in detail in Chapter 8.

Example 3.1. *2-by-2 tables of availability of HDL and LDL by CHD status in a random and balanced two-stage sample from the Framingham cohort at visit 3.*

Availability of HDL and LDL by case status:

	Full CHD Yes	Full CHD No		Random CHD Yes	Random CHD No		Balanced CHD Yes	Balanced CHD No	
Available Yes	777	2249	**3026**	777	777	**1554**	651	900	**1551**
Not Available	0	0	0	0	1472	1472	126	1349	1475
	777	2249	3026	777	2249	3026	777	2349	3026

TABLE 3.2: *Odds ratio estimates (with p-values) from logistic regression of the full sample and weighted logistic regression of the two-stage samples.*

	Full Sample ($n = 3026$)	**Random Two-stage** (1554)	**Balanced Two-stage** ($n = 1551$)
LDL			
Mod	1.50 (0.14)	1.37 (0.35)	1.40 (.32)
High	1.93 (0.02)	1.94 (.052)	1.93 (.05)
V.High	2.18 (.004)	1.96 (.05)	1.97 (.04)
HDL			
Borderline	1.16 (0.24)	1.18 (0.26)	1.16 (0.33)
Low	1.86 (<.001)	1.88 (<.001)	1.88 (<.001)
Female	0.54 (<.001)	0.52 (<.001)	0.54 (<.001)
Hypertension	2.35 (<.001)	2.32 (<.001)	2.34 (<.001)

3.2.3 Computation of sampling fractions

In the illustrative example above, the numbers of subjects selected at the second stage were simple fractions, whose reciprocals could be readily assigned as the weight in the logistic regression. However, for real applications, where the strata are more numerous, or the sampling more complex, there are custom-written software tools, such as the **twophase** command in the **Survey** package in R and the **meanscor** command in

Example 3.1 (continued). *Odds ratio estimates (with 95% confidence intervals) from two-stage design with smaller second-stage sample sizes.*

	Full Sample (n=3026)	Two-stage Half of cases (388+388)	Balanced Two-stage (n=777)
LDL Mod	1.49	1.39(0.62,3.12)	1.52(0.58,4.00)
V.High	2.07	1.64(0.75,3.62)	2.18(0.84,5.64)
HDL Borderline	1.17	1.41(0.92,2.16)	1.24(0.80,1.91)
Low	1.88	2.28(1.44,3.62)	2.14(1.33,3.42)
Female	0.55	0.50(0.36,0.68)	0.55(0.40,0.77)
Hypertension	2.36	2.41(1.75,3.33)	2.34(1.75,3.13)

Stata, that compute the weights and implement the weighted regression. In Stata, the user specifies the variables defining the sampling strata (or a stratum variable constructed from the combinations of those variables), the second-stage (incomplete) variable(s), and the model to be fit. For example, the ectopic pregnancy example described in Section 3.1.1 is used as an illustrative example in the help files for the **meanscor** command in Stata. The objective of the analysis is to estimate the association between ectopic pregnancy and chlamydia antibody (which is only available at the second stage) where the second-stage subjects are assumed to be randomly sampled from strata defined by gonorrhoea, contraceptive use and number of sexual partners. The command is called by simply specifying the logistic model for the outcome Y (ectopic pregnancy), exposure X (chlamydia) and other covariates Z (gonorrhoea, contraceptives) in the usual way, with the stratum (or its component variables: gonorrhoea,contraceptive use, sexual partners) as the first-stage variable(s), and declaring the variable that is only available at the second stage (chlamydia):

```
meanscor y gonn contra chlam,first(gonn-sexptn) second(chlam)
```

3.2.4 Two-stage survey of H. Pylori in school-children

As a result of the two-stage sampling in the survey of H. Pylori infection in Stockholm schoolchildren introduced in Section 3.1.1, blood samples were available from a majority (83%) of the families of infected children, but only from 19% of the families of non-infected children. In addition, the non-infected children whose families were approached were pupils at just 4 of the 11 schools and those 4 schools were selected for their low SES and high proportion of children of immigrant background. From the details of the data collection [106], the second-stage sampling fraction was shown to depend on socioeconomic status and the H. Pylori prevalence in the immigrant's country of origin, with no additional predictors identified. Thus, for the first-stage variables in the two-stage weighted regression analysis, the authors used the binary indicators for low SES and high H. Pylori prevalence in the country of origin.

The results of the two-stage analysis are presented in Table 3.3, with minor differences from the published paper [106] due to how different software packages handle second-stage observation with a missing value recorded for one or more variables.

Using the children from one-child families with uninfected mothers and fathers as reference, the highest risks are to children with an infected mother or infected sibling, with no significant contribution from the father. The very high risks from infected mother or siblings are consistent with an earlier report of a lack of evidence for child-to-child transmission outside the family [216]. These high estimates from the weighted regression are similar to those from standard logistic regression of the data from the four completely sampled schools, with the weighted regression of the full dataset providing improved precision as expected. The effect of the child being born in a high prevalence country is larger in the complete case analysis (6.7 vs. 3.6), reflecting the biased sampling: the four schools that were completely sampled were those with highest H. Pylori prevalence, which is also associated with immigrant background. In fact, for the non-case children in the other schools, the investigators targeted families of immigrant background and lower SES for sampling, in order to enrich the sample with infected relatives.

The weighted analysis accounts for the different intensity of sampling of non-infected children in the strata defined by SES and immigrant background, which the standard logistic regression does not. If the effect of either of these factors is of interest, it should only be interpreted from the two-stage analysis which reweights the available data to remove the

TABLE 3.3: *Odds ratio estimates (with 95% confidence intervals) from analysis of the H.Pylori data in [106], using standard logistic regression for the four completely sampled schools, and weighted* regression for the full data.*

	Complete data (four schools)	Weighted (correct)	Weighted (only SES)
Mother Infected	11.6 (2.0,67.9)	12.7 (3.1, 51.6)	8.9 (2.3, 34.2)
Absent	- -	3.6 (0.4, 31.4)	3.7 (0.4, 33.5)
Father Infected	1.4 (0.2, 9.8)	1.7 (0.5, 6.4)	1.3 (0.4, 4.7)
Absent	1.4 (0.2, 10.8)	1.3 (0.3, 6.7)	0.99 (0.2, 5.2)
Sib(s) infected	8.1 (1.8, 37.3)	10.3 (2.8, 38.4)	10.0 (2.7, 36.0)
No sibs	5.2 (0.7, 38.1)	5.9 (1.3, 27.6)	5.7 (1.1, 29.1)
SES	2.6 (0.6, 12.1)	2.1 (0.8, 5.9)	2.3 (0.9, 6.0)
High prev origin	6.7 (1.7, 25.7)	3.6 (0.9, 14.0)	2.9 (0.8, 10.4)
Antibiotics	0.6 (0.2, 2.3)	0.5 (0.2, 1.6)	0.6 (0.2, 1.8)

**The weights are the inverse sampling fractions in strata defined by SES and country or origin (reflecting the correct sampling), and defined only by SES.*

bias due to the sampling design. From such analysis, we can conclude that there is a significant effect of SES on the child's risk when adjusted for other factors. The third column of Table 3.3 presents the results from an analysis that assumes the families were targeted based only on SES (and not on high prevalence in their country of origin). The omission of this important factor in the actual sampling design results in reduced magnitude of the effects of mother's infection status and high prevalence in the child's country of origin.

The bias described in this example serves to illustrate the importance of careful documentation of the design that is implemented in a research study, if the full potential of the data are to be realised as new methodology becomes available. Such detailed sampling plans are known for clinical trials, as the definition and implementation of inclusion and exclusion criteria are routinely documented. While this has not been a feature of observational epidemiological studies, investigators are now adopting a number of recognised standards for reporting, such as the STROBE (STrengthening the Reporting of OBservational studies in Epidemiology) statement (https://www.strobe-statement.org) and associated checklist that is requested by many journals, and the STRATOS (STRengthening Analytical Thinking for Observational

Studies) initiative (http://www.stratos-initiative.org). By ensuring more careful documentation of how study data were collected, these initiatives will contribute to optimal use of those data as new methodology is developed.

3.2.5 Unintentional two-stage design

In the ectopic pregnancy study and the H. pylori study, investigators deliberately sampled more intensely from strata in the study populations that they deemed to be more informative for the research question at hand. For both of these examples, the second-stage data collection was planned, and on careful reading of how the study was conducted, the strata could be defined by just a few variables. However, incomplete data will not always be gathered from well-planned subsampling, but may arise from various efforts to make use of existing cohorts or case-control samples to address new research questions. For example, as the capacity for measuring genetic and molecular biomarkers becomes more advanced and affordable, it is common to find studies where biomarkers are measured in various subsets of individuals from well-defined cohorts or case-control studies where demographic and baseline characteristics have already been gathered. The analysis will usually include only the chosen subset of individuals on whom the new (incomplete) variable was obtained, so that the findings are relevant to a restricted 'target population'. However, even where the subset seems complex and rather ill-defined, it can nonetheless often be regarded as a two-stage sample, which would enable a valid analysis using all the available data. This has not only the advantage of greater generalisability, but also improved precision and thus a more cost-efficient study.

A typical example of such 'unintentional' two-stage design is the investigation of the role of the CHEK2 gene in the risk of post-menopausal breast cancer [55]. This study used a previous population-based case-control study that had collected questionnaire information on women aged 50–74 concerning their reproductive history, use of postmenopausal hormone replacement therapy (HRT) and various lifestyle factors. From 3345 cases and 3454 controls, the investigators sampled cases and controls in several steps, the first two of which involved randomly sampling 1500 cases and 1500 controls (frequency matched on age) and subsequently included any remaining women (191 cases and 108 controls) who had reported high exposure (4 or more years) to HRT. The decision for this second selection, and other subsamples described in the paper, may have been taken a priori, but it could also have resulted from the investigators having surplus funds after the first round of random sampling and the perception that women with longer HRT exposure were more informative. In any case, the sample after the two steps described here (1691 cases and 1608 controls) would have the desired effect of increased statistical power for the analysis of the subgroup of HRT-exposed women.

Although the sampling of cases and controls described above was conducted in two steps, the simple sketch in Figure 3.2(Top) reveals that it can actually be viewed as a two-stage design, where for simplicity of presentation the matching on age is ignored. Since case/control status and HRT exposure is known for all subjects, the design is equivalent to one where this information defines four first-stage strata, that are sampled at different intensity for genotyping, thus providing four weights: a weight of 1 for women in the two strata with high exposure to HRT since they were all sampled, and the reciprocal of the appropriate case and control sampling fractions for the other two strata.

In studies involving expensive laboratory measurements, sampling decisions may be made sequentially as budgets allow. As an example, let us suppose that in the previous example, the original plan was to genotype a random sample of 1000 cases and 1000 controls, and that after this was complete, sufficient funds remained for further sampling. The perception that HRT-exposed women were more informative would then lead to investing in the genotyping of all women with high exposure to HRT. If the investigators still had some funds remaining, they might then select a further random sample of 500 from cases not yet genotyped and likewise 500 controls. This somewhat *ad hoc* sampling scheme can be represented by the modified sketch in Figure 3.2(bottom). It should again become clear that this is equivalent to a two-stage design, which differs from the design above it in the weight given to women with low HRT use, since these now have two opportunities to be sampled.

3.2.6 Summary of two-stage studies

In a two-stage design, whether intentional or unintentional, the total study sample, whether cross-sectional, cohort, or case-control, is the individuals who have their outcome status recorded, together with some other explanatory variables. In a designed two-stage study, these individuals will be identified at Stage 1. If an important exposure measurement

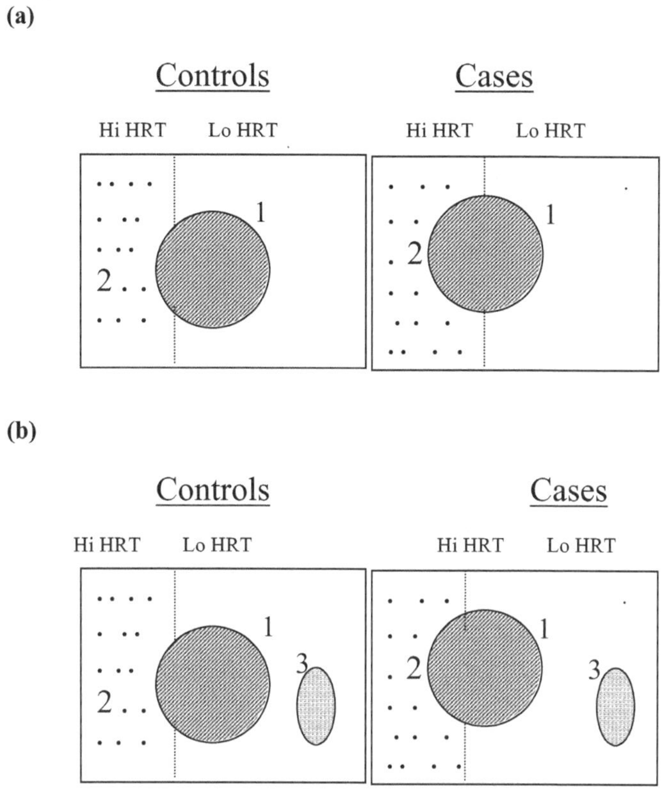

FIGURE 3.2: ***Top:*** *Schematic representation of sampling of breast cancer cases and controls for genotyping in [55]. 1 (shaded disc) = random sample of 1500 cases, and 1500 controls, 2 (dotted area) = include all with high exposure to HRT and not yet sampled.* ***Bottom:*** *Modification to the sampling above if subjects were selected at three stages: 1 = random sample of 1000 cases, and 1000 controls, 2 = include all with high exposure to HRT, 3 (small shaded oval) = random sample of 500 cases and 500 controls from the remainder.*

is obtained for a subsample of the individuals, these 'complete cases' are referred to as the 'second-stage' sample in the designed study. Provided the second-stage subjects can be regarded as a random sample within each of the strata defined by the outcome and some categorical first-stage variable(s), a valid analysis can be conducted using weighted logistic regression. By using the inverse of the sampling fractions in the strata as the weights, the bias from the sampling design is overcome, so that the available complete data (i.e. the second-stage individuals) are made representative of the entire study sample.

3.3 Secondary Analysis of Case-control Data

There are numerous examples of the reanalysis of case-control data to address secondary hypotheses about the disease of interest. For example, a Swedish population-based case-control study of gastric cancer that collected data from 1989 to 1995, found an association between occupational exposure to the metal industry and herbicides [57]. This case-control data enabled a number of further research findings, including the protective effect of aspirin on gastric cancer [3], differing effects of alcohol and smoking by subsite and histology [239], and the role of H. Pylori infection [58]. More recently, the same case-control dataset was used in the study of genetic markers [169] and a study that found serum antibodies against H. pylori to be associated with risk of non-cardia gastric adenocarcinoma [199].

The cases collected in a case-control study can also be followed up to study the short-term or longer-term patient outcomes [80]. Occasionally, the controls from a case-control dataset might be reanalysed to address some health research question for which they are an appropriate study sample. All of these types of subsequent analyses can be implemented with standard statistical tools, since each involves a clear design: case-control, a cohort of cases, or a (sub)sample of controls, where adjustment for any matching factors can be accommodated in regression analyses.

However, when rich data have been gathered in a case-control study, it is natural to ask if we can explore additional questions not just about predictors of case status or prognosis, or relationships between those predictors in the control individuals, but also about the relationship between a new 'outcome' (which was an explanatory variable in the case-control study) and an 'exposure' (which was also also an explanatory variable). From the following examples from the author's own collaborations, it will be clear that this is a common problem.

Case-control study of tubal infertility

In a case-control study of infertility conducted in Kenya in 2000, 47 women with tubal infertility were compared to 46 fertile controls for potential risk factors, including HLA type and evidence of chlamydia infection as measured by antibodies to Chlamydia trachomatis (CT) [37]. Investigators noted a higher rate of Chlamydia-associated infertility in women with specific HLA-types (DQA*0101 and DQB*0501) and wished to re-analyse the data with CT as the outcome and a specific HLA-type as the exposures. A standard logistic regression is not appropriate as the sample is clearly biased, with a ratio of fertile:infertile women of 1:1, while the prevalence of infertility in the population at that time was estimated to be approximately 15%.

Case-control study of cervical cancer

Human papilloma virus (HPV) is no longer considered to simply contribute to the risk of cervical cancer, but has been established as a necessary factor, with HPV vaccination now predicted to be capable of eliminating this cancer [26]. At the time when HPV was being recognised as a causative agent for cervical cancer, a case-control study was conducted in a population of screened women in Uppsala [241], where in addition to HPV, investigators found an association with smoking. The question arose as to whether the available case-control data could be used to provide valid estimates of the association between HPV and smoking, with particular interest in persistent smoking. The study of the relationship between these two factors is not only complicated by the fact that they were explanatory variables in a case-control study, but that the sampling was conducted in a rather complex way.

The cohort from which the study subjects were selected consisted of women born in Sweden with at least one smear registered in the period 1969–1995, and whose first smear was taken before age 50. For each case of cervical cancer, 5 potential controls were identified from the cohort, matched on year of birth and date of entry into the cohort. Controls should have no record of cervical cancer at any time prior to the date of diagnosis of their case. The first smear of the case and first smear of a randomly chosen one of their controls were reviewed: only cases with a normal first smear were retained in the study. If the selected control did not have a normal first smear, they were replaced by another control chosen randomly from the five. Following the publication of the paper, the research group discussed an additional step in control selection, where a control with only one stored smear would be replaced with another randomly sampled control from the remaining five, in order to provide information on smear and smoking at two time points. .

With this complex sampling scheme, the apparently simple question of the association between smoking and HPV infection would have been challenging to address. Today, the association with smoking is accepted, and the WHO 'fact sheet' about HPV and cervical cancer lists smoking as a risk factor for the persistence of HPV infection and the development of cervical cancer [238].

The New Zealand cot death case-control study

The example used in the detailed exposition below is from a New Zealand study of Sudden Infant Death Syndrome (SIDS), also known as 'cot death'. A paper in 1997 [150] reported a case-control study of SIDS, where data were collected on many potential risk factors, including mother's marital status and whether the child was immunised. In a subsequent paper [117], these data were used to address a secondary research question concerning the association between mother's marital status and failure to immunise the infant. Both of these variables were explanatory variables in the original study, but now the authors wished to regard the failure to immunise as the outcome and the mother's marital status as the exposure of interest. They developed a maximum likelihood method and compared to other methods.

3.3.1 What standard analysis is valid/invalid, and when?

Standard analysis of the data available, disregarding the original case-control design, can clearly be biased by the over-representation of cases and the association between the new outcome variable and the case-control status. Valid estimates are only obtained under very strict conditions [158]. If the controls in the case-control study are representative of the non-diseased population, then a cross-sectional analysis of the controls can address questions of prevalence of the new outcome and its association with other exposures measured in the original study. If one wishes to estimate an association in the overall population and not just in non-diseased individuals, this 'controls only' analysis will only be meaningful when the disease is rare. The analysis will sacrifice statistical power, as the sample analysed is only a fraction (usually half or less) of the total sample size in the original study. A more important problem is that this approach may not provide the required estimates if the case-control study had selected controls that were matched to cases on important confounding variables. If the new exposure of interest was a matching factor in the original study, then a valid estimate of its effect cannot be retrieved, although the matching variable can be used to adjust the estimates of other effects. These adjusted estimates may also be of limited generalisability if the matching has resulted in a control group that differs substantially from the study population.

A possible approach to including all cases and controls in the new analysis is to adjust for the original case-control status by including it in the logistic regression model with other potential confounders, and thus 'adjust' for its effect. However, prior to conducting such analysis, careful thought must be given to whether it is valid and meaningful. For the case-control study of fertility mentioned previously [37], adjusting for fertility in estimating the association between HLA type and chlamydia infection is not meaningful, as infertility may be a consequence of Chlamydia infection: the authors refer to 'Chlamydia-associated infertility' in the original paper, and in a subsequent paper they limited their investigation of HLA-type to just the infertile women [36]. However, the question regarding the association between HLA-type and Chlamydia infection in the population remained unanswered .

In the proposed study of the association between smoking and HPV infection using the case-control study of cervical cancer, a model for the risk of the new outcome (HPV) and its dependence on smoking cannot include a simple adjustment for cervical cancer status, since it is known that HPV influences cervical cancer risk (i.e.relative to the HPV measurement, the cancer outcome is in the future). If HPV also influences smoking habits, adjustment for cervical cancer will result in collider bias [86]. Even if the data had been obtained from a cross-sectional prevalence study, analysis of the association between smoking and HPV that adjusts for cervical cancer status would not be biologically meaningful since HPV is not only a well-known risk factor for cervical cancer, but is on the 'causal pathway'.

The inclusion of the original case-control status as a simple adjustment in a logistic model will also be invalid if the case status modifies the effect of (the new) exposure on (the new) outcome. Technically, this can be resolved by inclusion of interaction terms, although interpretation of any finding will then be more complicated.

It is clear from the many examples provided, that secondary analysis of case-control data requires something more than standard methods. The following section will demonstrate that this problem fits neatly into the context of two-stage designs, so that valid estimates can be obtained from an appropriately weighted logistic regression model using standard software tools. These estimates are essentially the same as those obtained from more complicated likelihood-based methods [117] which require specialised software commands that are not readily available to potential users.

3.3.2 Two-stage approach to reusing case-control data

If the relationship between two or more of the explanatory variables in a case-control study is to be investigated, then the available data is clearly a biased representation of the underlying population from which they were obtained, as the cases are over-represented. In the infertility study [37], 50% of the sample are infertile, while the prevalence in the study population is approximately 15%. The imbalance is often more extreme as case-control is often the design of choice for studying a rare outcome. Since case-control studies often include all cases, then the cases in the population are fully represented, but the controls selected for the study are a random sample who constitute only a small fraction of all the non-diseased in the population. In a matched study, controls are sampled within confounder strata, so that what is available is a random sample from each of those strata. If the numbers of individuals in these strata in the population are known, then these background population frequencies can be considered as the 'first stage' data, and the (randomly sampled) individuals in the case-control study as the 'second stage' sample. By upweighting the case-control data to represent the population, unbiased estimates of the required association can be obtained.

The available case-control data can thus be represented in the same way as the two-stage design, where now the population counts provide the 'first-stage' information. The top row of Figure 3.3 depicts the situation of a simple (i.e. unmatched) case-control study, where a binary explanatory variable, coded (0,1), is now of interest as the new 'outcome', denoted by Y, while the original case-control status is represented by the variable CC. Using similar notation to before, the N_{1j} denote the numbers of cases in the population of the original disease studied and N_{0j} the number of controls, with the subscript j denoting whether Y is 0 or 1. The small n_{ij} denote the numbers of subjects in each of the four strata that were sampled into the original case-control study.

The New Zealand Cot Death study[117] was a case-control study of cot death (SIDS) that sampled all cases and a random sample of controls. Subsequently, investigators wished to assess the association between mother's marital status and failure to immunise the infant, two characteristics that had been recorded as explanatory variables in the

	Y=1	Y=0
CC=1	N_{11}	N_{10}
CC=0	N_{01}	N_{00}

1st Stage

Population

Y=1	Y=0
n_{11}	n_{10}
n_{01}	n_{00}

2nd Stage

Case-control sample

	Y=1	Y=0
CC=1	268	68
CC=0	?	?

sample all cases $\longrightarrow$

Y=1	Y=0
268	68
1259	140

FIGURE 3.3: ***Top row:*** *illustration of a case-control sample (on the right) as second-stage data and the study population (on the left) as the first-stage data (CC: case/control indicator; Y: binary explanatory variable).*
Bottom row: *numbers of cases and controls in the New Zealand cot death study (on the right) and where known in the population (on the left) for immunised (Y=1) and non-immunised (Y=0) infants.*

original study. The information provided in Table 1 of the paper enables the table of sample sizes on the bottom right of Figure 3.3 to be completed: 268 of the 336 cases, and 1259 of 1399 controls had immunised their infant. Since all cases of SIDS in the population were included in the case-control study, the top row of the table describing the population is the same as for the sample. Thus, the only remaining count needed is the number of non-SIDS in the population. In the text of the article, the authors report that the 1399 controls were sampled from a population of 137,000. Thus, by assigning a weight of 1 to cases and a weight of 137,000/1399 to controls, the data can be used to obtain valid estimates for the population. From the data reported in Table 1 of the New Zealand cot death study, a simple dataset with three binary variables (SIDS, marital status, immunisation) can be constructed for the 1735 study subjects. Table 3.4 compares the OR from a weighted logistic regression of immunisation (as outcome) and marital status (as exposure) to the estimates previously reported [117] from a naive logistic regression, analysis of controls only, the Palmgren model [167], and the method proposed in the paper. The estimates from the weighted analysis and the Palmgren model are practically identical, despite the weighted regression being simpler to implement, as it does not require the relationship between the old and new outcomes to be modelled. Both estimates are very similar to those from analysis of only the controls, which

TABLE 3.4: *Odds ratio estimates and 95% confidence intervals from analysis of the New Zealand cot death data, using naive logistic regression of the case-control sample, logistic regression of the controls, the Palmgren model, the conditional likelihood developed in [117] and weighted logistic regression that treats the available data as a second-stage sample from the population.*

Method of analysis	OR estimate	95% confidence interval
Naive	1.649	(1.313, 2.071)
Controls only	1.087	(0.736, 1.606)
Palmgren	1.096	(0.744, 1.613)
Lee *et al.*	1.394	(1.023, 1.899)
Weighted	1.096	(0.744, 1.613)

is unsurprising for such a rare event, as the cases will receive a very small (relative) weight in the weighted regression. The estimates from the model-based analysis proposed by [117] differ markedly from the other non-naive methods, which might be due to an inadequate model, e.g. there was an interaction between marital status and immunisation in their effect on SIDS.

In the previous example, the weights were obtained from the population counts. However, many case-control studies are conducted in a setting where such information is not available. Such was the case for the tubal infertility study, where the only information available was the estimate of the prevalence of infertility in the study population. However, using the inverse of the prevalence a weight, valid estimates can be obtained. A weighted analyses of the infertility data to assess the effect of a specific HLA-type is left as an exercise for the reader.

3.4 Reusing Controls from Case-control Data

In addition to the relatively small case-control study (approximately 200 cases) described in Section 3.3 above that found H. Pylori to be a risk factor for gastric cancer [58], another larger case-control study (approximately 500 cases) conducted around the same time reported H. Pylori as *protective* against oesophageal cancer [240]. These studies resulted in a total of approximately 700 cancer-free individuals in which risk factors for H. Pylori could be investigated. The study bases consisted of all native Swedes aged 40–79 years, who lived in five counties in central and northern Sweden in 1993–1994 (Study A: [58]) and all native Swedes below 80 years who lived in Sweden in 1995–1997 (Study B: [240]). The controls in both studies were randomly sampled from the Swedish Population Register to correspond to the age- and sex distributions among the cancer patients. After some exclusions, there were 234 controls from study A and 495 controls from study B available for analysis of risk factors for H. Pylori. The description of these individuals in Table 3.5 indicates a similar median age, but different male/female balance in the two studies. Although the potential confounding by sex and age could be adjusted by inclusion of these variables (and study) in standard logistic regression, the effect of these characteristics could not be estimated, nor could the potential additional information they carried about the population be exploited.

To eliminate the effect of the non-representative sampling, weighted analyses were performed, where the weights took into account the probability of being sampled as a control. These weights were based on the size of the population in the strata defined by sex and 10-year age groups in the five Swedish counties for study A, and in all of Sweden for study B, respectively. These population counts

TABLE 3.5: *Characteristics of the controls from study A [58], study B [240] and overall. Those who were Immunoblot-positive were defined as currently or recently infected with H. pylori; ELISA-positive and/or immunoblot-positive and/or CagA-positive was considered as evidence of H. pylori infection at some point during life (ever infected).*

Participant characteristics	**Study A** ($n = 234$)	**Study B** ($n = 495$)	**Overall** ($n = 729$)
Male	70.1%	82.6%	78.6%
Median age	68	69	69
Antibodies to H. pylori			
ELISA	46.2%	40.2%	42.1%
Immunoblot	59.0%	49.9%	52.8%
Antibodies to CagA	65.8%	58.8%	61.0%

are openly available from Statistics Sweden, whose 'population' link at https://www.statistikdatabasen.scb.se/pxweb/en/ssd/ provides such data from 1968. Some results from a weighted analysis of these controls are presented in Table 3.6.

Individuals who grew up in rural areas and in large families had higher prevalence of H. pylori infection, but infection was not significantly associated with the place of residence in adult life. While the denser social network of an urban environment might be considered a risk factor for contracting the infection, work cited earlier in this chapter suggests transmission to schoolchildren occurs mostly within the family [216], and there are molecular studies that support this hypothesis. [107]. There was a trend, though not statistically significant, for consumption of *fil* (A Swedish sour milk with live bacterial cultures) to be protective against current or recent infection, but no such evidence for lifetime infection risk. This suggests that the protection may be against the persistence of the bacteria rather than against (childhood) acquisition, consistent with work reporting an inhibitory effect of lactic acid bacteria on the growth of H. pylori [41].

TABLE 3.6: *Odds ratio estimates (with 95% confidence intervals in parentheses) for factors associated with H. Pylori, using a weighted logistic regression of the controls enrolled in two case-control studies. The weights are the inverse of the ratio of the numbers of controls and the numbers in the source population in the strata defined by sex and 10-year age groups.*

	Current or recent infection OR (95% C.I.)	Ever Infected OR (95% C.I.)
Female	10.6 (0.3-1.0)	0.7 (0.4-1.3)
Age		
40–50	1.2 (0.4-4.0)	1.7 (0.6-5.0)
51–60	Ref	Ref
61–70	2.5 (1.3-4.6)	1.7 (1.0-3.2)
71–80	3.7 (2.0-6.9)	2.5 (1.4-4.5)
Number of siblings		
1–2	Ref	Ref
3–4	0.9 (0.6-1.6)	0.9 (0.5-1.6)
5–6	1.9 (1.0-3.4)	1.9 (1.0-3.6)
≥7	1.5 (0.8-2.7)	1.4 (0.8-2.6)
Childhood residence		
Rural	Ref	Ref
Urban or densely populated	0.6 (0.4-1.0)	0.6 (0.4-1.0)
20 years before interview		
Rural residence	Ref	Ref
Urban or densely populated	1.0 (0.5-1.7)	0.9 (0.5-1.7)
Intake of sour milk		
≤0.5 times/month	Ref	
0.51–4 times/month	1.1 (0.6-2.1)	
4.01–14 times/month	0.9 (0.5-1.7)	
>14 times/month	0.6 (0.3-1.1)	

3.5 Exercises

1. This exercise concerns the case-control study of ectopic pregnancy described in Section 3.1.1 of Chapter 3. The dataset **ectopic.dta** contains a total of 979 observations with the following variables:

   y a binary indicator for case (i.e. ectopic pregnancy) or control

   gonn history of gonnorhea infection

   contr use of contraception

   sexptn multiple sex partners

   chlam positive for chlamydia antibody
   (only available for 327 individuals)

   z stratum variable constructed from **gonn**, **contr** and **sexptn**

   The purpose of analysis is to estimate the effect of exposure to chlamydia antibody on the risk of ectopic pregnancy, adjusted for the other variables.

   (i) From the total number and number with chlamydia information in each stratum, derive the weights for the complete (second-stage) individuals.

   (ii) Run a weighted logistic regression on the second-stage data, to get the following adjusted ORs

	OR	p-value	95% Conf. Interval
gonn	.9496	0.863	(.5266, 1.712)
contr	.0944	$\leq$ .001	(.0654, .1362)
sexptn	2.099	0.002	(1.324, 3.329)
chlam	2.472	0.004	(1.331, 4.591)

   (iii) Repeat the analysis using a purpose-built package/command, such as **meanscor** in Stata or **Survey** in R.

2. In this exercise, you will sample a two-stage study from a cross-sectional sample of individuals from the Framingham cohort. The dataset `Framingham_HDL.dta` consists of information on 3,026 cohort members who had HDL and LDL measurements

taken at their third visit. The outcome of interest is any coronary heart disease (CHD), with 777 cases and 2249 non-cases. Variables in the data include:

randid (individual identification number)

anychd indicator for any CHD during follow-up

sex 1=male, 2=female

cursmoke 0=not current smoker, 1=current smoker

prevhyp indicator for prevalent hypertension

ldlc low-density lipoprotein cholesterol, mg/dL

hdlc high-density lipoprotein cholesterol, mg/dL

`ldlc_cat` categorical LDL: desirable ≤ 100 mg/dL, moderate $101-159$ mg/dL, high $160-189$ mg/dL, very high ≥ 190 mg/dL

`hdlc_cat` categorical HDL: low ≤ 40 mg/dL, borderline 41-59mg/dL, desirable ≥ 60 mg/dL

`hdlc_cat2`: `hdlc_cat` levels rearranged ('desirable' as reference)

The objective is to estimate the effect of HDL and LDL on any CHD, adjusted for sex and hypertension.

(i) Run a logistic regression analysis on the full cross-sectional sample with **anychd** as outcome and covariates `ldlc_cat`, `hdlc_cat2`, **sex**, and **prevhyp**, to estimate adjusted ORs for HDL and LDL.

(ii) This step will mimic a two-stage study where HDL and LDL were considered as 'expensive' covariates, but only measured for a second-stage subsample and were missing for the other individuals. To mimic a situation where the second-stage sample consists of all 777 cases and an equal number of controls, select a subsample of 777 controls (using a random number generator) whose HDL and LDL variables will be left unchanged and set the values of these 'expensive' covariates to missing for all the other controls. Add a second-stage indicator to the dataset. (**Note:** set a "seed" when creating the random number so that the exact same data can be reproduced if necessary).

(iii) Create a weight variable that is 1 for all cases and 2249/777 for each of the second-stage controls (those with HDL and LDL). Verify that running a weighted logistic regression (with robust standard error) of just the second-stage data gives similar estimates to the full cohort results.

(iv) Repeat the logistic regression analysis of all the data from (iii) (i.e. keeping first stage and second stage observations in the data) using the **meanscor** command in Stata or the **Survey** package in R and compare your results to what you obtained with weighted regression.

3. Repeat the analysis in the previous Exercise using a two-stage case-control study with 777 randomly sampled men and 777 randomly sampled women selected at the second stage.

4. Conduct a two-stage sampling experiment as in the previous two exercises but this time taking a second-stage sample of 1554 (i.e. 2×777) that is "balanced" (i.e. equal numbers) across the eight strata defined by the variables **anychd**, **sex** and **prevhyp**, using the following two approaches: (a) select one-eighth of the 1554 (195) from each stratum, taking all if the stratum has fewer; (b) where strategy (a) results in fewer than 1554, select the "surplus" from the strata larger than 195 to yield a sample of size 1554 that is as "balanced" as possible.

   (i) Re-run the weighted logistic regression analysis of the second-stage data for designs (a) and (b), using the appropriate weights. Compare your estimates to those in Exercise 2 above.

   (ii) Sampling strategy (b) is just one way of allocating "surplus" records to achieve a given total sample size. However, these could have been chosen from any stratum/strata, provided they are chosen randomly: explain how this would impact on the analysis and suggest why an investigator might wish to take an "unbalanced" sample.

5. The dataset `Hpylori_extract.dta` contains information for families from low prevalence countries, extracted from the full data that was analysed for the example presented in Table 3.3 in Chapter 3. The information in the extracted data includes

the HP status of the child and mother (variables **hpproband** and **hpmother** respectively), SES category, and an indicator variable (**stage2**) for children whose mother's status is known.

Use a two-stage analysis to estimate the effect of a positive mother on the child's risk, adjusted for SES. Compare your results to Table 3.3 in Chapter 3.

6. The dataset **infertility.dta** contains the unintentional second-stage observations (47 cases and 46 controls) from the study of tubal infertility described in Section 3.3 of Chapter 3, with variables:

   cc: case-control status (1=case, 0=control)

   age: age (in years)

   sexplife: lifetime sexual partners (numeric)

   ctyn: chlamydia (CT) antibodies 1=yes, 0=no

   dqa10151 and **dqa10262** (indicator variables for HLA types)

   (i) Estimate the association between chlamydia and HLA type **dqa10151** using only the controls from this study.

   (ii) Use the information given in Section 3.3 of Chapter 3 to reuse all the data to estimate the association between chlamydia and HLA type **dqa10151**.

   (iii) How would you interpret the difference in the estimates obtained from (i) and (ii)?

7. The study of breast cancer described in Section 3.2.5 is a simplification of the actual study *Linkage disequilibrium mapping of CHEK2: common variation and breast cancer risk* by Einarsdottir et al, PlosMed, 2006 (PMC1457009) where (1) random sampling of 1500 cases and 1500 controls was followed by (2) all remaining women with high exposure to HRT, (3) all cases and controls with diabetes, and (4) controls that had been included in a previous study in the same cohort. In addition, stored samples for the genotyping analysis were not available for all women. For each of the following, explain why or why not you could conduct a valid analysis:

   (i) For the simple two-stage design using just individuals sampled in (1) and (2), what assumption is necessary for valid analysis of the available genotype data?

(ii) Explain why or why not you could conduct a valid two-stage analysis of the combined data from (1), (2) and (4), making the same assumption about the available specimens as in (i). If valid analysis is possible, explain in detail how to obtain appropriate weights.

(iii) Suggest a situation where the inclusion of (3) would not result in bias. Could the available data be used to assess if this is realistic in the study population?

8. (i) For the study of breast cancer by Einarsdottir et al in the previous exercise, sketch a diagram like Figure 3.2 in Chapter 3 to describe the 3345 cases and 3454 controls in the cohort and the 1691 cases and 1953 controls who would have been selected by steps 1, 2 and 4 (i.e. ignoring diabetes) if the cohort of 6799 women had 338 cases and 196 controls with high exposure to HRT and assuming that none of the controls from step 4 had already been selected in steps 1 or 2.

(ii) The simulated dataset `sim_freq_HRT_BrCa.dta` has been generated to represent a cohort of 6799 women with indicator variables for case-control status, high exposure to HRT, diabetes, and selection at steps 1,2,3,4 as in Einarsdottir et al. Verify your frequencies in (i) using cross-tabulation commands (for Stata, the **coding** function that is available with **meanscor** could be used with case-control status as dependent variable and high HRT exposure as the first stage covariate).

(iii) If genetic information was available for all women selected, what are the appropriate weights for the individuals in the sample of 3644 women in (i)?

9. The simulated data in `sim_freq_HRT_BrCa.dta` has an indicator variable for diabetes (DB) for all members of the cohort.

(i) Obtain the correct frequencies for the 4-step sampling that was conducted for the paper by Einarsdottir et al described above.

(ii) Using the indicator variable `sampled1234` to identify the individuals sampled, compute the appropriate weights if all 1800 sampled cases and 2058 sampled controls had genetic data available.

10. (i) Verify that in the simulated data in `sim_freq_HRT_BrCa.dta` there are 110 cases and 104 controls with diabetes that are not selected in steps 1 and 2 (and thus selected at step 3).

    (ii) If the purpose of the research study was to investigate genetic biomarkers for breast cancer among non-diabetic women, could this be addressed by dropping the 110 cases and 104 controls? Why/why not?

    (iii) Using the simulated data, calculate the weights for an analysis to estimate the association between the genetic markers and breast cancer for non-diabetic women, assuming all sampled women had genetic data available.

4

Including Time: Cox Regression and Related

4.1 Inclusive, Exclusive, Concurrent Sampling

In the previous chapters, the RR, IRR and OR were introduced as measures of the effect of an exposure on a (disease) outcome. The RR from a cross-sectional or cohort study is simply the ratio of the risk in the exposed and unexposed individuals. For a cross-sectional study, the measure of risk used is the prevalence, while in a cohort study it is the proportion of the cohort members who develop the disease over the study period (i.e. the cumulative incidence). We will refer to these two measures as the **prevalence relative risk (PRR)** and the relative risk (RR), respectively. The IRR can also be estimated from a cohort study that records the person-time contributed by each participant. The OR from a cross-sectional or cohort study is similarly calculated as the ratio of the odds of disease in the exposed and unexposed individuals, with the **prevalence OR** and **OR** corresponding to the prevalence relative risk and RR.

When estimating a RR or IRR for a cohort, it may be sufficient to have a random subsample of the cohort, perhaps stratified by exposure status. The population OR can also be estimated from a random subsample, but unlike the RR and IRR, a valid OR can also be obtained from a sample that is stratified on the outcome. This is because the OR of exposure in cases compared to controls is the same as the OR of disease in exposed compared to unexposed. Depending on when we sample the cases and controls, the OR may represent the population at a specific time, or the experience of the population over a time period. If cases and controls are sampled at a specific time (e.g. in a given calendar year), the OR is a **prevalence OR**. A more common comparison is between a sample of the cases that occur during a period of follow-up and a sample of the individuals who remain disease-free during this period, which we will refer to as the classic case-control design. This design is common for clinical studies, which are often conducted in patient cohorts that are being followed up for outcomes of interest, and thus the natural comparison group consists of those patients that have not had the event by the end of follow-up. In case-control studies of a rare disease, it is common to include all cases but to subsample a small fraction of the non-cases.

It is clear that the OR for an exposure-disease association in a population can be estimated from all three major study designs (cross-sectional, cohort, case-control), but it is commonly perceived that *only* the OR can be estimated from a case-control study. However, depending on *when* the controls are sampled, different measures of association can be obtained from case-control data. This will be illustrated with the cohort displayed in Figure 4.1, where 10,000 unexposed and 10,000 exposed individuals are followed up for 10 years. If during this time, the rate of new cases (i.e. the proportion of non-cases who become cases) was exactly 5% per year among the exposed individuals and 1% among the unexposed, this would result in a total of 4013 cases among the exposed and 956 cases among the unexposed.

The year-by-year counts of the population at-risk (i.e. non-cases) are presented in Table 4.1, with 5987 (10,000−4013) and 9044 (10,000−956) non-cases in the exposed and unexposed individuals after 10 years. This numerical example will be used to illustrate how the timing of control selection can enable different population parameters to be estimated. These illustrations will consider 1:1 case-control studies, i.e. the number of controls selected will be equal to the number of cases observed.

The total numbers of exposed cases (4013) and unexposed cases (956) after ten years follow up provide the estimates of RR and OR (see Table 4.2) that were presented in Chapter 1. The population relative risk for disease in the 10-year period is RR = 4.2 and the population odds ratio is OR = 6.3. This OR could be estimated by comparing all the cases to a sample from the non-cases at the *end* of follow-up, which is referred to as **exclusive sampling**. From Figure 4.1 and Table 4.1, there are 15,031 non-cases at the end of follow-up (5987 exposed and 9044 unexposed). Thus, if a random sample of 4969 non-cases was selected to compare to the 4969 cases, we would expect a fraction $\frac{5987}{5787+9044}$ to be exposed(i.e., 1979 individuals) and the remainder to be unexposed (Table 4.3). If instead, the cases were compared to a sample taken from the whole cohort at the *start* of follow-up (**inclusive sampling**), the sample OR would provide an estimate of the population RR rather than the OR. In this example, the odds of exposure in the cases is 4013/956=4.2 and the odds of exposure at baseline is 1 (equal numbers of exposed and

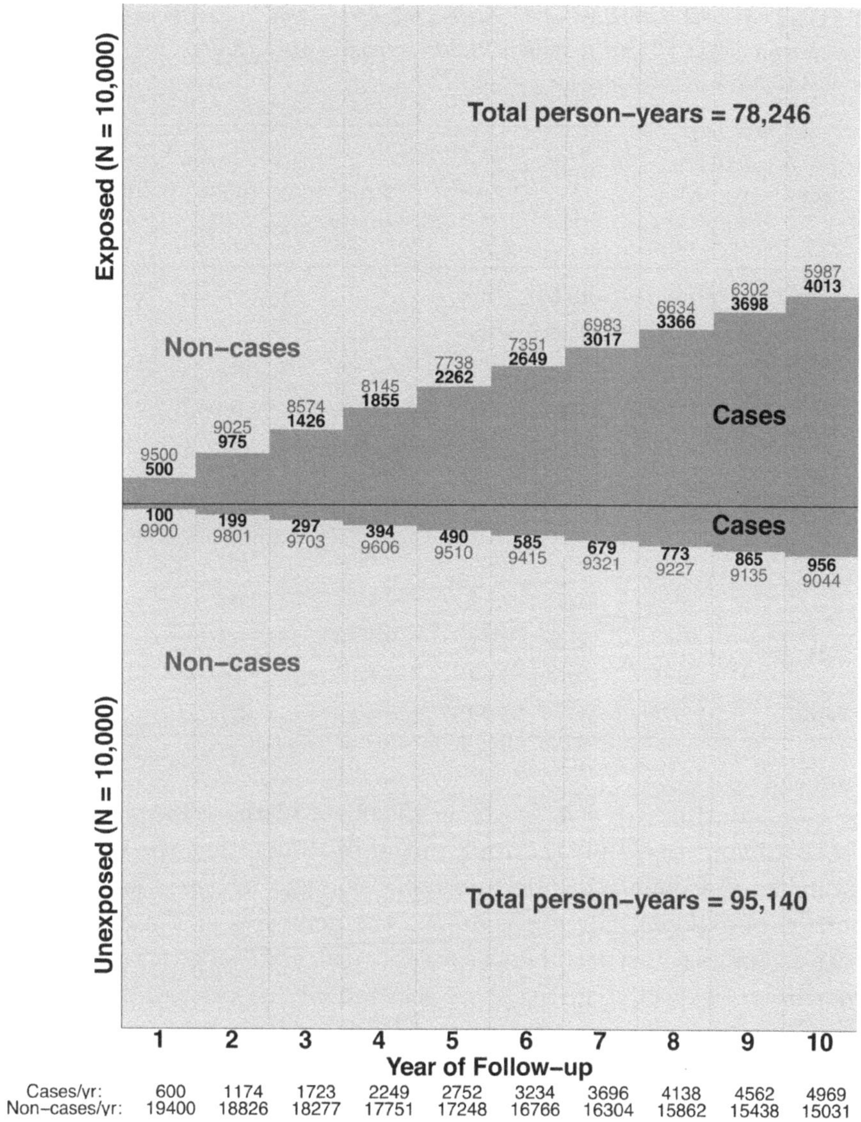

FIGURE 4.1: *Annual number and person-years of cases and non-cases followed-up for 10 years, stratified by exposure status.*

unexposed, i.e. 2485 exposed and 2485 unexposed in a sample of 4969), so that the OR from inclusive sample is expected to be 4.2 (Table 4.3).

There is another option for the timing of control selection that enables the IRR to be estimated without having to record the follow-up times of all individuals in the cohort. If at each time a case occurs, one

TABLE 4.1: *Illustration of inclusive, exclusive and concurrent sampling in a cohort of 20,000 individuals: 10,000 exposed and 10,000 unexposed, with incident rates of 5% and 1%, respectively.*

	Exposed		Unexposed				
Year	At risk	Mid-yr pop	At risk	Mid-yr pop	Prop non-cases exposed	Incident cases	Exposed concurrent controls
0	10,000		10,000				
1	9500	9750	9900	9950	0.4897	600	294
2	9025	9263	9801	9851	0.4794	574	275
3	8574	8799	9703	9752	0.4691	549	258
4	8145	8359	9606	9654	0.4589	526	241
5	7738	7941	9510	9558	0.4486	503	226
6	7351	7544	9415	9462	0.4384	482	211
7	6983	7167	9321	9368	0.4283	462	198
8	6634	6809	9227	9274	0.4183	442	185
9	6302	6468	9135	9181	0.4083	424	173
10	5987	6145	9044	9089	0.3983	406	162
Total		**78,246**		**95,140**		**4969**	**2223**

or more controls are selected from members of the cohort still under observation at that time (**concurrent sampling**), then the sample OR estimates the population IRR. In the example in Table 4.1 the proportion of exposed individuals among the non-cases at the end of each year (column 6 in the table) is used to calculate how many exposed controls are expected among those selected for the cases that year (column 7): among the total 4969 controls (chosen for comparison with the 4969 cases), the expected number exposed is 2223. Thus the odds of exposure in the controls is $\frac{2223}{4969-2223}$, which compared to the odds in the 4969 cases (4013/956), is an OR of 5.185, very close to the calculated IRR in the population (IRR=5.1, see Table 4.2). The small difference is due to the way time is handled: the concurrent controls would not be selected from individuals who are still non-cases at the end of each year as in our calculations, but at the actual time the case occurred during that year. To approximate cases (and thus controls) being sampled uniformly throughout the year, assume all were selected from the mid-year population at risk, then the total person years accumulated over the 10 years follow-up is 95140+78246, and the proportion of exposed

TABLE 4.2: *Cumulative incidence, odds, and incidence rates of disease in exposed and unexposed individuals in the population in Table 4.1, together with the corresponding RR, OR and IRR.*

	Exposed	Unexposed	Estimate
Cum. incidence	4013/10000 = 0.40	956/10000 = 0.096	RR = 4.2
Odds	4013/5987 = 0.670	956/9044 = 0.106	Incident OR = 6.3
Incidence rate	4013/78246 = 0.05	956/95140 = 0.01	IRR = 5.1

person-years is $\frac{78246}{95140+78246} = 0.4513$. This results in $4969(0.4513) = 2242$ exposed controls among the 4969 selected (odds=$\frac{2242}{4969-2242} = .822$) and comparing to the odds in cases (4013/956), an odds ratio of 5.1, equal to the IRR. The concurrent sampling that results in this important property is also known as **risk-set sampling** or **incidence density sampling**, since the controls from which the selection is made at each event time are those still *at risk* and the relative numbers (density) at each time depend on the incidence of disease in the cohort at that time. The OR calculated from the different sampling designs are summarised in Table 4.3.

TABLE 4.3: *Odds of exposure and odds ratios for different types of sampling of 4969 controls (equal to number of cases) from the cohort in Table 4.1.*

	Exposed		Odds of	
	Yes	No	exposure	OR
Cases	4013	956	4.1977	
Controls:				
Exclusive	1979	2990	0.6619	6.3
Inclusive	2485	2485	1	4.2
Concurrent (end of year)	2223	2746	0.8095	5.2
Concurrent (person-years)	2242	2727	0.8221	5.1

4.2 Time-to-event Data

Chapter 1 introduced two measures for the rate at which a disease occurs in the population, namely the *incidence rate* and the *hazard rate.* The incidence rate measures the risk to an individual over a specified time period (e.g. per year) while the hazard rate is the risk *at* any time point, i.e. the instantaneous risk. Where data are only available on the total numbers of cases in a given time interval, then an incidence rate is reported, as in Table 4.2 above. However, where the time of disease onset is known for each case, the more precise hazard rate can be estimated. Such data, known as **time-to-event data** are available from cohort studies and randomised clinical trials (RCTs), where study participants are followed from a well-defined starting time to an endpoint. The methods for analysis of such data are known as **survival analysis**, as they were originally developed for studying mortality of populations. For presenting the survival experience of a population, age is the time scale of interest, so that the implicit starting time point is birth. Survival analysis tools are applicable to any time-to-event data and any time scale, for example:

- age at death for members of a population
- time (in years) from cancer diagnosis to death
- time (in months) from first to second mammography screening
- age (in weeks) at first infant vaccination
- time (in days) from admission to discharge of hospital patients

Figure 4.2 illustrates the features of time-to-event data using a mini cohort of just 15 individuals followed for up to 15 years. In time-to-event data, the outcome of each individual has two components: the time for which they were followed, and whether or not they had the event of interest. In the figure, these two components are represented by the length of the 'time-lines' and whether they end in a black dot (event) or are **censored** (short vertical bar), which is explained in more detail in the following paragraph. The individuals still in follow-up at an event time are called the **risk set**.

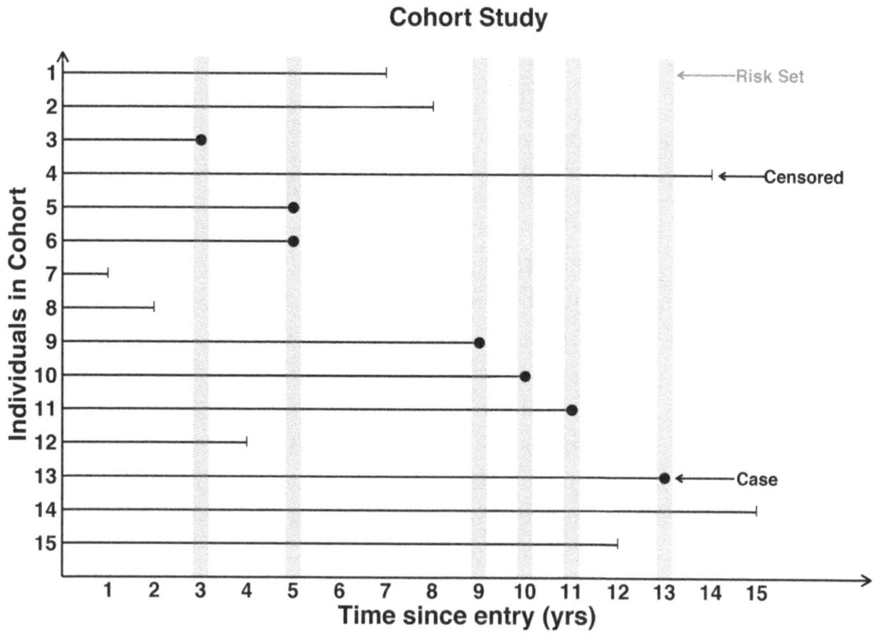

FIGURE 4.2: *Representation of a cohort showing the features of time-to-event data.*

An important feature of time-to-event data is **censoring**. If subjects enter the study at different times, this is known as **left censoring**; if subjects have been observed only for part of the study period (as for individuals 1, 2, 4, 7, 8, 12, 14 and 15 in the figure), so that their outcome status at the end of the study is unknown, this is known as **right censoring**. Individuals who were followed for the entire study period and remained event-free (only one in the figure, individual 14) are also defined as censored, and such censoring is known as **administrative censoring**. Censoring leads to differences in follow-up time between individuals, so that a simple risk measure (e.g. the proportion of individuals who have the event during follow-up) does not make use of the time information in the data. A more efficient use of this information is to use the time-at-risk (follow-up time) of each individual to obtain the total **person-time** and thus compute an incidence rate. This was illustrated in Chapter 1 in the line-plots in Figure 1.1. In settings where the follow-up time has been rounded, it is reasonable to assume that the events occur uniformly in the rounded time interval, so that the total person time is approximated by the number of individuals at-risk at the mid-point of the interval, e.g.

the use of the mid-year population in Table 4.1 to approximate person-years of follow-up during the year.

4.2.1 Hazard and survival

The hazard rate, or instantaneous incidence rate, at a specific time t, was introduced in Chapter 1 and is defined as the risk that a person who has not had the event prior to a specified time t will develop the event in the next instant. The shape of the hazard rate over time is usually denoted by $h(t)$ and sometimes called the hazard function to emphasise the dependence on time. For example, the hazard function for the mortality of a population is a function of age and is usually approximated by the ratio of the number of deaths at each age divided by the number of individuals in the mid-year population of that age. This function is plotted for the Swedish males in Figure 4.3a and shows the typical 'bathtub' shape for human populations: following the 'hazards' of infant mortality and very low risk of death in childhood, there is a period of constant and low risk of death in young adults (from age 20) before the steady rise in mortality with ageing, from about 40 years.

The plots in Figure 4.3 do not follow cohorts of the same individuals from birth to death, but actually present cross-sectional information: each age is represented by different individuals from the population in a single year. However, for an individual of a specific age in the living

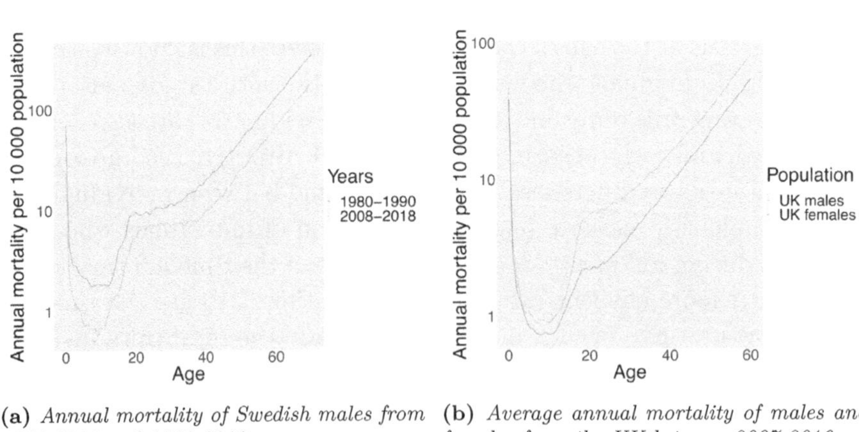

(a) *Annual mortality of Swedish males from 1980-1990 and 2008-2018*

(b) *Average annual mortality of males and females from the UK between 2007-2016*

FIGURE 4.3: *Population hazards for* **(a)** *Swedish males and* **(b)** *UK males and females.*

population, the hazard can be interpreted as the mortality rate that they will experience as they grow older (i.e. over time), if the current age-specific rates do not change.

Formally, the hazard rate at time t is defined as the probability of the event at time t for an individual who has not had the event before t

$$h(t) = \text{probability}(Y(t) = 1|Y(t) = 0 \text{ for } T \leq t) \tag{4.1}$$

Those who have not had the event prior to t are called the **risk set** at time t (see Figure 4.2) since all of these individuals are said to be *at risk* of the event as they approach time t. Thus, the hazard rate at times 3, 5, 9, 10, 11 and 13 in the figure would be estimated as 1/13, 2/11, 1/7, 1/6, 1/5 and 1/3, the probability of the event at time t for those at risk. In this simple example, none of the censoring times coincide with an event, but where this occurs, the inclusion/exclusion of the censored individual in the risk set depends on whether they can be considered to be in follow-up *at* time t, i.e. whether the censoring occurred just before or just after. The formal criterion for inclusion of an individual in the risk set is that, *had the event occurred for them at that time*, it would have been identified. For a specific cohort, this will depend on the protocol for their follow-up.

If the hazard function is known, then the probability of surviving up to any specific time can be computed. For example, Figure 4.4a displays the cohort of 15 individuals from Figure 4.2 rearranged from top to bottom (and renumbered) based on their follow-up time. This arrangement helps to clarify the computations in Figure 4.4b: the survival probability up to any time point is the probability of *not having* the event at any of the prior times, i.e. the product of the separate probabilities.

The plot of these survival probabilities, known as a **Kaplan-Meier plot**, is a 'step function' (see Figure 4.4c) as the estimate only changes when an event occurs. The equivalent information can be presented as **cumulative hazard** (see Figure 4.4d), which is the complement of the Kaplan-Meier plot. The steps in a Kaplan-Meier plot will be less visible for larger cohorts or higher event rates. For example, in the Kaplan-Meier curves in Figure 4.5, the cohort of Titanic survivors is rather small (n=435) and the curve is not as smooth as the plots for the Swedish and US comparison groups, which are based on large populations [79].

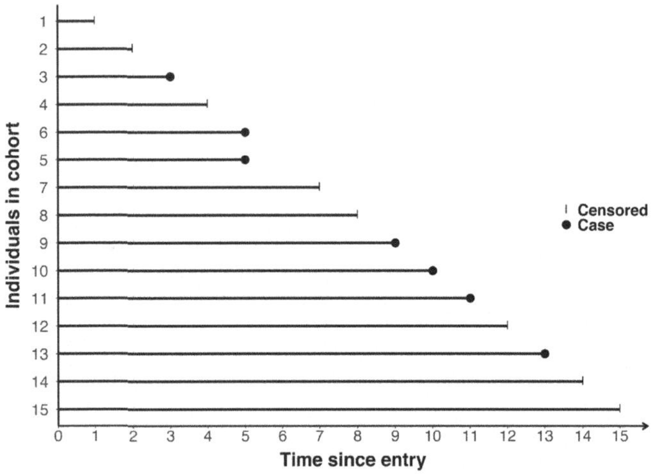

(a) *Line plot of simulated mini-cohort of 15 individuals*

Time t	t_0	t_3	t_5	t_i
No. at risk	$n_0 = 15$	$n_3 = 13$	$n_5 = 11$	n_i
Survival				
probability at t	$P_0 = \frac{n_0 - 0}{n_0}$	$P_3 = \frac{n_3 - 1}{n_3}$	$P_5 = \frac{n_5 - 2}{n_5}$	$P_i = \frac{n_i - d_i}{n_i}$
Estimate of S(t)	1	$P_3 = \frac{12}{13}$	$P_3P_5 = (\frac{12}{13})(\frac{9}{11})$	$P_3P_5 \dots P_i$

(b) *Risk sets and survival probabilities for mini-cohort in part (a)*

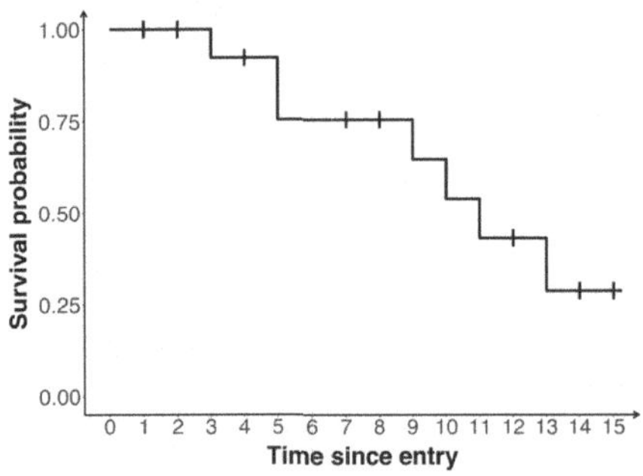

(c) *Kaplan-Meier curve for mini-cohort*

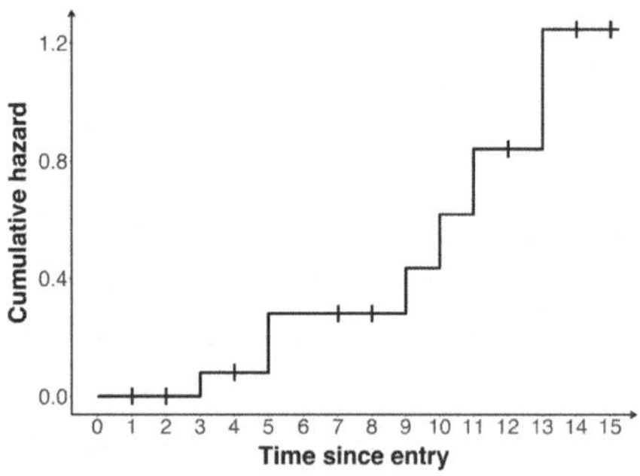

(d) *Cumulative hazard for mini-cohort*

FIGURE 4.4: *(a) Line plot, (b) Risk sets and survival probabilities, (c) Kaplan-Meier plot and (d) Cumulative hazard curve, for mini-cohort of 15 individuals*

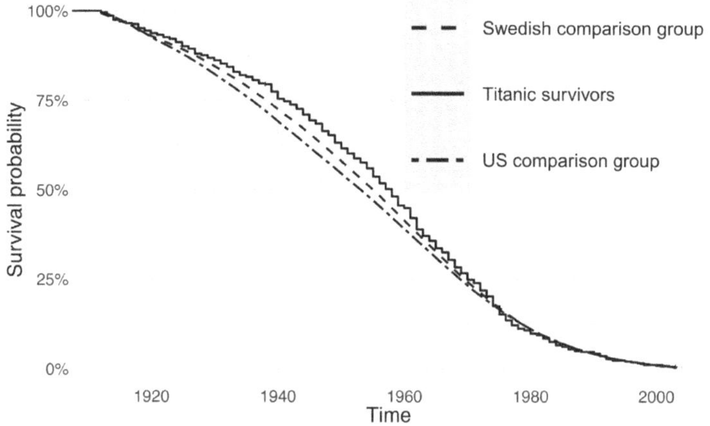

FIGURE 4.5: *Survival as a function of calendar year for Titanic survivors compared to Swedish and white Americans matched for age and sex [79].*

The Kaplan-Meier plot of the experience of a cohort sampled from a population is an *estimate* of the 'true' survival curve of the population. In the absence of any acute disaster, the population survival is a smooth curve (beginning at 100% and dropping to the percentage that are censored at the end of follow-up. The larger the sample size, the closer the estimate will be to this smooth curve. It will be clear by now that the shape of a survival curve depends on the hazard function, with a steeper drop in the survival curve whenever there is larger hazard. Figure 4.6 presents a simple example of four populations where the hazard

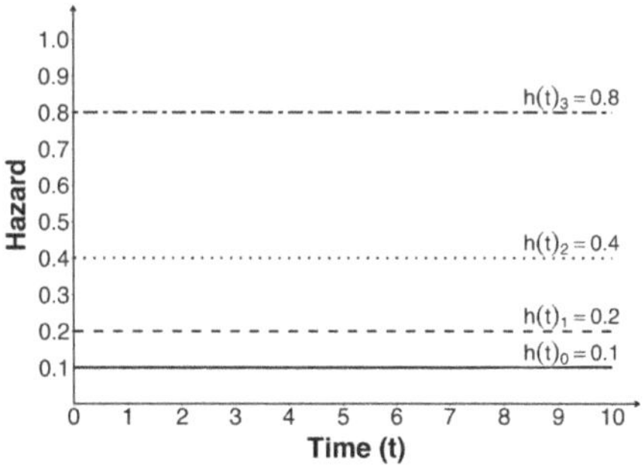

(a) *Four constant hazard functions*

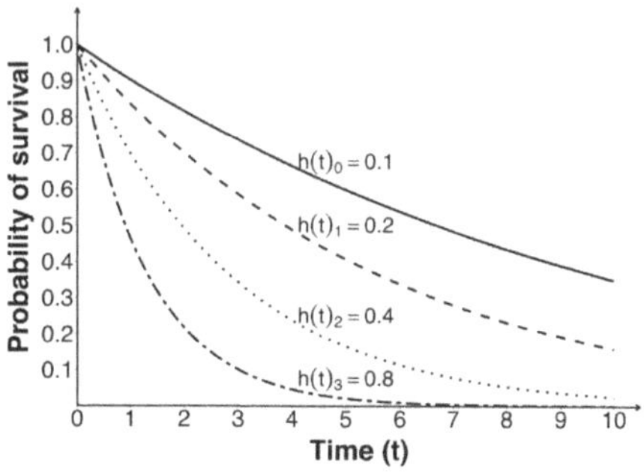

(b) *Survival curves corresponding to the hazard functions*

FIGURE 4.6: ***(a)*** *Example of four hazard functions with different constant intensity over time and* ***(b)*** *the corresponding population survival curves.*

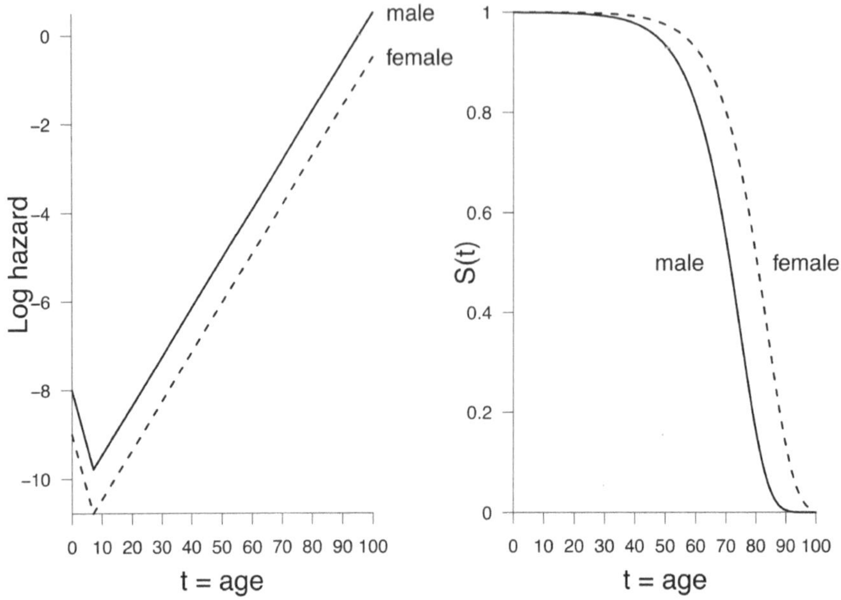

FIGURE 4.7: *Illustration of the survival curves (on the right) corresponding to simplified population hazards for males and females (on the left) with linear decline in infancy followed by linear increase thereafter.*

is constant over time (unlike human life expectancy!) and the resulting survival curves that would result. However, these examples are simplistic, as a realistic hazard function will not be constant, but depend on time, as in Figure 4.3. Simplifying this population hazard function to a linear decline in infancy followed by a linearly increasing hazard over age thereafter (left panel of Figure 4.7), the corresponding survival curve is shown on the right of the figure. So even with steadily increasing hazard, the survival curve is a smooth sigmoidal shape.

4.2.2 Proportional hazards

In addition to estimating the survival curve(s) for a population, survival analysis will often be concerned with examining how the time-to-event depends on an exposure of interest. For example, the plot on the right of Figure 4.7 demonstrates a small survival advantage for females from about age 40. A formal test of the male-female difference is provided by the 'log-rank test', which is offered by most software packages as an option with Kaplan-Meier analysis. However, to *quantify* the difference, and to adjust for potential confounding effects, we need to model survival as we did for binary outcomes using logistic regression. The usual regression model for survival data is the **Cox proportional hazards model** which:

- models the hazard h(t), i.e. the instantaneous rate at time t
- assumes for an individual with exposure X:

$$h(t|X) = h_0(t)e^{\beta X} \tag{4.2}$$

$$ln(h(t)) = ln(h_0(t)) + \beta X \tag{4.3}$$

where $h_0(t)$ is the hazard when X=0, called the **baseline hazard**. For a binary exposure X, coded as 1 (exposed) and 0 (unexposed), comparing the hazard at time time t for an exposed and unexposed individual:

$$h(t|X = 1) = h_0(t)e^{\beta} \tag{4.4}$$

$$h(t|X = 0) = h_0(t) \tag{4.5}$$

$$\frac{h(t|X = 1)}{h(t|X = 0)} = e^{\beta} \tag{4.6}$$

$$= \text{hazard ratio } (\mathbf{HR}) \tag{4.7}$$

$$\implies \beta = ln(HR) \tag{4.8}$$

Note the similarity to the logistic model and the odds ratio (OR). As with the logistic model, if the exposure X is continuous, e^{β} is the **hazard ratio per unit increase** in X. Table 4.4 highlights the similarities in the linear, logistic and Cox regression models.

While a linear regression analysis models Y as a function X and logistic regression models the ln(odds) of a binary event (Y=1), Cox regression models the ln(hazard) as a 'baseline' function of time (also on the log scale) plus an additional component due to the explanatory variables, for example β for a single binary exposure X or βX for a continuous exposure. This additional component does not depend on time, which for a binary exposure means that the plot of the hazard functions for exposed and unexposed individuals on the natural log scale has a constant 'gap', i.e. the hazards are parallel. This constant difference

TABLE 4.4: *Comparison of the relationship between exposure (explanatory variable) and outcome (dependent variable) in linear, logistic and Cox regression.*

Outcome (Y)	**Model**	**Linear Predictor**	**Measure of Association**
Continuous	**Linear**	$Y[X] = \alpha + \beta X$	Slope (β)
Binary	**Logistic**	$\text{logit}(Y=1) = \alpha + \beta X$	Odds Ratio (e^{β})
Time	**Cox**	$ln(h[(t\|X]) = ln(h_0(t)) + \beta X$	Hazard Ratio (e^{β})

between the hazards on the log-scale is a consequence of the model assumed in Equation 4.2, from which it can be seen that the *hazards* over time for individuals with $X = 1$ and $X = 0$ are *proportional*, differing by a constant *factor*, e^{β} at each time point. For a continuous exposure, the hazards at any time point for individuals with exposure values X and $X + 1$ differ by this constant factor.

It is important to note that Equation 4.2 places no restriction on the baseline hazard, but only requires the hazards for any level/value of exposure to be proportional (over time) to the baseline hazard and thus to each other. It now becomes clear why the simple Cox model introduced here is known as the **Cox proportional hazards model**. Returning to the simple settings in Figure 4.6, if the group with lowest hazard $h_0(t) = 0.1$ is taken as reference, then the hazard ratios for the other three groups are:

$$\text{HR}_{1 \text{ vs. } 0} = h_1(t)/h_0(t) = 2 \tag{4.9}$$
$$\text{HR}_{2 \text{ vs. } 0} = h_2(t)/h_0(t) = 4 \tag{4.10}$$
$$\text{HR}_{3 \text{ vs. } 0} = h_3(t)/h_0(t) = 8 \tag{4.11}$$

In the more realistic setting of Figure 4.7, despite the actual shape of the hazard functions for males and females, there is a constant gap between the log-hazards, supporting the proportional hazards assumption. For proportional hazards, there is a simple mathematical relationship between the hazard function and the survival function:

$$h(t|X) = h_0(t)e^{\beta X}$$

is equivalent to

$$S(t|X) = [S_0(t)]^{e^{\beta X}} \tag{4.12}$$

From this it is clear that:

- if β **is positive**, then larger values of X (and thus larger $e^{\beta X}$) are associated with *lower* survival. i.e. X **is a risk factor**
- if β **is negative**, then larger values of X (and thus smaller $e^{\beta X}$) are associated with *higher* survival. i.e. X **is a protective factor**.

This is illustrated graphically in Figure 4.8.

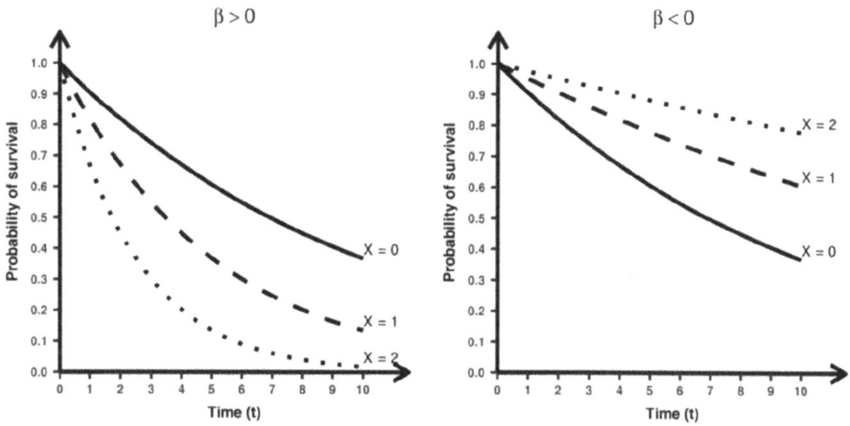

FIGURE 4.8: *Pattern of survival with increasing level of exposure X when the ln(HR) is positive and negative.*

4.3 Cox Regression

As for logistic regression, maximum likelihood methods are used to find a β that provides the best-fitting' model for time-to-event data. Assume for simplicity that each event time is unique (i.e. the units of time are sufficiently precise that there are no co-incident events). As mentioned earlier and illustrated in Figure 4.2, the individuals under observation at any time point, and thus at risk of having the event, are called the 'risk set'. But only one of these actually has the event at that time and Cox regression maximises the likelihood that it is *this* individual (rather than any of the others). Thus the likelihood component at any event time is the ratio of the hazard of the case to the total hazard of all members in the risk set. Denoting the time of the ith event as t_i, the risk set at this time as R_i and the exposure value of this case as X_i, then the ratio to be maximised is

$$\frac{h_0(t_i)e^{\beta X_i}}{\sum_{j \in R_i} h_0(t_i)e^{\beta Xj}} \tag{4.13}$$

$$= \frac{e^{\beta X_i}}{\sum_{j \in R_i} e^{\beta Xj}} \tag{4.14}$$

as the baseline hazard $h_0(t_i)$ cancels (see Figure 4.9). The likelihood over all event times is then:

$$L(\beta) = \prod_{t_i} \frac{e^{\beta X_i}}{\sum_{j \in R_i} e^{\beta X_j}} \tag{4.15}$$

which is a partial likelihood since the baseline hazard is not modelled.

4.3.1 Adjusted hazard ratio

The introduction to Cox regression above assumes that only a single exposure, X, is of interest. A Kaplan-Meier plot can display the survival curves for different levels of a categorical exposure. While the exposure variable X in the Cox regression model can be a binary, categorical, or continuous variable, the interpretation of the HR provided above assumes a binary exposure: the hazard of an exposed individual is higher by a factor e^β *at all follow-up times*. For a categorical exposure with more than two levels, the data analyst (or the software!) will choose one level as the reference against which the others are compared for their HR, similar to the approach for logistic regression. For a continuous exposure variable, the HR, like the OR from logistic regression, is the increased risk per unit change in exposure. It is left as an exercise for the reader to verify that these interpretations of the HR for different types

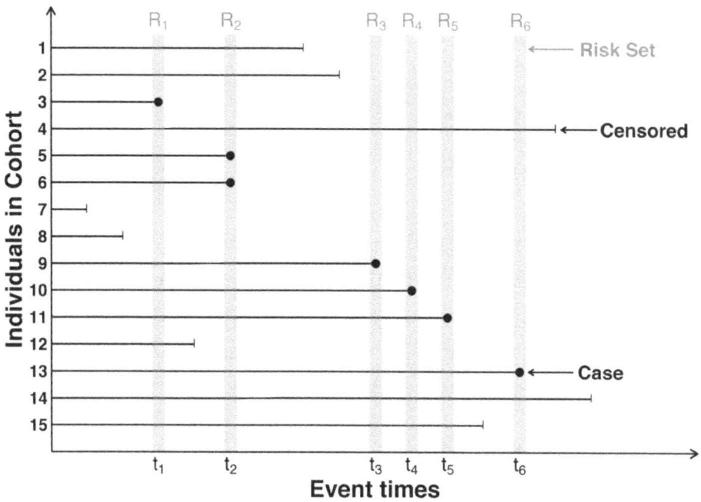

$$\textbf{Hazard for case } i = \frac{h_0(t)e^{\beta X_i}}{\sum_{k\in R_i} h_0(t)exp^{\beta X_k}}$$

$$\textbf{Total hazard for risk set } i = \frac{h_0(t)e^{\beta X_i}}{\sum_{k\in R_i} h_0(t)e^{\beta X_k}}$$

$$\textbf{Likelihood at } t_i = \frac{e^{\beta X_i}}{\sum_{k\in R_i} e^{\beta X_k}} \quad \begin{matrix}\leftarrow \textbf{baseline} \\ \textbf{hazards} \\ \leftarrow \textbf{cancel}\end{matrix}$$

$$\textbf{Likelihood for all events} = \prod_{t_i} \frac{e^{\beta X_i}}{\sum_{k\epsilon R_i} e^{\beta X_k}}$$

FIGURE 4.9: *Schematic drawing of a cohort study, with hazards and likelihood for the Cox proportional hazards model.*

of explanatory variables follow from the likelihood in Equation 4.15 in the same way as done for logistic regression in Chapter 2, Section 2.5.

In real analyses of time-to-event data, a Cox regression model with a single exposure might be conducted as a preliminary analysis, to estimate the crude HR. While this provides a quantitative risk measure to complement the qualitative information in a Kaplan-Meier plot (for categorical exposure), the research question will typically require further analysis to adjust for confounding and to understand the independent contribution of a number of risk factors. For example, if there are two risk factors of interest, X_1 and X_2, and a confounder Z, the simplest model extends Equations 4.2 and 4.3 to accommodate these three explanatory variables as follows:

$$h[t|X_1, X_2, Z] = h_0(t)e^{\beta_1 X_1 + \beta_2 X_2 + \beta_3 Z} \tag{4.16}$$
$$ln\{h[t|X_1, X_2, Z]\} = ln\{h_0(t)\} + \beta_1 X_1 + \beta_2 X_2 + \beta_3 Z \tag{4.17}$$

so that the joint effects of these variables are assumed to be additive on the log-hazard scale. Another assumption of this model is that there is no effect modification, as the hazard ratios for X_1 and X_2 (at each level of Z) are e^{β_1} and e^{β_2}. To test for effect modification, the data analyst includes interaction terms in the same way as seen for logistic regression.

Example: risk of postpartum venous thromboembolism

To illustrate the application of the Cox regression model, we will analyse the time from delivery to a diagnosis of postpartum venous thromboembolism (VTE). In particular, we will investigate the hazard ratio for pregnancies with vs. without preeclampsia (PE), a rare but serious form of gestational hypertension. Since both VTE and preeclampsia are known to have a risk of recurrence, we limit the analysis to pregnancies of women with no previous diagnosis of VTE or PE. The data available for analysis are 970,778 deliveries recorded in the Swedish Medical Birth register from 2002-2012, of which 27,028 (2.8%) were complicated by preeclampsia.

The definition of postpartum VTE varies, but is generally defined as occurring within six weeks of delivery. In this illustration, we will extend the follow-up time to one year. As VTE incidence and risk factors are different for the ante-partum, peri-partum and postpartum periods [226], we will censor any pregnancies of mothers who conceived again within one year of delivery. Since the main focus is on the increased risk of postpartum VTE associated with preeclampsia, the analysis will be conducted in three steps: an examination of the Kaplan-Meier curves, a univariable Cox regression to estimate the crude HR for PE, and finally fitting a multivariate Cox model with other known risk factors and potential confounders. Figure 4.10 presents the Kaplan-Meier curves for time from delivery to VTE, stratified by PE status of the pregnancy.

In agreement with published results, the cumulative incidence of VTE over one year is very low, but there is a clear separation between the survival curves, indicating that preeclampsia is associated with higher risk (Log-rank test χ^2=59.2, p<0.001). From the simple Cox model with only preeclampsia as exposure (see Table 4.5 first row), the crude

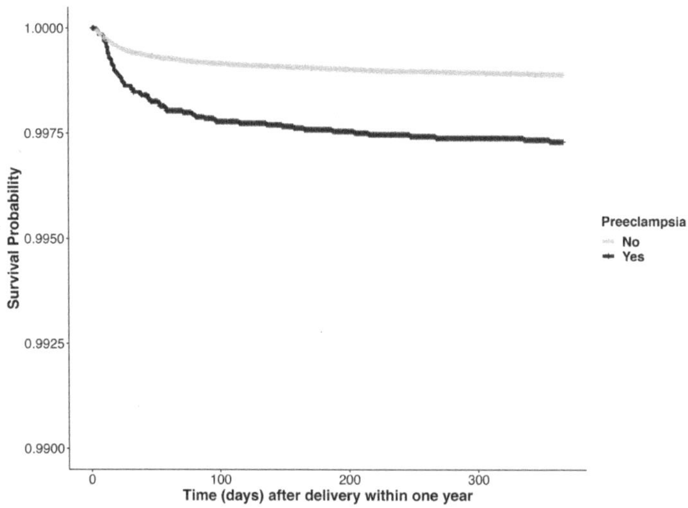

FIGURE 4.10: *Kaplan-Meier plots of time from delivery to postpartum VTE in a large cohort of Swedish pregnancies.*

hazard ratio indicates that for a woman who had preeclampsia during pregnancy, the hazard of VTE at any time during the first year postpartum is approximately two-and-a-half times higher than for a woman

TABLE 4.5: *Hazard ratio estimates and 95% confidence intervals from univariable analysis of the crude effect of preeclampsia (first row) and multivariable analysis including other risk factors and potential confounders.*

Risk factor	HR	95% CI	p-value
PE (Crude effect)	2.55	(2.03, 3.20)	<.001
PE	1.83	(1.43, 2.33)	<.001
Maternal age	1.02	(1.02, 1.04)	<.001
BMI Overweight	1.60	(1.39, 1.83)	<.001
Obese	2.16	(1.84, 2.53)	<.001
Caesarean delivery	1.75	(1.53, 2.01)	<.001
First birth	1.14	(1.00, 1.29)	0.01
Smoker	1.62	(1.35, 1.95)	<.001
Transfusion*	2.68	(2.10, 3.41)	<.001

* *Transfusion around delivery*

whose pregnancy was not complicated by preeclampsia. While some of this raised risk can be attributed to other characteristics of the women and pregnancies with preeclampsia (see Table 4.5), even after adjustment for those factors, the hazard ratio still represents almost a two-fold risk for preeclampsia: HR=1.81 (95% C.I. 1.40 to 2.33).

4.3.2 Stratified Cox regression

Until now we have assumed that there is an underlying 'baseline' hazard for individuals in the study population and that this hazard is increased or decreased by a constant factor (the HR) at all time points for individuals with a specific exposure value relative to the reference level. Although we considered only a simple additive model for the log-hazard above, this can be extended with interaction terms, in the same way as the logistic model, if the effect of exposure is *not common* across strata defined by the confounder(s). The data analysis proceeds in the same way as for logistic regression with interaction terms and the HRs have similar interpretation to the ORs. However, the Cox regression models presented so far have another important assumption, i.e. that there is a 'baseline hazard' function over time that is relevant for all individuals in the study population. This assumption of a *common baseline hazard* enabled the $h_0(t)$ to be cancelled from the Cox likelihood above (see Figure 4.9), resulting in a simplified partial likelihood. However, the assumption of a common baseline hazard will be unreasonable in situations where there are strata in the population that are understood to have a different hazard profile. In such cases, a **stratified Cox regression** should be conducted, with the survival experience of each stratum represented in the likelihood with their own baseline hazard, event times and risk sets. This is presented graphically in Figure 4.11, where yet again the similarity to stratified logistic regression will be noticed. The implementation of a stratified Cox regression resembles a conditional logistic regression of matched data, as the data analyst simply needs to specify the stratum variable in the call to the regression command.

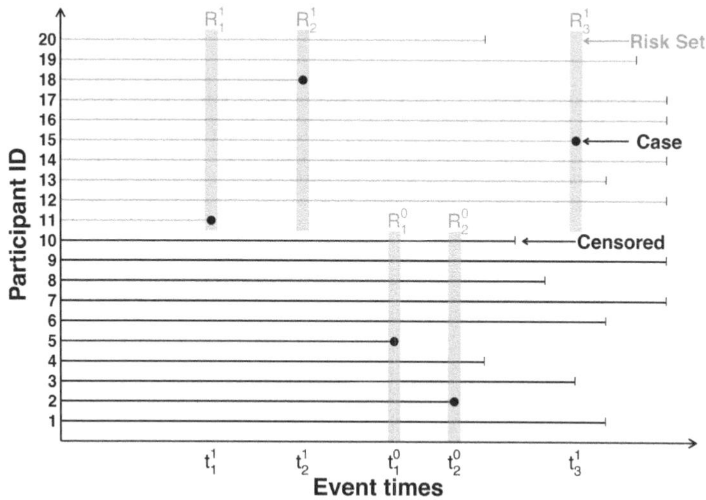

$$\text{Likelihood for stratum 1} = \prod_{t_i^1} \frac{e^{\beta X_i^1}}{\sum_{k \epsilon R_i^1} e^{\beta X_k^1}}$$

$$\text{Likelihood for stratum 0} = \prod_{t_i^0} \frac{e^{\beta X_i^0}}{\sum_{k \epsilon R_i^0} e^{\beta X_k^0}}$$

$$\text{Likelihood for all events} = \prod_{s} \prod_{t_i^s} \frac{e^{\beta X_i^s}}{\sum_{k \epsilon R_i^s} e^{\beta X_k^s}}$$

FIGURE 4.11: *Cox proportional hazards likelihood for stratified sampling from a cohort, where t_i^s and R_i^s denote the time and risk set for the ith event in stratum s.*

4.4 Nested Case-control Sampling

For the Cox partial likelihood for a cohort study (see Figure 4.9), the contribution to the likelihood at each event time is the ratio of the hazard of the case to the total hazard of the risk set. In most applications, the number of non-cases in a cohort will far outnumber the cases, which raises the question as to whether it is necessary to have *all* the non-cases in the denominator at every event time. If the cohort is very large, it seems that we could represent the hazard information at each event time using a subsample of the individuals at risk at that time point.

This is the idea of the **nested case-control** design, first proposed by Thomas in 1977 [215].

Using a subsample of non-cases at each event time to represent the risk set can result in significant savings in cost and time compared to collecting information on all cohort members. It is common to select just a few controls per case, as the efficiency relative to the whole cohort is approximated by the simple 'M/(M+1) rule' [218], which states that a study with 3 controls per case can achieve approximately three-quarters of the power of the full cohort study. However, for less costly data such as electronic records, investigators may select many more controls per case to ensure sufficient power for subgroup analyses.

Figure 4.12 illustrates a nested case-control study with two time-matched controls per case. Since the controls at each event time are selected randomly from those that are still at risk, a control may be chosen more than once (e.g. individual 19 in the figure) and a control may later become a case (e.g. individual 15). In much of the epidemiological literature, if case-control data is sampled within a well defined cohort, the study is described as a 'nested case-control' study. Indeed it is true that all case-control studies can be viewed as nested' within some cohort or population, but in this book, nested case-control sampling will be understood to be matched on time, which is also known by the more specific **incidence density sampling** or **concurrent sampling**. Earlier in this Chapter, we demonstrated that the odds ratio from concurrent sampling provides an estimate of the IRR in the cohort, so it should not be too surprising that this sampling design for controls in a case-control study can provide an estimate of the HR.

Assuming the Cox proportional hazards model, the hazard for each of the cases can be compared to the total hazard in the *sampled* risk sets, i.e. the cases and their time-matched controls (see Figure 4.12). These sampled risk sets are denoted by R_i^* in order to distinguish them from the full risk sets R_i in the cohort. Using R_i^* instead of R_i in the expressions from Equations 4.14 and 4.15 results in a partial likelihood [165] such as Equation 4.19.

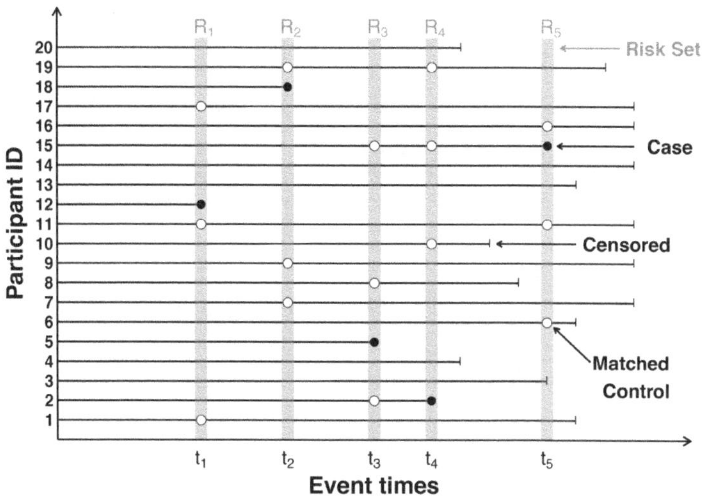

$$\begin{array}{r}\text{Hazard for case } i\rightarrow\\ \text{Total hazard for } \textbf{\textit{sampled}} \text{ risk set } i\rightarrow\end{array}\ \frac{h_0(t)e^{\beta X_i}}{\sum_{k\in R_i^*} h_0(t)e^{\beta X_k}}$$

$$\textbf{Likelihood at } t_i = \frac{e^{\beta X_i}}{\sum_{k\in R_i^*} e^{\beta X_k}}$$

$$\textbf{Likelihood for all events} = \prod\nolimits_{t_i} \frac{e^{\beta X_i}}{\sum_{k\epsilon R_i^*} e^{\beta X_k}}$$

FIGURE 4.12: *Likelihood for nested (time-matched) case-control sampling from a cohort, where R_i^* denotes the* ***sampled*** *risk set at event time t_i (i.e. the case and their matched controls.*

$$\textbf{Likelihood at } t_i = \frac{e^{\beta X_i}}{\sum_{k\in R_i^*} e^{\beta X_k}} \tag{4.18}$$

$$\textbf{Likelihood for all events} = \prod_{t_i} \frac{e^{\beta X_i}}{\sum_{k\epsilon R_i^*} e^{\beta X_k}} \tag{4.19}$$

For a 1:1 nested case-control study, where the exposure of the case and their control at time t_i are denoted by X_{i1} and X_{i0}, the likelihood in Equation 4.19 reduces to Equation 4.20.

$$\prod_{t_i} \frac{e^{\beta X_{i1}}}{e^{\beta X_{i1}} + e^{\beta X_{i0}}} \tag{4.20}$$

If a case and control have the same exposure value, the pair does not contribute to the likelihood for β as the ratio of the numerator and denominator reduces to $\frac{1}{2}$. For a 1:K matched study, the likelihood is:

$$\prod_{t_i} \frac{e^{\beta X_{i1}}}{e^{\beta X_{i1}} + \sum_{k \in R_i^*} e^{\beta X_{ik0}}} \tag{4.21}$$

where X_{ik0} for $k = 1, 2, \ldots K$ denotes the explanatory variables of the time-matched controls for case i. Again, any sets where the case and all their matched controls have the same exposure value do not contribute to the likelihood. These expressions for the matched (on time) risk sets are identical to those seen earlier for conditional logistic regression for a matched design (Equations 2.53 and 2.57).

It should now be clear that a conditional logistic regression of the time-matched pairs will provide the estimate of the HR in a Cox model. This equivalence is made clear by some software packages, where the same command is used for nested case-control data as for case-control data that is matched on factors other than time. However, in the first setting (i.e., with time-matching and assuming the Cox model), the β that is estimated is the ln(HR), while in the second, it is an estimate of the adjusted ln(OR) of the binary outcome. This was already demonstrated in the numerical example in Tables 4.1– 4.3 earlier in this chapter, where the odds ratio from concurrent sampling estimated the IRR in the population, while the OR from exclusive sampling estimated the population OR.

4.4.1 Illustration: Cox and conditional logistic regression

As an illustration of the relationship between Cox and conditional logistic regression that was described in the previous section, we return to the analysis of postpartum VTE risk that was presented in Section 4.3.1. The outcome is a very rare event (only 1088 cases of VTE among the 970,778 deliveries) but since the data was obtained from a linkage of national health registers, there would be no cost savings from using a smaller number of non-cases. However, if exposure information had to be retrieved from medical charts or from laboratory records, this is a typical situation where a nested case-control study would offer a huge efficiency gain over a cohort study. As an illustration, we sampled concurrent controls for the 1088 cases in the cohort, and conducted conditional logistic

TABLE 4.6: *Adjusted* hazard ratio estimates (with 95% confidence intervals) of the effect of preeclampsia on postpartum VTE, from full cohort analysis and nested case-control studies with 1, 5 and 10 controls per case.*

	Cohort	1:1 NCC	1:5 NCC	1:10 NCC
PE	1.8(1.4,2.3)	2.4(1.4,4.1)	1.5(1.1,2.0)	1.9(1.4,2.5)
Maternal age	1.0(1.0,1.0)	1.0(1.0,1.1)	1.0(1.0,1.0)	1.0(1.0,1.0)
BMI				
Overweight	1.6(1.4,1.8)	1.9(1.5,2.3)	1.8(1.5,2.1)	1.6 (1.4,1.9)
Obese	2.2(1.8,2.5)	2.2(1.6,2.9)	2.4(2.0,2.9)	2.3(1.9,2.7)
Caesarean	1.8(1.5,2.0)	1.9(1.5,2.4)	1.9(1.6,2.2)	1.8(1.5,2.1)
First birth	1.1(1.0,1.3)	1.4(1.1,1.7)	1.1(0.98,1.3)	1.2(1.0,1.4)
Smoker	1.6(1.3,2.0)	1.8(1.3,2.5)	1.6(1.3,2.0)	1.7(1.4,2.1)
Transfusion	2.7(2.1,3.4)	3.9(2.2,7.1)	2.7(1.9,3.7)	3.0(2.2,4.0)

* *mutually adjusted for all variables shown and for age.*

regression analysis of the time-matched sets using the same model as used for the full cohort in Table 4.5. Three different study sizes were conducted, with 1, 5 and 10 controls per case, and the results are presented in Table 4.6.

The estimates from the 1:1 case-control study are very close to the true' estimates from the whole cohort, and with reasonable precision despite being based on sampling only 1088 controls from almost one million available. As the ratio of controls to cases is increased to 5 and 10, the estimates (and their standard errors) become closer to the cohort values. For the 1:10 sample, the results are almost indistinguishable from the cohort results: the small differences are expected due to the random sampling, which was implemented just once for this illustration.

While conventional wisdom suggests that there is little or no gain in efficiency from sampling more than 5 controls, that general rule of thumb does not take account of the effect of a very rare exposure in the matched analysis. In our example, the exposure (PE) is extremely rare, affecting only 2.78% of all deliveries. As a result of this, many matched pairs in the 1:1 design will consist of a case and control who are both unexposed, and as shown in Equations 4.20 and 4.21, these do not contribute to the conditional logistic regression. By sampling larger risk sets (i.e., more controls per case), it becomes less likely that *all* members of the set have the same exposure value, and so the risk set enters the analysis. In the implementations above, the very rare exposure resulted in a large majority of the matched pairs (998 out of 1088) with concordant exposure for case and control, so that the analysis was based on just 90 cases and their matched controls. In contrast, more than twice as many cases were retained in the 1:5 case-control study and more than three times as many in the 1:10 design (see Table 4.7).

TABLE 4.7: *Number of records included in each of the regression analyses in Table 4.6. The cohort of 970,778 deliveries includes a total of 1088 cases (72 exposed).*

	Cohort (970,778)	**1:1 NCC (n=180)**	**1:5 NCC (n=1266)**	**1:10 NCC (n=3432)**
Total controls	969,690	1088	5440	10,880
Controls exposed	26956	28	154	305
Concordant sets				
all exposed		5	0	0
all non-exposed		993	877	776
Discordant sets		90	211	312
Sample size	970,778	180	1055	3120

4.5 Case-cohort Sampling

From the previous section, it is clear that it is not necessary to follow all cohort members to estimate a hazard ratio. In the nested case-control design, the subsample of non-cases selected at each event time are used to represent all non-cases in the full risk set at that time. An alternative approach is to select a representative subsample of the whole cohort at the start of follow-up and use these individuals to represent the experience of the cohort at each event time. This is the idea of the case-cohort design, where a small **subcohort** is selected at baseline and followed up over time (not to be confused with a cohort of cases!). Like the nested case-control design, the case-cohort design often includes all cases in the cohort, so the sample for analysis consists of the subcohort and any additional cases that occurred outside the sub-cohort. This is presented graphically in the top panel of Figure 4.13 for a cohort of 30 individuals, 10 of whom (marked by solid black 'life-lines') were selected into the subcohort at the beginning of follow-up. The cases inside and outside the subcohort are indicated by square and round markers respectively. The case-cohort sample for analysis in this illustration thus consists of 12 individuals, represented by the grey shading.

In the 1986 paper where Prentice first proposed the case-cohort design [172], the risk-set for each case that occurs, whether inside or outside the sub-cohort, consists of the members of the subcohort at risk at that time (and the case, if outside the subcohort). A member of the subcohort who becomes a case during follow-up, such as individuals numbered 2, 18 and 25, will no longer contribute to the risk sets at later time points: for example, individual 2 will only contribute to the risk sets for events at times t_1 (in the subcohort), t_2 (outside the subcohort) and t_3 (their own event). Cases that occur outside the subcohort will only contribute to their own event time. Thus the contribution to the likelihood at each event time is given by Equation 4.22, where S_i denotes the members of the subcohort still at risk at time t_i. Since the same subcohort of individuals is used at each event time, this is an estimated (not exact) likelihood, referred to as a pseudo-likelihood. The likelihood over all event times is given by Equation 4.23

$$\textbf{Likelihood for event } i = \frac{e^{\beta X_i}}{\sum_{j \epsilon S_i} e^{\beta X_j} + I[i \notin S_i] e^{\beta X_i}} \tag{4.22}$$

$$\textbf{Likelihood for all events} = \prod_{t_i} \frac{e^{\beta X_i}}{\sum_{j \epsilon S_i} e^{\beta X_j} + I[i \notin S_i] e^{\beta X_i}} \tag{4.23}$$

On comparing with Equation 4.15, it can be seen that Equation 4.23 (or equivalently the Prentice likelihood in the bottom panel of Figure 4.13) is a Cox likelihood, where the individuals being followed include the members of the subcohort (from the start of the follow-up) and the additional cases outside the subcohort (from just before the time of their event). Thus, if the entry time for the additional cases is set to any time

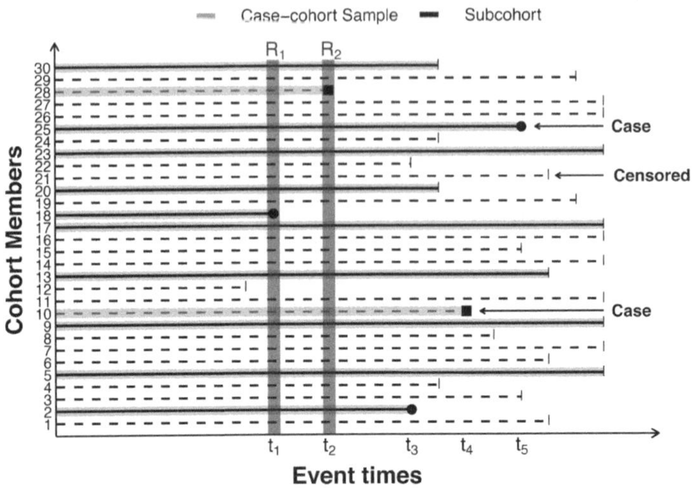

$$\textbf{Hazard for case } \boldsymbol{i} = h_0(t)e^{\beta X_i}$$

$$\textbf{Hazard for subcohort at } t_i = \textstyle\sum_{j \in S_i} h_0(t)e^{\beta X_j}$$

S_i is the subcohort at risk at t_i

$$\textbf{Likelihood (Prentice)} = \prod_i \frac{e^{\beta X_i}}{\sum_{k \epsilon S_i^*} e^{\beta X_k}}$$

S_i^* is the subcohort (and the case) at risk at t_i

$$\textbf{Likelihood (IPW)} = \prod_i \frac{e^{\beta X_i}}{\sum_{k \epsilon S_i^{\#}} e^{\beta X_k} w_k}$$

$S_i^{\#}$ is the subcohort and *all* cases at risk at t_i

$w_k = 1$ for cases and $\frac{1}{\pi}$ for controls

FIGURE 4.13: *Illustration a case-cohort sample (grey shaded life lines) from a cohort of 30 individuals, of whom 12 (solid black lines) were selected as a sub-cohort at the start of follow up. Cases occurring inside and outside the sub-cohort are indicated by ● and ■ respectively. The Prentice and weighted likelihoods are presented.*

very close to, and before, their event time, a simple Cox regression command in any software can be used to estimate the HR. This simple 'trick' means the HR can be readily estimated with any standard statistical software. However, due to this estimate being from a pseudo-likelihood, there was initially no simple expression for its standard error.

4.5.1 Approaches to case-cohort analysis

In the years following the introduction of the case-cohort design, there were many statistical publications investigating its properties and suggesting various modifications. This work was focused on efforts to derive an expression for the standard error of the ln(HR) and to characterise the most efficient design. Although the statistical methods are beyond the scope of this book, the many approaches proposed can be easily appreciated intuitively, as they all concern if/how the cases outside the subcohort should contribute to the risk sets. Theoretical work by Prentice and Self in 1988 developed an estimator of the standard error for a modified version of the likelihood in Equation 4.23 where cases outside the subcohort were *not* allowed to contribute to the risk set at their own event time. Thus, these individuals would appear only in the numerator of the likelihood component at their own event time, but not the denominator. While this facilitated the development of an expression for the standard error, it would seem that the HR estimate obtained would be inefficient, as the likelihood does not use all the information available in the data. Indeed, the original pseudo-likelihood of Prentice also does not make use of all available information from cases outside the subcohort, as they only 'enter' the analysis at their own event time, and their prior information is ignored.

A number of scientists suggested that cases outside the sub-cohort should also contribute to the risk sets *before*, and not just *at*, their own event time. This clearly uses more information, as it means that in contrast to the Prentice likelihood where cases in the sub-cohort only contribute to the risk set at their own event time, all individuals in the case-cohort sample (i.e., those whose life-lines have grey shading in Figure 4.13), whether they are inside or outside the sub-cohort, now contribute to the risk sets. As a result, the risk sets are no longer representative of the background cohort, as they have been 'enriched' with (future) cases. To overcome this bias, some kind of re-weighting is needed to estimate the total hazard in each risk set and it is the choice of this weighting that discriminates between the various methods that have been proposed. A few of these will be summarised here for the setting of a case-cohort study where all cases in the cohort are to be included, and a proportion π of the cohort has been selected as the subcohort.

The simplest idea is to assign a weight of 1 to cases (whether they occur inside or outside the sub-cohort) and a weight of $\frac{1}{\pi}$ (the inverse of the sampling fraction) to the non-cases (see lower panel of Figure

4.13). Readers will recognise the close similarity to the weighting used in the two-stage designs of Chapter 3. To analyse this design, which was proposed in 1992 [14], the user simply assigns a weight of 1 to all the cases in the case-cohort sample, a weight of $\frac{1}{\pi}$ to the controls, and then runs a weighted Cox regression. Since the weights are the inverse of the probability an individual is selected into the case-cohort sample, this approach is known as **Inverse Probability Weighting (IPW)**. As with the conditional logistic regression encountered in Chapter 3, the naive standard error is too small as it does not adjust for the uncertainty in the weights, so the robust standard error should be used.

One of the weighting proposals of Borgan and co-authors in 2000 [15] is a very similar IPW approach, with a weight of 1 for all cases, but the weight for non-cases is the ratio of the number of non-cases in the cohort to the number of non-cases in the subcohort, i.e. the inverse of the sampling fraction of cohort *non-cases*. Again, once the sampling fraction is known, the HR (and its standard error) can be easily obtained from this likelihood using a weighted Cox regression (and robust standard errors). For a rare disease, the non-case sampling fraction will be very close to π and there will be no meaningful difference in the results obtained from the two IPW methods. Another weighting strategy for the cases outside the sub-cohort was proposed by Barlow [9], where a weight of $\frac{1}{\pi}$ is assigned to these cases at times prior to their own event time, so that they are treated like subcohort members while they are still at risk and there is no 'borrowing' of information from the future concerning their ultimate case status.

The flurry of activity in researching these variations of the case-cohort design, and the claims and counter-claims regarding efficiency, probably contributed to the lack of adoption of this design for many years. Epidemiologists may have perceived it as not only more complicated than the widely-used case-control design, but a design whose properties were not fully understood. Added to this was the lack of any special command in major statistical software packages for running a case-cohort analysis as existed for other analyses. However understandable these perceptions might be, they are also very unfortunate: the case-cohort design is very straightforward to implement and the analysis using any weighting system is extremely simple. In a comparison of the different weighting systems in the 2015 paper by Kim [102], the actual weighting used makes very little difference, provided the cohort is reasonably large and the subcohort is at least equivalent in size to a 1:2 case-control study. Software packages that now have custom-built

TABLE 4.8: *2-by-2 table of case-cohort sample drawn from the postpartum VTE dataset by sampling with probability 0.56% from the whole cohort.*

	Subcohort Yes	No	
Case (VTE)	4	1084	1088
Control (no VTE)	5382	964,308	969,690
	5386	965,392	970,778

commands for analysing case-cohort data will use one of these weighting systems as default, and may or may not offer options. However, the analyst can always run their own weighted Cox regression, after some simple data organisation.

4.5.2 Illustration: nested case-control and case-cohort designs

To illustrate the application of the case-cohort design, we use the same postpartum VTE data as in Tables 4.5 and 4.6. In the cohort of 970,778 deliveries, there were 1088 cases, a proportion of 0.112%, so to correspond to the number of controls in the 1:5 nested case-control study, a subcohort was selected by random sampling from the cohort with probability 5(1088/970778)= 0.56%. This resulted in a subcohort of 5386 deliveries, only 4 of which had a VTE event during follow-up. Thus the remaining 1084 cases outside the subcohort are combined with these sub-cohort members to form the case-cohort sample of 6470 deliveries. The numbers of cases and non-cases inside and outside the sub-cohort are presented in Table 4.8. These data were analysed for the joint effects of the same factors as in 4.5 and 4.6 using two methods: the Prentice method and a weighted Cox regression. For the weighted analysis, the cases were assigned a weight of 1 and controls were weighted by the inverse of their sampling fraction from all non-cases, i.e.

$$\pi = 5382/969,690 = 0.00555$$

This **Borgan II** weight is almost identical to the simple subcohort sampling fraction (.0056) in this example. The estimates and confidence intervals from these analyses of the case-cohort sample are presented in Table 4.9, where the weighted analysis uses robust standard errors. The

TABLE 4.9: *Adjusted hazard ratio estimates (with 95% confidence intervals) of the effect of various risk factors on postpartum VTE: NCC 1:5 is the 1:5 nested case-control study from Table 4.6; CCH 1:5 is the case-cohort study described above with a sub-cohort approximately 5 times the number of cases.*

	NCC 1:5 CLR	CCH (1:5) IPW	CCH (1:5) Prentice
Preeclampsia	1.49 (1.10, 2.01)	1.50 (1.17, 1.91)	1.62 (1.19, 2.22)
Maternal age	1.02 (1.00, 1.03)	1.01 (1.00, 1.03)	1.03 (1.01, 1.04)
BMI			
Overweight	1.76 (1.50, 2.06)	1.75 (1.52, 2.00)	1.54 (1.32, 1.80)
Obese	2.40 (1.98, 2.90)	2.23 (1.90, 2.62)	2.03 (1.69, 2.45)
Caesarean	1.86 (1.58, 2.19)	1.77 (1.53, 2.03)	1.72 (1.46, 2.02)
First birth	1.13 (0.98, 1.31)	1.11 (0.97, 1.26)	1.09 (0.95, 1.26)
Smoker	1.63 (1.30, 2.03)	1.57 (1.30, 1.89)	1.49 (1.19, 1.85)
Transfusion	2.66 (1.93, 3.66)	2.47 (1.93, 3.16)	2.54 (1.83, 3.51)

CLR: Conditional logistic regression
IPW: Inverse probability weighting (Borgan II weights)
Prentice: Prentice option in **cch** command in R

results from the 1:5 nested case-control study in Table 4.6 are provided in the first column of the table for comparison.

For the analysis of the 1:5 case-cohort sample, the weighted Cox method is slightly more efficient, with narrower confidence intervals, but the differences are very small. The choice of method for case-cohort analysis becomes less important for low incidence, so that the close agreement of the two methods here is to be expected since we are studying an extremely rare outcome. Comparing the 1:5 case-cohort study to the 1:5 nested case-control study, the case-cohort study has better precision for most of the hazard ratio estimates. For a binary predictor, the case-cohort design is known to be more powerful than a nested case-control design analysed with conditional logistic regression. This is unsurprising, especially for rare (or common) exposures, as there is a loss of the concordant risk sets in the analysis. This is especially marked for the main exposure of interest (preeclampsia) in our example, where the nested case-control sample was concordant for 877 of the 1088 risk sets, so that only 211 sets (1266 individuals) contributed to the estimation of that hazard ratio. Thus it is noteworthy that despite the loss of these data from the analysis, the precision of the estimates is very similar to those from the case-cohort design. This relative efficiency of the nested case-control and case-cohort designs will be discussed further in the next section when the strengths of the two designs are compared, and again later in the book when alternative methods of analysing nested case-control data are introduced.

4.6 Comparison of Risk Sets

The association between a time-to-event outcome and an exposure X (and other explanatory variables Z) can be estimated from the whole cohort, a nested case-control sample or a case-cohort sample. The likelihoods for these three designs are presented in Table 4.10. The feature that distinguishes the nested case-control and case-cohort designs is *when* the controls are sampled, but the objective is the same, i.e. to *estimate* the contribution of the full risk set R_i at each event time t_i from a representative sample. When the full cohort is available, the risk set R_i consists of the case at that time and all members of the cohort still at risk. In the nested case-control study, this full risk set is represented by the *sampled* risk set, R_i^* consisting of the case and the (small number of) controls sampled at that time. In contrast to this concurrent sampling, the case-cohort design selects a sub-cohort of individuals at the start of follow-up (i.e., inclusive sampling) which provides the controls for the risk set at each event time. All cases, whether inside or outside the sub-cohort, are included in the case-cohort sample, and at event time t_i the full risk set R_i is represented by $S_i^{\#}$ which consists of all sub-cohort members who are still at risk at that time, augmented by all at-risk cases.

Unlike the R_i^* from nested case-control sampling, the controls in the $S_i^{\#}$ from case-cohort sampling are not representative of the non-cases in the full cohort at time t_i, since in addition to the sub-cohort members who have not yet had the event, it contains *all cases outside the sub-cohort* who are still at risk (and will later have the event). Thus the sample at any event time has an over-representation of cases, since all cases in the full cohort may contribute, whereas only sub-cohort controls are included. This imbalance can be quite dramatic: for example, in the illustration in Table 4.8, the 1:5 case-cohort sample had only 4 cases in

TABLE 4.10: *Comparison of likelihoods and risk sets for cohort, nested case-control and case-cohort designs.*

Study Type	**Likelihood**	**Risk Set**
Cohort	$\prod_{t_i} \frac{e^{\beta X_i + \gamma Z_i}}{\sum_{k \epsilon \boldsymbol{R_i}} e^{\beta X_k + \gamma Z_k}}$	$\mathbf{R_i}$: All individuals still at risk at time t_i, when case i develops the outcome, are included in the risk set.
Nested Case-control	$\prod_{t_i} \frac{e^{\beta X_i + \gamma Z_i}}{\sum_{k \epsilon \boldsymbol{R_i^*}} e^{\beta X_k + \gamma Z_k}}$	$\mathbf{R_i}^*$: At time t_i when case i develops the outcome, a *sample* of controls who are still at risk are chosen from that risk set. The sampled controls can continue through follow-up and be chosen as controls again, or become cases themselves. This type of sampling is also referred to as *incidence density sampling* or *concurrent sampling.*
Case-cohort	$\prod_{t_i} \frac{e^{\beta X_i + \gamma Z_i}}{\sum_{k \epsilon \boldsymbol{S_i^{\#}}} w_k e^{\beta X_k + \gamma Z_k}}$	$\mathbf{S_i}^{\#}$: All members of the sub-cohort and cases outside the sub-cohort who are at risk at t_i. $\mathbf{w_k}$: Since all cases in the full cohort are included in the case-cohort sample, the case sampling fraction = 1. For non-cases, the sampling fraction is <1, and so these individuals must be upweighted to be representative of the non-cases in the full cohort. $\mathbf{w_k}$ represents the weight of individual k.

the sub-cohort, but 1084 outside the sub-cohort. To correct for this bias, the controls are 'upweighted' by the inverse of the sampling fraction. Some methods use the inverse of the sampling fraction for selecting the sub-cohort from the full cohort, which in the example is 0.0056, and some use the sampling fraction of non-cases, i.e. the proportion of non-cases in the sub-cohort to non-cases in the full cohort (.00555 in the example). The latter, known as the Borgan II method, will be used in this book.

4.7 Comparison of Nested Case-control and Case-cohort

From the previous sections it is clear that the HR in a cohort can be estimated without following up the entire cohort. Two designs were presented where all the cases, but only a small proportion of the controls, were sampled: the nested case-control study and the case-cohort study. The nested case-control design has long been recognised for its efficiency and is widely used in epidemiological research. In contrast, the adoption of the case-cohort design has been much slower despite its similar efficiency. Some of this delay may be due to reluctance of epidemiologists to trust a design for which the statistical properties and numerous modifications had generated much debate in the statistical literature, including claims and counter-claims of superior efficiency. The 2015 paper by Kim [102] provides a welcome summary of the bias, power and efficiency in a range of simulation studies, and concludes that there is rarely any notable difference between the nested case-control design analysed with conditional logistic regression and the case-cohort design using weighted Cox regression. Although the weighted Cox regression can today be readily implemented after some small data organisation tasks, the lack of special software commands for case-cohort analysis until recently was likely a discouragement to potential users.

The feature that distinguishes these designs is *when* the controls are sampled. Table 4.11 outlines the many differences between these two designs that are consequences of this simple difference, and might determine which design is most appropriate in a given research situation.

TABLE 4.11: *Comparison of advantages (+) and disadvantages (−) of nested case-control and case-cohort designs.*

Differences	**Nested case-control**	**Case-cohort**
Biased controls	+ Controls are sampled from the full cohort at the event times so are not in active follow-up that might change their behaviour	− Subcohort members that are followed rigorously have potential for being biased as representatives of the full cohort
Outcome(s)	− Only the outcome that defines the cases can be studied	+ Any outcome can be studied, provided the subcohort can be augmented with events that occur outside the subcohort
Exposures	− Exposures ascertained at or prior to the time of selection. Time dependent exposures not accommodated	+ Retrospective and time-varying exposures can be accommodated
Data collection	− Information on cases and controls obtained at the same time, requiring effort and expense throughout follow-up + This however has the advantage of a case and their controls being comparable for the methods of measurement	+ The sub-cohort is identified at the start of follow-up, so data collection can start immediately and be conducted in a short time − This however has the potential disadvantage of different methods of measurement for some cases

Continued

TABLE 4.11: *Continued. Comparison of advantages (+) and disadvantages (−) of nested case-control and case-cohort designs.*

Differences	**Nested case-control**	**Case-cohort**
Censoring	+ Since controls are chosen at each event time from the full risk set, the design ensures controls are available for all cases	− The sub-cohort may become 'thin' later in follow-up, especially if there is heavy censoring or fine stratification, resulting in some events for which there are no controls
Time scale	− Controls are matched to cases on a specific time-scale (time on study, attained age, ...) and the HR estimated from the conditional logistic regression pertains to that time scale	+ The sub-cohort is representative of the full cohort, so that analysis is not limited to a single time-scale
Extend follow-up	− New cases will need new controls identified, enrolled and measured	+ No new enrolments necessary as sub-cohort can be used for extended follow-up time
Model	− Matched sets analysed by conditional logistic regression	+ Flexible with respect to model used and method of analysis
Risk measures	- Only a relative risk measure (the HR) can be estimated from the matched data as the baseline hazard cancels in conditional logistic regression	+ The sub-cohort reflects the full cohort, so in addition to the HR, it is possible to estimate the prevalence, RR and cumulative incidence/hazard

Continued

TABLE 4.11: *Continued. Comparison of advantages (+) and disadvantages (−) of nested case-control and case-cohort designs.*

Differences	**Nested case-control**	**Case-cohort**
Matching/ Stratification	− Effects of matching factors cannot be estimated from the conditional logistic regression	+ Stratification factors can be included in the model
Software	+ Standard well-known software commands	− Some standard commands, less widely-available and less well-known
Missing data	− An exposure or confounder variable missing for a case will result in the loss of the risk set	+ Only the individual with the missing data is lost from analysis
Timing of specimens	+ Collection and/or measurement at the same point in time may be very important, as the matching will overcome biases from changes in technology or storage time effects	− Trade off between effects of storage time and technological drift: for long follow-up time, effect of technological changes could be minimised by analysing all specimens at the end of follow-up, but subcohort specimens gathered at the start of follow-up may be compromised by storage time
Efficiency	Similar efficiency for the same sample size −however, for rare exposures, risk sets may be lost from analysis due to concordance	+ All sampled subjects retained in analysis

4.8 Exercises

1. This and subsequent exercises makes use the dataset `full_cohort.dta`, which is a simulated dataset similar to that used in the paper *Comparisons of risk prediction methods using nested case-control data* by Salim et al in Stat Med 2017 (PMID 27734520), consisting of 50,000 cohort members where the outcome of interest is time from enrolment to coronary heart disease, with event indicator 1=coronary heart disease, 0=censored. The variables recorded for this cohort include:

   t time (in years) from enrolment to coronary heart disease(CHD)

   censored event indicator (0=CHD, 1=censored)

   Age age in years

   Gender 1=Male, 0=Female

   Chol cholesterol in mg/dL

   HDL high-density lipoprotein in mg/dL

   SBP systolic blood pressure in mmHg

   Treat antihypertensive treatment (1=Yes, 0=No)

   Smoke smoking status (1=Yes, 0=No)

   (i) Create a categorical variable for age: < 50, 50-59, 60-69, 70-79, 80+.

   (ii) Center each of the other continuous covariates (cholesterol, HDL, and SBP) at their mean values by subtracting the mean.

   (iii) Run a Cox regression analysis of the whole cohort with the new variables from (i) and (ii) and the remaining binary variables (gender: 1=Male, 0=Female, Treat: 1=Yes, 0=No, Smoke: 1=Yes, 0=No).

   (iv) Run a logistic regression of the binary outcome and compare the ORs to the HRs from (iii).

   (v) Draw a 1:1 case-control sample that is matched on sex and age category. Save a copy of this dataset for the remaining tasks in this exercise and for Exercise 2 below.

(vi) Run a conditional logistic regression analysis of the data from (v) and compare the results to the full cohort.

(vii) Re-run the logistic regression analysis of the data from (vi), this time using an *unconditional* model and verify that you get valid ORs for all variables except the matching factors (sex and age category), provided you adjust for the matching factors.

2. Where sampling fractions are known or can be estimated, a weighted analysis of case-control data will provide valid estimates of the effects of the matching factors. In practice, the sampling fractions might be obtained in two different ways:

   (a) where each member of the cohort has information on the matching factors and on whether or not they were sampled into the case-control study, the sampling fractions can be readily computed

   (b) where the individual cohort data is not available, but the numbers of individuals in the strata can be obtained from an external source (e.g. population counts by age and sex are available for many countries and regions)

   (i) Arrange (or re-create) the case-control sample from Exercise 1 (vii) in a dataset with one record for cohort member, with an indicator variable identifying those who were sampled. Use these data to verify that a weighted logistic regression recovers the cohort ORs from Exercise 1 (iv).

   (ii) From the full cohort data used in Exercise 1, create a summary dataset containing only the variables sex and age group, together with the number of cohort members in each of these strata (this will mimic the summary population data that many government authorities make available). Now merge your case-control dataset from Exercise 1 to this summary data and verify that a weighted analysis provides valid ORs.

3. Run a Cox regression analysis of the whole cohort described in Exercise 1, to obtain the crude HR for Gender and the HR adjusted for age-category.

Note: If the following steps take a long time to run, you could use a smaller cohort (e.g. a random 10,000 from the 50,000).

(i) Draw a *nested* (i.e. matched on time) case-control sample, with 5 controls for each case, using simple random sampling. Run a conditional logistic regression of **event** and **Gender** using your nested case-control sample and compare the results with the crude HR for gender obtained from a Cox regression analysis of the whole cohort.

(ii) Draw a nested case-control sample that is matched on age category. Compare the OR for gender from a conditional logistic regression analysis to the age-adjusted HR from the Cox regression of the whole cohort.

(iii) Use the data from (ii) to run the full model in Exercise 1, and compare the results to the Cox regression of the whole cohort.

4. (i) Select a random sample of the full cohort used in the previous exercises, with sample size equal to the number of controls in the 1:5 case-control study in Exercise 3. Create an indicator variable that marks these individuals as members of a subcohort.

(ii) Cross-tabulate the subcohort indicator and case indicator to get the sampling fraction for controls in the subcohort.

(iii) Generate a weight variable =1 for cases and the inverse of the sampling fraction for non-cases.

(iv) Run a weighted Cox regression to obtain the age-adjusted HR for gender and request the robust variance estimates.

(v) Compare your results to those from the Cox regression of the full cohort and the conditional logistic regression of the nested case-control data in Exercise 3.

(vi) Repeat the weighted Cox regression of the case-cohort data with the full model and compare the results to those from the full cohort and from the nested case-control sample.

(vii) Repeat the selection and analysis of a case-cohort sample using purpose-built commands.

5

Estimates Available from Standard Designs

All of the designs presented so far are associated with a specific estimate of disease occurrence or risk. For example, the classic case-control study provides an odds ratio, and the nested case-control study provides a hazard ratio. The cohort study, with its detailed information provides both of these measures, as well as estimates of the actual hazard rate (not just ratio!) and cumulative risk at any point in time during follow-up. Since the case-cohort study includes a subsample of the whole cohort (called the 'subcohort'), this subsample can also be used to estimate the same quantities as can be estimated from the full cohort. However, the nested case-control study does not have a representative sample from the full cohort, so in studies where the absolute risk is of interest, this design has not been used.

The standard designs are also associated with a specific method of analysis: logistic regression for case-control data, Cox regression for cohort data, conditional logistic regression for nested case-control data, and (weighted) Cox regression for case-cohort data. However, there are many more estimates available from standard designs than those that are routinely reported. Some of these can be obtained from the models used for the standard analysis, and some become accessible by applying a familiar method of analysis to data from a design for which it is not the standard approach. Thus, armed with the designs and methods of analysis from Chapters 1–4, it is possible to estimate many other features of risk than first thought, with some requiring just some 'sleight of hand' with rearranging the data to capitalise on existing software that was written for other purposes! The following sections will introduce a selection of these, and outline how they can be estimated using standard software tools, or purpose-built commands or packages.

5.1 Measures of Exposure Impact

In addition to the relative risk measures introduced so far (RR, OR, HR), there are other measures that provide information about the *impact* of an exposure in a way that is more amenable to health policy and planning, and that are directly parallel to concepts that are used to communicate the effectiveness of medical treatments. The most widely-used measure of the effectiveness of a treatment for a disease or an intervention to prevent disease is the **Number Needed to Treat (NNT)**. In the simplest setting of the treatment of a disease that is fatal if untreated, the NNT is the number of patients that need to be treated to achieve one cure. The ideal treatment has a NNT of 1 (i.e. 100% success rate), but where a treatment is only successful in a proportion π of patients, then the NNT=$\frac{1}{\pi}$. The assessment of medications in real life is more complex than this trivial example, since patients may recover spontaneously or there may be other treatments available that have some benefit. In a randomised placebo-controlled clinical trial, where the patients on treatment and placebo are similar, the NNT is the number of patients that need to be treated to achieve one additional cure compared with those in the placebo group. For example, if the recovery rate is 15% in the placebo group and 25% in the treatment group, this means that for every 100 patients, there are 10 additional patients who recover, which is one additional recovery in every ten, so the NNT=10. Thus the NNT is the reciprocal of the difference between the risks in the treated and untreated:

$$NNT = \frac{1}{\pi_1 - \pi_0} \tag{5.1}$$

where π_1 and π_0 are the proportions of events in the treated and untreated.

In describing an intervention to *prevent* disease, such as prophylaxis medication or screening, the NNT is defined as the expected number of patients that would need to be treated to prevent one additional case, compared to those who received a control intervention or none. This is sometimes written NNTH, to indicate that it is the number that need to be treated for one (additional) person harmed, and again it is the reciprocal of the difference in the proportions harmed in the two groups. An example that has been much discussed is the effectiveness of breast cancer screening. A UK panel reported in 2013 [142] that for every 10,000 women who would be screened, 43 deaths from breast cancer would be prevented, an NNT of 233. The cost of such a screening programme is more complex than the simple financial resources of screening 233 women to prevent one breast cancer death. The same paper reported that in every 10,000 screened women, 129 would be over-diagnosed with a breast cancer that they did not have or that would not have manifest clinically in their lifetime. Thus, the policy-makers were faced with a NNTH of 10,000/129 = 78, which corresponds to approximately three women harmed for every one who is helped. These benefits and harms would be expected to change over time due to improved accuracy of the screening examination and improved prognosis for treated tumours. Most importantly, the performance of a screening programme depends on the risk factors of the women targeted. This is borne out by the American College of Physicians guidance for clinicians concerning breast cancer screening [175]. Firstly, the guidance is for 'average-risk women' (a difficult concept in itself) and secondly, there are three different guidelines proposed for three different age groups. While age is an obvious risk factor, women and populations will also differ with respect to other important risk factors such as family history of cancer and childbearing patterns. The participation in screening, and adherence and response to treatment, will all impact on a summary estimate such as NNT for a population. This 'profile' of the population with respect to their risk factors is also an important consideration for calculating and interpreting the effects of an exposure, as we will see in the following section.

5.1.1 Number needed to be exposed, NNE

The impact of an exposure on a population that is known as the **Number Needed to be Exposed (NNE)**, is an exact parallel of the NNT. Where the exposure of interest is harmful, the NNE is sometimes written as **NNEH**, to emphasise that it is the number that need to be exposed for one additional adverse outcome (i.e. 'harm') compared to those who are unexposed. In the same way as for an intervention, the NNE can be estimated as the reciprocal of the difference in the event rates in the exposed and unexposed. This difference is also known as the **risk difference** or **excess risk**, but perhaps the clearest terminology is **absolute risk increase**, which emphasises that it involves *absolute* (i.e., actual) risks, not relative risks, and that interest is focused on the magnitude by which this is increased by the exposure. Thus, denoting the risks in the exposed and unexposed individuals as π_1 and π_0:

$$NNE = \frac{1}{\pi_1 - \pi_0} \tag{5.2}$$

$$= \frac{1}{ARI} \tag{5.3}$$

where ARI is the absolute risk increase
in exposed compared to unexposed individuals.

The NNE can also be expressed in terms of the RR (see Equation 5.4 by simply dividing the numerator and denominator of Equation 5.2 by π_0. To express that NNE in terms of an OR > 1 (Equation 5.5) requires somewhat more algebraic manipulations [10] and is left as an exercise for the reader. For a protective exposure, the OR will be < 1, but if the *benefit* of the exposure is defined as the outcome of interest, then the OR will be > 1 and formula 5.5 can still be used to estimate the number needed to be exposed for benefit: in such situations, the NNE is sometimes written as **NNEB**.

$$NNE = \frac{1}{\pi_0(RR - 1)} \tag{5.4}$$

$$= \frac{1}{(OR - 1)\pi_0} + \frac{OR}{(OR - 1)(1 - \pi_0)} \tag{5.5}$$

π_0: risk of the event in the unexposed

Example 5.1, presents the association of BMI with CHD and stroke in the cross-sectional sample from visit 1 of the Framingham study. The two exposures considered are Overweight (BMI $\geq$ 25) and Obesity (BMI $\geq$ 30) The NNE is reported to the nearest integer value and the reader can verify that it can be obtained from the ARI, the RR or the OR. There are some interesting differences in the impact of these exposures on the two outcomes. The impact of overweight or obesity on CHD is similar, with one additional case expected for every 8 or 9 persons exposed, consistent with the recognition of BMI as an important risk factor for CHD. In contrast, for stroke, obesity has a greater impact than overweight, with NNE 18 compared to 27.

Example 5.1. *Illustration of computation of NNE from ARI, RR or OR, using the cross-sectional data from visit 1 of the Framingham study. Estimates of the NNE for overweight (BMI≥25) and obesity (BMI≥25), for one additional case of CHD or stroke to be attributable to the BMI level.*

	CHD		Stroke		
	Yes	No	Yes	No	Total
BMI<25 (Ref)	421	1572	146	1847	1993
BMI 25–29.9	596	1249	184	1661	1845
BMI≥30	218	359	82	495	577

	CHD		**Stroke**	
	BMI≥25	BMI≥30	BMI≥25	BMI≥30
π_1	0.336	0.378	0.110	0.142
π_0	0.211	0.265	0.073	0.086
ARI	0.125	0.113	0.037	0.056
NNE	8	9	27	18
RR	1.59	1.43	1.50	1.65
OR	1.89	1.68	1.56	1.76
NNE (Equation 5.4)	8	9	27	18
Adjusted*				
OR	1.58	1.67	1.31	1.62
NNE (Equation 5.5)	12	9	46	21

* *Adjusted for age and sex*

5.1.2 Adjusted NNE

If the exposure is assigned in a randomised trial, then it is meaningful to estimate the population NNE from the simple expressions presented above. However, for an observational study, the NNE will depend on the characteristics of the participants, which may be associated not only with an individual's risk of the adverse outcome, but also with their exposure.

Such characteristics are the confounders that have been discussed at length in Chapter 2. Thus, a more appropriate measure of the impact of an exposure from an observational study is the *adjusted* NNE, which can be estimated from an adjusted OR that is > 1 using Equation 5.5. The adjusted OR can be obtained by logistic regression, or where there are only a few binary or categorical confounders, the Mantel-Haenszel OR can be calculated. In the last two rows of the table in Example 5.1, the odds ratios for the associations of BMI with CHD and stroke have been adjusted for sex and age (dichotomised at 50 years) and an interaction between these two factors. The adjusted NNE for the impact of overweight on stroke is 49, almost twice the unadjusted value of 27, while the adjustment did not result in much change to the NNE for obesity (from 18 to 22), reflecting the larger confounding due to age and sex on the effect of overweight.

Interpretation of adjusted NNE

It is important to realise that an adjusted NNE depends on the risk factor profile of the unexposed individuals in the sample, as the π_0 term in the denominator is the risk of the event in this group. Thus the interpretation of an adjusted NNE of 10 is that for every 10 exposed individuals in a population *with the same distribution of risk factors as the unexposed population under study*, one additional event would be expected. If the continuous risk factors have been centred at their means, and the categorical risk factors have all been coded as zero for the reference level, then the NNE refers to a group that can be easily described. However, some specific group may be of greater interest, in which case the NNE needs to be calculated at the value(s) of the risk factor(s) of interest. For example, if the impact of BMI in males of a specific age was of interest in the simple example above, then males should be defined as reference and continuous age centered at the average male age. If a logistic model has been fitted to cohort or cross-sectional data to obtain the adjusted OR, then the model can be used to calculate the probability of the event in the exposed and unexposed members of the sub-population of interest [10]. The difference in the expected proportion of events is the estimate of the ARI, whose reciprocal is the NNE (Equation 5.2). An alternative method [11] is to use the logistic model to calculate the risk difference obtained by adding the exposure to each of the unexposed individuals, and using the average risk difference to estimate the ARI. This method performs best if there is very wide variation in the distribution of a continuous confounder, but otherwise gives similar results.

Another quantity that can also be a useful measure of impact is the average risk difference obtained by *removing* the exposure from all *exposed* individuals. This is known as the **Exposure Impact Number (EIN)** and is the average number of exposed persons among whom one additional case can be attributed to the exposure.

Estimation of NNE from case-control studies

All the measures of exposure impact involve risks, which can be estimated from cohort and cross-sectional studies but not from case-control studies. Although the NNE can be expressed in terms of the OR, which is available from case-control data, the expression also involves the risk of the event in the unexposed population, π_0 (see Equation 5.5). This cannot be estimated from a case-control study, and thus an external estimate would be needed in order to make use of Equation 5.5 with a crude or adjusted OR from a case-control study to estimate the NNE. An external estimate is also useful where it is of interest to obtain the NNE corresponding to a published OR (from any study design): for example, the use of the UK published annual CHD death rates for smokers and non-smokers to obtain the NNE from a published OR associated with smoking in the UK population [85]. Where the sampling fraction for selecting the controls from the population is known, a weighted logistic regression model can also provide valid estimates for the probabilities used to compute the ARI in Section 5.1.2 above.

5.1.3 Attributable risks and impact numbers

Numerous other measures of disease impact have been presented in the scientific literature [81] but we will focus on the proportions that represent the concept of 'attributable risk' and their associated impact numbers: the **Population Attributable Risk (PAR)** and **Population Attributable Fraction (PAF)**. The PAR is the difference between the risk of disease in the whole population and the risk in the unexposed population, which can be expressed as a proportion, or as numbers of cases per 100,000 population or other denominator. The PAF is the PAR expressed as a proportion of the risk in the whole population and is interpreted as the proportion of the risk in the population that could be eliminated by eliminating the exposure. If the exposure is protective, then the research question can be reversed as before to consider the 'preventable fraction'. Attributable risks are commonly used in the assessment of a public health intervention, as they reflect not only the strength of association between a risk factor and disease, but also the prevalence of the risk factor in the population. To describe excess risk or attributable risk and their impact numbers in terms of the familiar measures of disease occurrence (risk of disease, prevalence of exposure), it is sufficient to have the following simple notation:

$$\begin{aligned}\pi &= \text{risk of the disease in the population}\\ \pi_1 &= \text{risk of the disease in the exposed}\\ \pi_0 &= \text{risk of the disease in the unexposed}\\ \Rightarrow RR &= \frac{\pi_1}{\pi_0}\end{aligned}$$

$$\begin{aligned}p_e &= \text{proportion exposed (prevalence of exposure)}\\ p_u &= \text{proportion unexposed}\\ \Rightarrow \pi &= p_e\pi_1 + p_u\pi_0\end{aligned}$$

Table 5.1 presents the various risks in terms of π_1 and π_0, which can be estimated from a cohort or cross-sectional study, and a description and interpretation is provided for each term in columns 3 and 4 of the table. The impact number in column 5 of the table is simply the reciprocal of the corresponding proportion, can be expressed in terms of the RR and prevalence of exposure by substituting π by $p_e\pi_1 + p_u\pi_0$ and p_u by $1 - p_e$. Careful consideration of the proportion makes it clear whether the impact number refers to the whole population, the population of cases, or the population of all exposed cases (see last column of Table 5.1) which is essential for communicating a clear message.

For rare outcomes, the RR describing the crude association between an exposure and outcome can be approximated by the OR from a case-control sample. If the controls are a (reasonable sized) random sample from the population, other components of the impact numbers in Table 5.1 can also be approximated, such as the prevalence of exposure in the population p_e. However, as already mentioned in section 5.1.1 above, a case-control study does not provide an estimate of the risk of disease in the unexposed, π_0, that is required for computing the NNE, so that even for a rare outcome, where $RR \approx OR$, an external estimate of π_0 would be required in order to estimate the NNE or PIN. For the estimation of the CIN, the prevalence of the exposure in the population, p_e, could be approximated by the prevalence in the controls, since the cases are rare.

TABLE 5.1: *Table of risks and the associated impact numbers in terms of RR and other quantities that can be estimated from cohort or cross-sectional studies.*

Term	Proportion	Meaning	Term interpretation	Impact number (RR)	Impact number (OR)	Impact number interpretation
ARI Absolute Risk Increase	$\pi_1 - \pi_0$	Absolute risk increase (excess risk) **in exposed compared to unexposed individuals**	Disease incidence **in the exposed** that would be eliminated if exposure was eliminated	NNE= $\frac{1}{(RR-1)\pi_0}$	NNE=$\frac{1}{(OR-1)\pi_0}+\frac{OR}{(OR-1)(1-\pi_0)}$	Number of **exposed individuals** in the population for one additional case due to exposure
PAR Population Attributable Risk	$\pi - \pi_0$	Absolute risk increase (excess risk) **in the population compared to unexposed individuals**	Incidence **in the population** that would be eliminated if exposure was eliminated	PIN=$\frac{1}{p_e\pi_0(RR-1)}$	$\frac{1}{\frac{OR*O_0}{1+OR*O_0}+\pi_0}$ $O_0=\frac{\pi_0}{1-\pi_0}$: odds of outcome in unexposed	Number of **individuals in the population** amongst whom one additional case is due to exposure
PAF Population Attributable Fraction	$\frac{\pi-\pi_0}{\pi}$	The proportion of incidence **in the population** (i.e. exposed and unexposed) due to exposure	Percent of incidence **in the population** that would be eliminated if exposure was eliminated	CIN= $\frac{1+p_e(RR-1)}{p_e(RR-1)}$	CIN $\approx \frac{OR}{(OR-1)p_e^1}$ p_e^1: prevalence of exposure in the cases	Number of **cases** in the population amongst whom one case is due to exposure
AF Aetiological Fraction	$\frac{\pi_1-\pi_0}{\pi_1}$	The proportion of incidence **in the exposed** due to exposure	Percent of incidence **in the exposed** that would be eliminated if exposure was eliminated	ECIN $=\frac{RR}{1-RR}$		Number of **exposed cases** in the population amongst whom one case is due to exposure

NNE: Number needed to expose
PIN: Population impact number, CIN: Case impact number, ECIN: Exposed case impact number
Expression for NNE is exact but CIN uses a rare-disease approximation

Adjusted impact numbers

The usual approach to adjusting for confounding factors is to use a multivariable logistic regression model, which yields an OR, not a RR. If impact numbers can be expressed in terms of OR rather than RR, then the adjusted impact of an exposure can be estimated using the adjusted OR from standard analysis. The expression for the NNE in terms of the OR [10] was already presented in Equation 5.5 and is provided again in column 5 of the first row of Table 5.1. An expression for the PAF (and thus for its reciprocal, the CIN) in terms of an OR has also been derived [65] that provides a good approximation for rare diseases (third row of Table 5.1). In addition to the OR, this expression includes a term for the prevalence of exposure among the cases, a quantity that can be estimated from cohort, cross-sectional or case-control studies.

Combined, sequential and average attributable fractions

In planning for public health policies, the reduction or elimination of harmful exposures or behaviours might be approached in various ways. Where there are several recognised risk factors, these may be addressed at the same time or in a gradual manner. The combined impact of several exposures can be assessed using the same methods as for a single exposure, with the only difference being the unexposed' reference group who will now be defined as unexposed to all factors. Unfortunately, the attributable fractions will not necessarily add up to the combined value [65]: in the case of a step-by-step intervention, the sequential attributable fractions can be calculated instead and these add up to the combined attributable fraction. For a three-step intervention, the three estimates represent

- the proportion of disease that would be eliminated by step 1
- the *additional* proportion of disease that would be eliminated by step 2 beyond that eliminated by step 1
- the *additional* proportion of disease that would be eliminated (beyond that eliminated by steps 1 and 2) by adding step 3

The sequential attributable fractions depend on the order in which the exposures are to be eliminated, which is useful when there is a clear order for the introduction of the policies: for example if smoking is first banned on public transport, followed later by a ban in public buildings and finally in restaurants and bars. However, in some situations, the exposure to be eliminated may have no clear order, or indeed may be removed simultaneously as in the case of lifestyle changes. In these situations, it would be useful to have estimates of the impact of each of the components that add up to the overall effect. This 'average attributable risk' can be computed by averaging over the different permutations of the order in which exposures are eliminated. Estimates of combined, sequential and average attributable fractions are provided by *averisk* [65] and graphPAF [93].

5.1.4 Confidence intervals for measures of impact

Since the NNE is simply the reciprocal of a difference in the proportions π_1 and π_0, then for cohort or cross-sectional data, the confidence interval for the crude NNE can be obtained by simply inverting the estimate and the confidence limits of the ARI. These can be computed from the proportions and the critical values of a standard normal distribution [85] or readily obtained from any statistical calculator that handles a difference in proportions. However, for a crude NNE from a case-control design or an adjusted NNE from any design, the NNE is not a simple reciprocal, but a more complex function of an (adjusted) OR as seen in Equation 5.5 and Table 5.1. Expressions for the standard error of this estimate were derived [10, 11] and computed using custom-written SAS code that is available at http://www.rbsd.de/softw.html, but estimates of adjusted NNE with confidence intervals are not available in the other packages widely used by epidemiologists. However, an approximate confidence interval can be obtained by simply using Equation 5.5 to compute the NNE values corresponding to the upper and lower limits of the confidence interval for the adjusted OR. This ignores the uncertainty in the estimate of π_0, but provided this estimate is reasonably precise, a good approximation to the confidence interval is readily obtained.

The estimates of NNE for the impact of obesity on CHD and stroke in the Framingham data described in Example 5.1 are presented in Table 5.2. The confidence intervals for the NNE calculated by substituting the OR and its confidence limits in the formula in Equation 5.5 are very similar to those obtained by inverting the confidence limits for the ARI (NNE and NNE* in rows 2 and 4). The closer agreement for the CHD estimates than for the stroke estimates is unsurprising, as the OR formula is approximate, disregarding the uncertainty in the proportion π_0: for stroke, this proportion, $\pi_0 = 0.086$, has an uncertainty of 10.4% (two standard errors) while for CHD, $\pi_0 = 0.265$ with an uncertainty of only

5.4%. The crude and adjusted estimates of NNE for CHD (and their confidence intervals) obtained from case-control sampling are also in close agreement with the estimates from the whole cross-sectional sample. For stroke, the estimates from the case-control sample are consistent with those from the full cross-sectional estimates, but with larger variation due to smaller sample sizes.

For the CIN, an estimate with confidence interval can be obtained by inverting the population attributable fraction and its confidence limits [85]. Two software packages developed in R for estimating the population attributable fraction (PAF) from various study designs are *AF* [43] and *graphPAF* [93] available on CRAN. The graphPAF package enables the estimation of a wide variety of alternative calculations for disease burden, including joint, sequential and average PAFs.

Table 5.3 presents the estimates of the PAF of CHD due to overweight and the PAF of stroke due to obesity from the Framingham data,

TABLE 5.2: *The impact of obesity on CHD and stroke in terms of NNE, crude and adjusted (for age and sex), estimated using the full cross-sectional data from Framingham visit 1 and from case-control samples of similar size for CHD and stroke.*

		CHD	**Stroke**
Cross-sectional			
(n=4415)	**ARI (%)**	11.3 (7.1, 15.5)	5.6 (2.63, 8.60)
	NNE	**9 (6, 14)**	**18 (12, 38)**
	OR	1.68 (1.40, 2.02)	1.76 (1.36, 2.28)
	NNE*	**9 (6, 14)**	**18 (11, 36)**
	Adj OR	1.67 (1.38, 2.02)	1.62 (1.24, 2.12)
	Adj NNE*	**9 (6, 15)**	**22 (12, 54)**
Case-control		Ratio 1:1 (n=2470)	Ratio 1:5 (n=2472)
	OR	1.59 (1.27, 1.99)	1.90 (1.44, 2.51)
	NNE*	**10 (7, 20)**	**15 (10, 30)**
	Adj OR	1.61 (1.28, 2.04)	1.84 (1.38, 2.46)
	Adj NNE*	**10 (6, 20)**	**16 (10, 35)**

* *NNE computed from the OR using Equation 5.5*

with the corresponding CIN (to the nearest integer) with confidence intervals. The estimates were obtained from the AF package, whose robust estimates can result in slightly different confidence intervals than those from *graphPAF*. The crude and adjusted estimates from the whole cross-sectional sample and from the case-control sub-samples are in good agreement.

TABLE 5.3: *The impact of overweight on CHD and of obesity on stroke, in terms of PAF and the corresponding CIN, estimated using the cross-sectional data from Framingham visit 1 and from case-control subsamples.*

	CHD		Stroke	
	PAF	**CIN**	**PAF**	**CIN**
		Crude estimates		
Full data	.245 (.194, .296)	4 (3 , 5)	.079 (.037, .120)	13 (8 , 27)
Case-control	.298 (.234, .362)	3 (3 , 4)	.094 (.009, .179)	11 (6 , 106)
		Adjusted estimates		
Full data	.216 (.164, .268)	5 (4 , 6)	.067 (.026, .108)	15 (9 , 39)
Case-control	.191 (.139, .242)	4 (3 , 5)	.073 (.035, .111)	14 (9 , 29)

5.2 Estimating RR from Logistic Regression

The example presented in Figure 4.1 and Table 4.3 of Chapter 4 illustrated how the OR from different sampling designs provides estimates of different measures of risk in a cohort. The OR from inclusive sampling, where the cases identified during follow-up are compared to controls selected at the start of follow-up, estimates the RR. In a cross-sectional study, the corresponding approach would be to compare a sample of cases at a given time to a sample from the entire population at that time. As early as 1982, Miettinen referred to this kind of sampling as 'replacement of the sample of non-cases by a sample of the base' [147], where the 'base' or 'study base' is the entire cohort or cross-section of the population under study. Using B_1 and B_0 to denote the numbers of exposed and unexposed individuals in the base, and C_1 and C_0 the total numbers of exposed and unexposed cases, then the relative risk is simply:

TABLE 5.4: *Doubling the cases in a simple 2-by-2 table of exposure and disease status.*

Original Data

	Case: Yes	Case: No
Exposed	a	b
Unexposed	c	d
		n

Modified Data

	Case: Yes	Case: No
Exposed	a	$b+a$
Unexposed	c	$d+c$
		$n*$

$$RR = \frac{C_1/B_1}{C_0/B_0} \tag{5.6}$$

$$= \frac{C_1/C_0}{B_1/B_0} \tag{5.7}$$

The second expression is the ratio of the odds of exposure in the cases to the odds in the base. These odds can be estimated either from the total cases and the full study base, or selected cases and a selected sample from the base.

5.2.1 Doubling the cases in cohort or cross-sectional data

In an incidence study, all cases that occur during follow-up will have been non-cases at baseline, so that together with the non-cases (at the end of follow-up) they constitute the study base'. Likewise, in a cross-sectional study, the base consists of all the individuals, cases and non-cases, in the population at the time of the survey. Thus, to enable a comparison of cases with the study base, the simple 2-by-2 table could be replaced by a modified table (see Table 5.4) where the cases are counted twice, once as a case and once as a non-case. The odds ratio from the modified table is $\frac{a/(a+b)}{c/(c+d)}$, i.e. the relative risk. But what about the adjusted RR and adjusted OR?

Mantel-Haenszel OR and RR as weighted averages

For a categorical confounder, the Mantel-Haenszel OR and Mantel-Haenszel RR are computed from the 2-by-2 tables in the strata defined by the confounder. For example, for two strata:

Stratum 1

	Case: Yes	Case: No	
Exposed	a_1	b_1	
Unexposed	c_1	d_1	
			n_1

Stratum 2

	Case: Yes	Case: No	
Exposed	a_2	b_2	
Unexposed	c_2	d_2	
			n_2

the Mantel-Haenszel OR and Mantel-Haenszel RR are:

$$OR_{MH} = \frac{\frac{a_1 d_1}{n_1} + \frac{a_2 d_2}{n_2}}{\frac{b_1 c_1}{n_1} + \frac{b_2 c_2}{n_2}} \tag{5.8}$$

$$RR_{MH} = \frac{\frac{a_1(c_1+d_1)}{n_1} + \frac{a_2(c_2+d_2)}{n_2}}{\frac{c_1(a_1+b_1)}{n_1} + \frac{c_2(a_2+b_2)}{n_2}} \tag{5.9}$$

For K strata, these formulae generalise to:

$$OR_{MH} = \frac{\frac{a_1 d_1}{n_1} + \frac{a_2 d_2}{n_2} + \cdots + \frac{a_K d_K}{n_K}}{\frac{b_1 c_1}{n_1} + \frac{b_2 c_2}{n_2} + \cdots + + \frac{b_K c_K}{n_K}} \tag{5.10}$$

or indexing the strata by i:

$$OR_{MH} = \frac{\sum \frac{a_i d_i}{n_i}}{\sum \frac{b_i c_i}{n_i}} \tag{5.11}$$

and similarly:

$$RR_{MH} = \frac{\sum \frac{a_i(c_i+d_i)}{n_i}}{\sum \frac{c_i(a_i+b_i)}{n_i}} \tag{5.12}$$

To see the effect of doubling the cases in each of the strata, it is helpful to recognise that the Mantel-Haenszel OR and Mantel-Haenszel RR are actually weighted averages of the separate ORs and separate RRs in the strata. For the OR_{MH} this can be seen by multiplying and dividing each component of the numerator in equation 5.11 by $c_i b_i$ so that it can be written:

$$OR_{MH} = \frac{\sum \frac{a_i d_i}{c_i b_i} \frac{c_i b_i}{n_i}}{\sum \frac{b_i c_i}{n_i}} \tag{5.13}$$

$$= \frac{\sum \frac{a_i d_i}{c_i b_i} w_i}{\sum w_i} \tag{5.14}$$

$$= \frac{\sum OR_i w_i}{\sum w_i} \tag{5.15}$$

$$\tag{5.16}$$

where $w_i = \frac{b_i c_i}{n_i}$ is the weight for stratum i.

In a similar way, the Mantel-Haenszel RR can be written as a weighted average of the stratum-specific RRs by multiplying and dividing each component of the numerator of Equation 5.12 by $(a_i + b_i)c_i$

$$RR_{MH} = \frac{\sum \frac{a_i(c_i+d_i)}{n_i}}{\sum \frac{c_i(a_i+b_i)}{n_i}} \tag{5.17}$$

$$= \frac{\sum \frac{a_i}{a_i+b_i} \frac{c_i+d_i}{c_i} \frac{(a_i+b_i)c_i}{n_i}}{\sum \frac{c_i(a_i+b_i)}{n_i}} \tag{5.18}$$

$$= \frac{\sum RR_i w_i}{\sum w_i} \tag{5.19}$$

where $w_i = \frac{(a_i+b_i)c_i}{n_i}$ is the weight for stratum i.

5.2.2 Mantel-Haenszel OR after doubling the cases

Returning now to doubling the cases, and writing the modified number of exposed and unexposed controls as B and D (i.e. $B = b + a$ and $D = d + c$), then if the Mantel-Haenszel odds ratio is calculated from these modified data, it will be the weighted average:

$$OR^*_{MH} = \frac{\sum \frac{a_i D_i}{c_i B_i} w_i^*}{\sum w_i^*} \tag{5.20}$$

where w_i^* denotes the weight for the modified table, i.e. $\frac{c_i B_i}{n_i + a_i + c_i}$ since the total number in each table will also have increased by $a_i + c_i$ from doubling the cases. Substituting for w_i^* in Equation 5.20 and replacing B_i by $b_i + a_i$ and D_i by $d_i + c_i$:

$$OR^*_{MH} = \frac{\sum \frac{a_i(d_i+c_i)w_i^*}{c_i(b_i+a_i)}}{\sum w_i^*} \tag{5.21}$$

$$= \frac{\sum RR_i w_i^*}{\sum w_i^*} \tag{5.22}$$

Thus the OR_{MH} calculated from the modified data is a weighted average of the stratum-specific *relative risks*, but the weight for stratum i is $\frac{c_i(b_i+a_i)}{n_i^*}$ which differs from the weight in Equation 5.19 above, i.e. $\frac{c_i(b_i+a_i)}{n_i}$. If the number of cases is small relative to non-cases, then $n_i \approx n_i^*$ and it is clear that the OR_{MH} calculated from the modified data will yield an estimate of the RR_{MH} of the original (unmodified) stratified data. However, this approximation does not only work for samples where cases are few: the net result of reweighting the different RR values with the weights that use n_i^* in place of n_i is close to the RR_{MH} from Equation 5.19. Some examples using the Framingham data will serve as illustration.

For the following stratified data from Table 2.6 in Chapter 2, the Mantel-Haenszel OR and RR are 2.126 and 1.48 respectively. These same results are obtained by calculating the weighted average of the separate ORs or RRs.

Male

	Antibodies Yes	Antibodies No	
Rural	36	14	50
Urban	50	50	100
	86	64	150

OR = 2.57
(wt= 4.67)
RR = 1.44
(wt= 16.67)

Female

	Antibodies Yes	Antibodies No	
Rural	24	126	150
Urban	10	90	100
	34	216	250

OR = 1.71
(wt= 5.04)
RR = 1.6
(wt= 6)

$$OR_{MH} = \frac{2.57 \times 4.67 + 1.71 \times 5.04}{4.67 + 5.04} = 2.126$$

$$RR_{MH} = \frac{1.44 \times 16.67 + 1.6 \times 6}{16.67 + 6} = 1.48$$

Doubling the cases in each table results in ORs of 1.44 and weights of 10.59 and 5.28, and a weighted OR of 1.49. A detailed illustration is provided in Example 5.2 using the data from Example 2.3 in Chapter 2.

Example 5.2. *Estimation of Mantel-Haenszel RR of diabetes associated with CHD in the Framingham data, by doubling the cases.*

Original data from Example 2.3 in Chapter 2:

Age 42–51 (Diabetes)

	Yes	No
Yes CHD	1	32
No CHD	28	1553

OR = 1.73 **(wt=.555)** **RR=1.711** **(wt=.57)**

Age 52–61 (Diabetes)

	Yes	No
Yes CHD	4	74
No CHD	47	1221

OR = 1.404 **(wt=2.58)** **RR=1.384** **(wt=2.72)**

Age 62–71 (Diabetes)

	Yes	No
Yes CHD	7	69
No CHD	29	440

OR = 1.538 **(wt=3.67)** **RR=1.49** **(wt=4.04)**

$$OR_{MH} = \frac{\sum OR_i w_i}{\sum w_i} = 1.504$$

$$RR_{MH} = \frac{\sum OR_i w_i}{\sum w_i} = 1.467$$

Doubling the cases results in the following tables:

Age 42–51 (Diabetes)

	Yes	No
Yes CHD	1	33
No CHD	28	1581

OR = 1.711 **(wt=.555)**

Age 52–61 (Diabetes)

	Yes	No
Yes CHD	4	78
No CHD	47	1268

OR = 1.384 **(wt=2.624)**

Age 62–71 (Diabetes)

	Yes	No
Yes CHD	7	76
No CHD	29	469

OR = 1.490 **(wt=3.793)**

from which the weighted average of the three ORs is:

$$OR^d_{MH} = \frac{\sum OR_i w_i}{\sum w_i} = 1.467 = RR_{MH}$$

5.2.3 Adjusted RR from logistic regression

The examples above illustrate that the Mantel-Haenszel OR calculated by doubling the cases is similar to the adjusted RR calculated from the same cohort or cross-sectional data. In fact, if the probability of disease in the population is described by a relative risk model (and not a logistic model), a logistic regression analysis of the modified data provides an unbiased estimate of the adjusted RR in a cohort. This was illustrated in a simulation study [109], where it was also shown that the naive standard error obtained from the logistic regression was reasonable only for low prevalence (up to 10% for a modest RR (1.5) and up to 15% for a larger RR (2.5). Otherwise the naive standard error is too large, which is unsurprising, since the doubled cases, with one record in the modified dataset having outcome $Y_{mod} = 1$ and the other $Y_{mod} = 0$, has increased the uncertainty compared to the original cohort data. An alternative corrected standard error that reflects the duplication in the data can be calculated from the logistic regression output but is not automatically provided by standard statistical software.

The somewhat surprising ability of the logistic regression model to estimate the adjusted RR can be understood theoretically from considering a cohort where the underlying risk follows a relative risk (not logistic) model. If the binary outcome Y in the underlying cohort follows a relative risk model, then the probability of the outcome for an individual will be the following function of their exposure X

$$P[Y = 1|X] = e^{\alpha+\beta X} \quad . \tag{5.23}$$

and e^{β} is the RR associated with exposure, i.e. the RR in exposed versus unexposed for a binary indicator of exposure, and the RR per unit of exposure for a numerical measure. Denoting the total number of individuals in the cohort as N and the total number of cases as N_1, then doubling the cases results in a dataset with an additional N_1 records, one for each case, where their outcome has been modified to $Y_{mod} = 0$. All other records in the modified dataset have their original outcome value, $Y_{mod} = Y$ (see Figure 5.1).

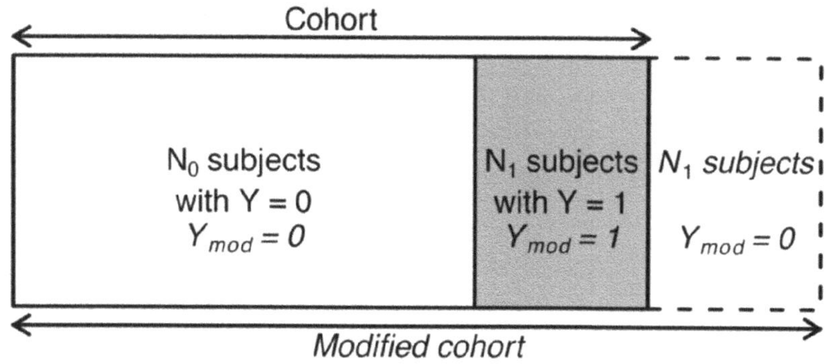

FIGURE 5.1: *Visualisation of a cohort of N_1 cases and N_0 non-cases, where the cases have been 'doubled'.*

The probability that an individual in this dataset has $Y_{mod} = 1$ is the proportion of records with $Y_{mod} = 1$:

$$P[Y_{mod} = 1] = \frac{N_1}{N_1 + N_0 + N_1} \tag{5.24}$$

$$= \frac{N_1}{N + N_1} \tag{5.25}$$

where N is the total size of the original cohort. Dividing numerator and denominator by N enables this probability to be written in terms of the probability of the original outcome in the cohort:

$$P[Y_{mod} = 1] = \frac{P[Y = 1]}{1 + P[Y = 1]} \tag{5.26}$$

For a binary exposure, the total number of exposed and unexposed individuals in the original cohort can be denoted by N_e and $N_{\bar{e}}$ respectively, so that if the risk of the outcome follows the relative risk model in Equation 5.23, the numbers of cases and non-cases arising in the exposed and unexposed members of the cohort will be described by the 2-by-2 table on the left in Figure 5.2.

(a) Original Cohort

	Y=1	Y=0
X=1	$N_e e^{\alpha+\beta}$	$N_e(1-e^{\alpha+\beta})$
X=0	$N_{\bar{e}} e^{\alpha}$	$N_{\bar{e}}(1-e^{\alpha})$

(b) Modified Cohort

	$Y_{mod}=1$	$Y_{mod}=0$
X=1	$N_e e^{\alpha+\beta}$	$N_e(1-e^{\alpha+\beta})+N_e e^{\alpha+\beta}$
X=0	$N_{\bar{e}} e^{\alpha}$	$N_{\bar{e}}(1-e^{\alpha})+N_{\bar{e}} e^{\alpha}$

FIGURE 5.2: *Relationship between (a) an original cohort and (b) 'cohort' obtained by doubling the cases, where the outcome is described by the relative risk model in Equation 5.23.*

The probability that $Y_{mod} = 1$ *in the modified dataset* for an exposed and unexposed individual is:

$$\text{exposed: } P[Y_{mod}=1|X=1] = \frac{N_e e^{\alpha+\beta}}{N_e + N_e e^{\alpha+\beta}} \tag{5.27}$$

$$= \frac{e^{\alpha+\beta}}{1+e^{\alpha+\beta}} \tag{5.28}$$

$$\text{unexposed: } P[Y_{mod}=1|X=0] = \frac{N_{\bar{e}} e^{\alpha}}{N_{\bar{e}} + N_{\bar{e}} e^{\alpha}} \tag{5.29}$$

$$= \frac{e^{\alpha}}{1+e^{\alpha}} \tag{5.30}$$

which is the familiar logistic regression model with $OR = e^{\beta}$ for exposed versus unexposed. For a categorical exposure with more than two levels, the probability that an individual with exposure level j in the modified dataset has $Y_{mod} = 1$ is:

$$P[Y_{mod}=1|X=j] = \frac{N_j e^{\alpha+\beta_j}}{N_j + N_j e^{\alpha+\beta_j}}$$

$$= \frac{e^{\alpha+\beta_j}}{1+e^{\alpha+\beta_j}} \tag{5.31}$$

and for a continuous X

$$P[Y_{mod}=1|X] = \frac{e^{\alpha+\beta X}}{1+e^{\alpha+\beta X}} \tag{5.32}$$

Thus when the outcome in the cohort is described by a relative risk model, doubling the cases results in a modified cohort where the probability that an individual with exposure value X has $Y_{mod} = 1$ is a logistic function whose ln(OR) parameter is the RR in the original cohort. As a result, the OR from logistic regression analysis of the modified cohort estimates the RR of interest.

Illustrative example (cross-sectional data)

Using data from a study of occupational exposure to cadmium and high levels of cadmium in the blood, an article titled A Practical Guide for Multivariate Analysis of Dichotomous Outcomes' [119] presented estimates of RR from several models for the association between a binary outcome and a three-level exposure variable, adjusted for age and sex. The odds ratios from a logistic regression were included to demonstrate that the OR cannot be interpreted as a RR in this example, which is not surprising as the outcome was not rare (prevalence 48.4%). We use these data to illustrate that by doubling the cases in the dataset, a simple logistic regression can provide an estimate of the RR comparable with other less familiar methods.

The data were collected in a cross-sectional survey from 124 workers who were occupationally exposed to cadmium. The duration of exposure is grouped into 3 categories: ≤ 1 year, 1 to 8 years, and > 8 years. The outcome, blood cadmium level, is dichotomised, with levels above 5 $\mu g/L$ being defined as elevated and lower levels as normal. The results from the logistic regression analysis after doubling the cases are presented in Table 5.5, where they are compared with the reported results from analysis of the unmodified data using logistic regression and Poisson regression. The estimates of RR and the 95% CIs from the doubling of cases are similar to those from the Poisson regression, the approach recommended by the authors of the paper. The confidence intervals obtained by using the naive logistic regression of the modified data are included in italics underneath the corrected confidence intervals, where it can be seen that they are much too wide.

Estimating RR from case-cohort data

The RR in an underlying cohort can be estimated from a case-cohort sample by doubling the cases [192]. The probability that an exposed individual *in the modified dataset* has $Y_{mod} = 1$ is now given by Equation 5.34, since now only a fraction f of the cohort has been selected into the sample as the subcohort.

$$P[Y_{mod}=1] = \frac{N_e e^{\alpha+\beta X}}{fN_e + N_e e^{\alpha+\beta X}} \quad (5.33)$$

$$= \frac{e^{\alpha+\beta X}}{f + e^{\alpha+\beta X}} \quad (5.34)$$

This can be rewritten as:

$$P[Y_{mod}=1] = \frac{e^{\alpha^*+\beta X}}{1 + e^{\alpha^*+\beta X}} \quad (5.35)$$

where $\alpha^* = \alpha - ln(f)$. Again, this is a logistic function of the exposure X, so that an estimate of the coefficient β can be obtained from a logistic regression analysis of the modified data. However, the intercept α^* now depends on the sampling fraction used for the subcohort, so that this needs to be taken into account if an estimate of the prevalence in the unexposed population, α, is required. This is the exact parallel of the logistic regression analysis of a simple case-control sample selected from a

TABLE 5.5: *Estimates of relative risk (with 95% confidence intervals) of elevated blood cadmium levels associated with duration of exposure, from 'doubling the cases' compared with other approaches.*

Duration (years)	Naive Logistic	Poisson regression	Doubling of cases*
Crude			
1 to <=8	5.51 (2.20, 13.82)	2.96 (1.53, 5.74)	2.96 (1.53, 5.74) *(1.25, 7.84)*
>8	24.08 (5.65, 102.57)	4.46 (2.33, 8.55)	4.46 (2.33, 8.55) *(1.65,12.07)*
Adjusted			
1 to <=8	6.55 (2.31, 18.59)	3.16 (1.60, 6.22)	3.13 (1.59, 6.19) *(1.25, 7.84)*
>8	23.76 (5.47, 121.46)	4.54 (2.33, 8.86)	4.53 (2.30, 8.89) *(1.57, 13.07)*

* *Naive confidence intervals in italics*

cohort (see Chapter 2), where the OR can be estimated but the intercept has been altered by the sampling.

5.2.4 Estimating RR from case-control ddata

In a case-control design, a random sample of cases is compared to a random sample of controls, often within strata defined by potential confounders. Considering the simplest case-control design, where all cases in a cohort are compared to a simple random sample of controls, it is clear that such data enables the estimation of the probability of exposure in a case (or in a control) but not the probability of the outcome in the exposed (or unexposed) persons in the cohort, as the exposed and unexposed groups have not been randomly sampled. As a result of the sampling design, the cases in the sample cannot be described in terms of the probability of $Y = 1$ in an exposed or unexposed person (which is needed for the relative risk model as in the previous section) but only in terms of the odds of $Y = 1$. For this reason, it is standard practice to use logistic regression to analyse case-control data and to report odds ratios.

However, we have seen in Chapter 3 that if the fraction of non-cases sampled as controls in a case-control study is known, a weighted analysis provides estimates of the population parameters. By weighting each control by the inverse probability that they were sampled, the data is effectively 'inflated' to represent all controls, and so it 'reconstructs' the whole cohort to provide unbiased estimates. This simple realisation is key to enabling the RR to be estimated from case-control data. Since the doubling-of-cases approach uses the standard logistic regression model, then provided the basic cohort information is available to enable the sampling weights to be computed, a weighted logistic regression of the modified data will provide an unbiased estimate of the RR in the cohort. The weight associated with each record in the modified data is the appropriate weight for the original case-control data: true controls ($Y = 0$ and $Y_{mod} = 0$) have a weight equal to the inverse of their sampling fraction, and both records created from a case ($Y = 1$), one with $Y_{mod} = 1$ and one with $Y_{mod} = 0$, have weight 1. The robust standard error obtained from the weighted logistic regression is too large but a corrected SE can be computed in a similar way to previously, using the residuals from the regression. These residuals must now be weighted to account for the doubled records.

Illustration (case-control data)

The feasibility of estimating a RR from case-control data by doubling the cases will be illustrated using data from a population-based study of hemolytic and non-haemolytic neonatal jaundice [118]. This illustration will focus on haemolytic jaundice, which accounts for 86% of the cases, and so will exclude alloimmunised pregnancies and pregnancies where the mother had a transfusion. Risk factors of interest are prematurity and obesity and the analysis is restricted to deliveries from 1992, when BMI information became available. The overall rate of jaundice among the neonates was 3.9%, with a crude RR of 16.5 and crude OR of 27.8 for those born preterm. Table 5.6 presents the adjusted RR from analysis of the full cohort and from a 1:2 case-control sample using the 'double-the-cases' approach. The case-control sample consisted of all 21,997 cases and a random sample of 43,994 from a total of 538,469 infants, so the weighted logistic regression following the doubling of the cases assigned a weight of 1 to all cases and a weight of $548469/43994 \approx 12.2$ to each control.

The OR estimates from standard (naive) logistic regression of the case-control data, which are provided for comparison in Table 5.6, are

TABLE 5.6: *Estimated adjusted RRs from doubling the cases for the analysis of association between preterm delivery and neonatal jaundice in a population-based cohort and in a case-control sample. Adjusted ORs from standard logistic regression are included for comparison. In addition to adjustment for all factors shown, estimates are adjusted for maternal age and smoking status.*

	Double the Cases		Logistic
	Cohort	Case-control	Case-control
	RR (95% C.I.)	RR (95% C.I.)	OR (95% C.I.)
Preterm	15.5 (15.1,15.9)	15.4 (14.7,16.1)	26.5 (24.6,28.5)
BMI <18.5	1.03 (0.96,1.12)	1.18 (1.06,1.31)	1.22 (1.07,1.4)
BMI 22.5-30	1.19 (1.16,1.23)	1.19 (1.14,1.25)	1.22 (1.15,1.29)
BMI $\geq$ 30	1.44 (1.38,1.50)	1.41 (1.33,1.5)	1.47 (1.36,1.59)
Multiparious	0.58 (0.56,0.60)	0.59 (0.57,0.61)	0.55 (0.53,0.58)
Female infant	0.80 (0.78,0.82)	0.8 (0.77,0.83))	0.78 (0.74,0.82)

similar to those from the whole cohort in the published paper [118], and the very large association with preterm delivery is well known. Similar estimates of adjusted RRs are obtained from doubling the cases in the whole cohort or in the case-control sample: the RR for preterm delivery is approximately 15.5 from both analyses, with slightly wider confidence intervals from the case-control data as expected (Table 5.6). It is clear that interpretation of the odds ratio from the standard logistic regression analysis as an approximate 27-fold increase in risk would be inappropriate, as this is almost twice the underlying adjusted relative risk. An inspection of the predicted values from the two logistic models (i.e. with and without doubling the cases) indicated a similar fit in the analyses, so it is reasonable to assume an underlying RR model.

Matched case-control data

Where controls are matched to cases on one or more confounders, the double-the-cases approach also provides valid adjusted RRs, provided each control is weighted to reflect the appropriate sampling fraction, i.e. the proportion of controls selected *in the same stratum*. The neonatal jaundice analysis above was repeated for a 1:2 matched case-control sample, where controls were matched to cases on two binary variables, sex of infant and advanced maternal age ($\geq$ 35 years). These two factors define four strata in the study population, so that each control is assigned one of four weights depending on the stratum to which they belong. The results from analysis of these data using a naive logistic regression and the double-the-cases approach are presented in Table 5.7. The estimates are very similar to those from the simple case-control sample, and again the naive logistic regression provides OR estimates close to those from the whole cohort. After doubling the cases, the weighted logistic regression provided adjusted RR estimates close to the cohort values reported in Table 5.6.

5.3 Risk of Transient Effects Using a 'Quasi-Cohort'

The quasi-cohort design was proposed as an efficient method for estimating the risk, relative risk and risk difference of acute and transient events in pharmacoepidemiology, such as adverse events from long-term medications [208]. The design assumes that data are systematically gathered

TABLE 5.7: *Adjusted OR from naive logistic regression and adjusted RR from doubling of cases, using 1:2 case-control sample, matched on sex of infant and advanced maternal age (dichotomised at 35).*

Variables	Naive logistic OR (95% CI)	Doubling of cases RR (95% CI)
Preterm	26.36 (24.5, 28.36)	15.64 (14.94, 16.36)
BMI $<$18.5	1 (0.86, 1.16)	1.02 (0.91, 1.14)
BMI 25–30	1.21 (1.14, 1.28)	1.18 (1.13, 1.24)
BMI $\geq$30	1.54 (1.42, 1.66)	1.46 (1.37, 1.55)
Multiparious	0.55 (0.53, 0.58)	0.59 (0.57, 0.61)

for the exposure and outcome of interest, as is commonly done in the large healthcare databases that are routinely used for monitoring the effects of many drugs. The idea is similar to a nested case-control design in that all cases are selected and only a random sample of non-cases, but with an important difference: the selected records for analysis are not individuals but 'person-moments' and the exposure is ascertained at, or shortly before, the person moment. The actual time duration of the person moment, and of the exposure period, will depend on the acute nature of the outcome and knowledge or biological hypotheses about how it may be triggered by the exposure. For the purposes of explanation, it will be assumed in the following that person days are the meaningful unit and that an exposure effect will be detected on the same day. The **quasi-cohort** *consists of all the person days contributed by the follow-up of the individuals in the cohort* and it is helpful to imagine the cohort data expanded to have one record per person per day, with each of these days classified as exposed or unexposed.

The quasi-cohort design involves selecting all 'event days' (person days when events occurred) from the quasi-cohort together with a random sample of person days from the quasi-cohort. This random sample can be selected by simple random sampling or by incidence density sampling based on the known event times. Nested case-control studies actually sample the person moment of each selected case (i.e., the time of their event, such as a diagnosis) and the corresponding person moment of their time-matched control (the moment that their matched case was diagnosed). These cases and controls are then compared for their exposure at the time of selection or in some time window before. While the OR from the time-matched analysis (i.e. conditional logistic regression) estimates the rate ratio, it does not provide estimates of the separate rates in unexposed and exposed individuals, nor the ability to estimate risk difference or absolute (cumulative) risk. As a result, the descriptive analysis is presented as a comparison of cases versus controls, rather than the more meaningful comparison of exposed versus unexposed. To borrow the subtitle from the original paper [208], these various shortcomings can be overcome by 'upgrading the nested case-control study' using the quasi-cohort design. The idea is very simple: the random sample of person days from the quasi-cohort are 'upweighted' to represent the total person days. The recovery of the full person-time experience of the cohort enables the estimation of risks in exposed and unexposed individuals.

The first two columns of Table 5.8 describe a cohort of individuals whose total follow-up time is N person-days, $N_{\bar{e}}$ of which are unexposed days and N_e are exposed. The total number of days when events occurred is x, with $x_{\bar{e}}$ of these events on unexposed days and x_e on exposed days. Thus the event rates in the cohort are $\frac{x_{\bar{e}}}{N_{\bar{e}}}$ for the unexposed days and $\frac{x_e}{N_e}$ for exposed (second last column of Table). To study these risks using a quasi-cohort design would involve choosing all the x event days and a sample of quasi person-days from the full quasi-cohort. As with case-control studies, this sample will usually be chosen to be equal to (a factor times) the number of cases. In Table 5.8, the size of the quasi-cohort sample is denoted by small n to distinguish it from the total size of the quasi-cohort, N. Once the quasi person-days are selected, they can be classified as unexposed $n_{\bar{e}}$ or exposed $n_{\bar{e}}$ (column 3 of the table). Since the sampling fraction of the quasi person-days is $f = n/N$, then the total number of unexposed and exposed person days in the cohort are found by simply multiplying the quasi person-days by a weight that is the inverse of the sampling fraction $w = \frac{1}{f} = \frac{N}{n}$ (last column of the table). With these denominators, the rate of events in the unexposed and exposed can be calculated, and thus the rate ratio or rate difference.

In the published paper proposing the quasi-cohort design [208], the author presents an example of the risk of pneumonia following inhaled corticosteroids using a large cohort of Canadian patients with COPD. The cohort of 163,514 patients contributed 304,646,593 person-days of follow-up and there were 20,344 patients hospitalised with pneumonia. These event days are classified by exposure status in the second column of Table 5.9. For the design in the top panel of the Table, an equal number

TABLE 5.8: *Outline of the quasi-cohort calculations that yield the event rates for unexposed and exposed person-days (p.days) in the cohort.*

	Full Cohort		Quasi	Event Rate	
	p.days	event days	p.days	Cohort	Quasi
Unexposed	$N_{\bar{e}}$	$x_{\bar{e}}$	$n_{\bar{e}}$	$\frac{x_{\bar{e}}}{N_{\bar{e}}}$	$\frac{x_{\bar{e}}}{n_{\bar{e}}.w}$
Exposed	N_e	x_e	n_e	$\frac{x_e}{N_e}$	$\frac{x_e}{n_e.w}$
Total	N	x	n		

$w = N/n$

TABLE 5.9: *Rates of serious pneumonia in COPD patients (events per 100,000 person days) following use of corticosteroids (from [208]).*

1-fold Quasi-cohort	p.days*	event days	Rate (per 100,000 p.days)
Unexposed	12201	9453	9453/(12201*w1) = 5.17
Current	4559	7636	7636/(4559*w1) = 11.18
Discontinued	3584	3255	3255/(3584*w1) = 6.06
4-fold quasi-cohort			
Unexposed	49267	9453	9453/(49267*w4) = 5.12
Current	18062	7636	7636/(18062*w4) = 11.28
Discontinued	14027	3255	3255/(14027*w4) = 6.19

* p.days = person days

$w1 = 14975$ for 1-fold
$w4 = 3744$ for 4-fold

of person days was selected from the quasi-cohort of size 304,646,593 (i.e. sampling fraction = .0006677, weight $w = 14975$) and classified by exposure status, while the design in the lower panel selected $4 \times 20,344$ person days, so that the sampling fraction is 4 times smaller and the weight is now 3744. Following Table 5.8, the event rates can be calculated and these are presented as events per 100,000 person days in the final column of Table 5.9. The small differences in the estimates from the two designs are due to the random sampling and will have somewhat more variability for the smaller sample.

From the crude rates estimated from the quasi-cohort as illustrated above, a rate differences can be readily computed and a confidence interval obtained using the usual method for a difference in proportions. The adjusted estimate of rate difference (RD) can be obtained by first conducting a logistic regression analysis of the quasi-cohort sample, and then using the adjusted OR as an estimate of the adjusted RR in Equation 5.36 which relates RD to RR.

$$RD = R_t(RR - 1)/(P_0 + P_1 RR) \tag{5.36}$$

where P_0 and P_1 are the prevalence of unexposed and exposed person-days in the selected quasi-cohort sample and R_t is the overall rate of the outcome in the full cohort, i.e. the number of events divided by the total person time. Where interest is focused on the rate difference between two levels of an exposure that has at least three categories, Equation 5.36 can be generalised, or the quasi-cohort data analysed using a suitable statistical model [208].

5.4 Modelling Complex Exposure measurements

There are many important exposures in epidemiology that cannot be represented by one of the simple types of variables that have been presented so far. A full description of the nature and extent of an exposure may involves several characteristics, such as dose, duration and recency. For example, researchers interested in the effects of smoking on health will typically gather information on current status (non-smoker, current smoker, ex-smoker), time since quitting for ex-smokers and the number of cigarettes smoked per day for smokers (and perhaps ex-smokers). Since these characteristics are correlated, their joint investigation in a logistic or Cox regression requires careful attention to how they are coded and modelled to ensure that the different effects can be estimated and interpreted. For example, even if we can fit a logistic model including a simple binary variable X_1 for ever/never smoker and a continuous variable X_2 for number of cigarettes per day, then the coefficient of X_2 does *not* provide an adjusted OR, nor does such adjusted OR (the common OR per cigarette in smokers and non-smokers!) make any sense. This problem would not arise if X_2 was a different exposure (e.g. daily alcohol intake), as then the effect of alcohol adjusted for smoking refers to the common effect of alcohol intake in smokers and non-smokers, which is reasonable and interpretable provided there is no evidence of effect modification.

Other examples of exposures that have more than one characteristic of interest are alcohol consumption, use of hormone replacement therapy (HRT), and reproductive history (including parity, age at first or last delivery, as well as other factors). In all these examples, use of the unexposed group as a reference category will lead to the same inconsistencies as in the smoking example above. Although this problem was presented in detail in 1999 [144] with suggestions for how to model and interpret the effects of such exposures, applications in the epidemiological and medical literature continue to use simplified measures of exposure to circumvent the pitfalls in interpretation. In the following subsections, we will summarise the details from the 1999 paper, explaining what can and cannot be estimated, and presenting exposure coding that leads to interpretations of interest. For the purpose of these explanations, it will be assumed that the exposure has the following three characteristics mentioned above for smoking: a binary indicator for ever/never exposed, and numerical variables for dose and duration, both of which are to be categorised. A real example will be presented from reproductive epidemiology, where several aspects of preterm history were of joint interest as risk factors for an adverse pregnancy outcome.

5.4.1 Estimating several aspects of the same exposure

For the purpose of illustration, we will consider an exposure for which three characteristics are of interest: a binary indicator of any exposure during a specified time, a variable classifying the level of intensity of the exposure into four categories (none, low, medium, high) and a variable classifying the duration of exposure into four categories (zero, short, moderate, long). The level of intensity classified as low, medium and high will depend on the nature of the exposure. Whether a duration is considered short or long will also depend on knowledge about the potential harm of the exposure and on the time-span for which the history is recorded. We will assume this exposure information is to be gathered for cases that occur in a cohort and for some or all of the non-cases at the end of follow-up, and that a logistic regression model is used to estimate the effects. As seen in Chapter 2, the selection of a sub-sample of exclusive controls will provide valid OR estimates for exposure effects, as the sampling only affects the intercept in the logistic model.

Table 5.10 shows the different strata defined by the three exposure variables. The unexposed group are marked as 'Ref' as this would usually be the choice of reference group, but we will shortly see that this is problematic in the setting where multiple characteristics of exposure are of interest. The strata marked with 'x' in the table are those for which no data are available: for example, there can be no unexposed individuals (those with level of exposure 'none') who have short, moderate or long duration of exposure, and equivalently, the individuals with zero duration of exposure cannot have a low, medium, or high level of exposure.

As already mentioned, the unexposed individuals, marked 'Ref' in the table, would seem to be the obvious reference group to which the other categories should be compared using adjusted odds ratios. However, keeping in mind that an adjusted odds ratio is the common odds ratio associated with a variable *for each combination of the other variables*, it is clear that we cannot estimate the (common) effect of any of the levels of exposure (vs. none) for the different duration values, since there are no unexposed individuals in any of the duration categories. Likewise, the odds ratio associated with any duration of exposure (vs. 0) cannot be estimated for any of the low, medium or high levels of exposure. In either case, an attempt to tabulate the three stratum-specific tables to compute a Mantel-Haenszel estimate would result in tables with empty cells. This logical problem arises from attempting to consider the unexposed individuals as the reference group. Overcoming this problem involves alternative coding that allows logical comparisons to be made between groups of interest.

TABLE 5.10: *Illustration of strata defined by three exposure variables: any/none, level of exposure and duration, with X indicating categories that cannot be observed.*

Duration of Exposure	**Level of Exposure**			
	none	**low**	**medium**	**high**
0	Ref	x	x	x
short	x			
moderate	x			
long	x			

5.4.2 Recoding the different measures of exposure

In addition to the indicator variable, X_E, for any exposure, two other variables, X_L and X_D, can be created to represent the same information as in the three levels of exposure and three duration categories:

$$X_E = \begin{array}{ll} 0 & \text{not exposed} \\ 1 & \text{exposed} \end{array}$$

$$X_L = \begin{array}{ll} 0 & \text{no exposure or low level} \\ 1 & \text{medium level of exposure} \\ 2 & \text{high level of exposure} \end{array}$$

$$X_D = \begin{array}{ll} 0 & \text{no exposure or short duration} \\ 1 & \text{moderate duration of exposure} \\ 2 & \text{long duration of exposure} \end{array}$$

Any cell in Table 5.10 can be represented by a combination of these variables. For a model with no interactions between the X_D and X_L variables (i.e. assuming a common effect of exposure level for each duration, and a common effect of duration at each exposure level), the ln(odds) of the outcome could be modelled as a simple linear function of the X variables as in Chapter 2. Since the variables X_D and X_L are categorical, the values 1 and 2 would be represented by binary dummy variables (either explicitly by the data analyst or implicitly by the software), so the logistic model can be written:

$$ln(odds) = \alpha + \beta_E X_E + \beta_{L1} X_{L1} + \beta_{L2} X_{L2} + \beta_{D1} X_{D1} + \beta_{D2} X_{D2} \quad (5.37)$$

where the variables are coded as follows:

		Code=1	Code=0
Level:	X_{L1}	medium	otherwise
	X_{L2}	high	otherwise
Duration:	X_{D1}	moderate	otherwise
	X_{D2}	long	otherwise

Although the variable X_E is a binary indicator for any exposure, its coefficient β_E is *not* the ln(OR) for exposure, as the unexposed individuals are also represented by the variables X_{L1}, X_{L2}, X_{D1} and X_{D2}. Using Equation 5.37 above, the ln(odds) for each combination of the exposure characteristics is given by the expressions in Table 5.11 and the estimates of the various β parameters from the logistic regression can be used to obtain the odds ratios of interest. Note that the OR of the outcome for low level and short duration of exposure compared to no exposure is:

$$OR = \frac{e^{\alpha+\beta_E}}{e^{\alpha}} = e^{\beta_E}$$

so the coefficient β_E does not represent the odds ratio for any exposure versus none, but for the least exposed category (low level, short duration) versus none.

The other β estimates provide the odds ratios for the effect of exposure level (within each duration stratum) and effect of duration (within each exposure level), i.e. the adjusted effects of exposure level and duration. For example, among individuals with a specific level, the odds ratio for moderate duration compared to short duration is:

$$OR = \frac{e^{\alpha+\beta_E+\beta_{D1}}}{e^{\alpha+\beta_E}} = e^{\beta_{D1}}$$

and the odds ratio for long duration compared to short duration is $e^{\beta_{D2}}$. Likewise, for individuals with a specific duration, the odds ratios for medium and high levels of exposure compared to low level are $e^{\beta_{L1}}$ and $e^{\beta_{L2}}$ respectively. Other odds ratios of interest can be obtained from sums or differences of parameter estimates: for example, the OR for a comparison of long versus moderate exposure is $e^{\beta_{D2}-\beta_{D1}}$ and a comparison of

TABLE 5.11: *Coefficients in logistic model (Equation 5.37) for each combination of exposure characteristics.*

Exposure	**Exposure Level**			
Duration	**none**	**low**	**medium**	**high**
0	α			
short		$\alpha + \beta_E$	$\alpha + \beta_E + \beta_{L1}$	$\alpha + \beta_E + \beta_{L2}$
mod		$\alpha + \beta_E + \beta_{D1}$	$\alpha + \beta_E + \beta_{D1} + \beta_{L1}$	$\alpha + \beta_E + \beta_{D1} + \beta_{L2}$
long		$\alpha + \beta_E + \beta_{D2}$	$\alpha + \beta_E + \beta_{D2} + \beta_{L1}$	$\alpha + \beta_E + \beta_{D2} + \beta_{L2}$

high versus medium level of exposure is $e^{\beta_{L2}-\beta_{L1}}$. A comparison of any group, except the low level short duration, to the unexposed, involves a sum of two or three estimates, and a comparison of any group to those with minimum level and duration involves a sum of two terms.

The presentation above assumes all characteristics of exposure are categorical variables. However, the level of intensity for many exposures is measured by a numerical quantity, such as number of cigarettes per day, radiation dose used for radiotherapy, concentration of coliform in drinking water or of harmful pesticides in vegetables, and many more. Where it is reasonable to assume a trend, the coding and logistic model are simplified, as there is no need to estimate the separate effects of each level of exposure. For example if we replaced the three-category exposure level above by a linear term for the numerical exposure level, the logistic model would contain just a single term for exposure level, $X_L\beta_L$ where X_L is the numerical value of the exposure and e^{β_L} is the OR per unit change in exposure for any duration. As before, we are assuming that a model without interaction terms is appropriate. To test for effect modification, the model would be expanded to contain interaction terms, as in the simpler cases presented in Chapter 2.

5.4.3 Coding interactions

The model presented above assumed that there was no effect modification between X_L and X_D, i.e, that the effect of a medium or high level of exposure was the same regardless of the duration, or vice versa (the duration of an exposure had the same effect for medium and high levels). This is unlikely to reflect the effect of exposures with a cumulative effect, of which there are many. To model a different effect for short and long duration of exposure of a specific level, the most general model for the ln(odds) in Table 5.11 (relative to unexposed) could be constructed using the indicator of any exposure X_E and eight indicator variables, X_{ij} where the suffix i, j denotes duration i and level j (i.e. cell (i, j) of the table. This coding is presented in Table 5.12 and the corresponding logit expressions in Table 5.13.

Any comparisons of interest can be obtained from the estimates of the parameters in Table 5.13 by taking the ratio of the appropriate odds ratios, as explained in the previous section.

TABLE 5.12: *Coding using indicator variables for all combinations of levels and duration versus the reference.*

$X_{01} =$	1	short duration, medium level
	0	otherwise
$X_{02} =$	1	short duration, high level
	0	otherwise,
$X_{10} =$	1	moderate duration, low level
	0	otherwise
$X_{11} =$	1	moderate duration, medium level
	0	otherwise
$X_{12} =$	1	moderate duration, high level
	0	otherwise
$X_{20} =$	1	long duration, low level
	0	otherwise
$X_{21} =$	1	long duration, medium level
	0	otherwise
$X_{22} =$	1	long duration, high level
	0	otherwise

5.4.4 Illustration of analysis of complex exposure

This example investigates different aspects of reproductive history for their contribution to the risk of cervical insufficiency [145]. The analysis

TABLE 5.13: *Most general logit model for each combination of exposure characteristics in Table 5.10 using an indicator for any exposure and eight binary binary variables as defined in Table 5.12.*

Exposure Duration	Exposure Level			
	none	low	medium	high
0	α			
short		$\alpha + \beta_E$	$\alpha + \beta_E + \beta_{01}$	$\alpha + \beta_E + \beta_{02}$
moderate		$\alpha + \beta_E + \beta_{10}$	$\alpha + \beta_E + \beta_{11}$	$\alpha + \beta_E + \beta_{12}$
long		$\alpha + \beta_E + \beta_{20}$	$\alpha + \beta_E + \beta_{21}$	$\alpha + \beta_E + \beta_{22}$

here is based on 29,103 deliveries to multiparous women recorded in the Swedish Medical Register between 1992 and 2012, among which there were 2,662 cases of cervical insufficiency. A history of preterm delivery is a recognised risk factor for this condition, and the purpose of this analysis is to jointly investigate two other aspects of preterm history: two or more previous preterm deliveries and the severity of preterm in the most recent delivery.

Using the approach introduced in the previous sections, the coding in Table 5.14 can be used for an indicator of any exposure, X_E (i.e. any history of preterm delivery), number of previous preterm deliveries, X_N, and number of weeks preterm of the most recent delivery, X_W. The variables X_E and X_N are already binary, and the variable X_W can be written in terms of indicator variables X_{W1} and X_{W2} (for 32–36 weeks and 22–31 weeks gestation in the most recent delivery) so that the logistic model for the probability, p, of the outcome is:

$$logit(p) = \alpha + \beta_E X_E + \beta_{W1} X_{W1} + \beta_{W2} X_{W2} + \beta_N X_N \quad (5.38)$$

and the parameters in Table 5.15 can be estimated.

TABLE 5.14: *Recoding of the 3-category variable for severity of preterm in the most recent delivery, and the 2-category variable for number of preterm deliveries.*

	0	never had a preterm
$X_E =$	1	ever had a preterm
	0	never had a preterm, or most recent delivery not preterm
$X_W =$	1	most recent delivery: 32–36 weeks preterm
	2	most recent delivery: 22–31 weeks preterm
$X_N =$	0	never had a preterm, or had 1 previous preterm
	1	≥2 previous preterms

TABLE 5.15: *Values of logit(p) for model in Equation 5.38.*

No. of weeks preterm	Number of previous preterms		
(most recent delivery)	None	1	2 or more
Never had a preterm	α		
Recent not preterm		$\alpha + \beta_E$	$\alpha + \beta_E + \beta_N$
32–36 weeks preterm		$\alpha + \beta_E + \beta_{W1}$	$\alpha + \beta_E + \beta_N + \beta_{W1}$
22–31 weeks preterm		$\alpha + \beta_E + \beta_{W2}$	$\alpha + \beta_E + \beta_N + \beta_{W2}$

Fitting a logistic model with the variables X_E X_{W1}, X_{W2} and X_N to the Swedish data described above, the following estimates were obtained for the β coefficients (with standard errors in parentheses):

$$\begin{aligned}
\alpha &= -2.48\ (0.03)\\
\beta_E &= \ 0.63\ (0.09)\\
\beta_{W1} &= \ 1.70\ (0.18)\\
\beta_{W2} &= \ 2.36\ (0.29)\\
\beta_N &= \ 1.39\ (0.24)
\end{aligned}$$

The odds of each of the events in Table 5.15 can be expressed in terms of these coefficients, and odds ratios calculated for comparisons of interest. For example, to compare any of the preterm history categories to those with no preterm history, the odds ratios are as in Table 5.16. These results suggest that among women with a history of preterm deliv-

TABLE 5.16: *Contributions of estimated coefficients in Equation 5.38 to the odds in each exposure category compared to the reference odds ($e^{\alpha} = e^{-2.48}$) (upper panel) and corresponding odds ratio estimates (lower panel).*

No. of weeks preterm	Number of previous preterms		
(most recent delivery)	None	1	2 or more
Never had a preterm	Ref*		
Recent not preterm		$e^{0.63}$	$e^{0.63+1.39}$
32–36 weeks preterm		$e^{0.63+1.70}$	$e^{0.63+1.39+1.70}$
22–31 weeks preterm		$e^{0.63+2.36}$	$e^{0.63+1.39+2.36}$

* *Reference group are those with no previous preterm*

ery, those whose preterm was on their most recent delivery are at much higher risk of cervical insufficiency, particularly if the recent delivery was extremely preterm, with odds ratios of $e^{1.7} = 5.5$ and $e^{2.36} = 10.5$, respectively. More specifically, for women with the same number of previous preterm deliveries, the odds of cervical insufficiency is approximately 5-fold higher ($e^{1.7}$) in those whose most recent delivery was 32–36 weeks compared to those whose most recent delivery was not preterm, with an approximate doubling of this OR if the most recent delivery was extremely preterm. The common estimates for the effect of the recent delivery, for mothers who had one or more than one previous preterm, are a consequence of the model in Equation 5.38, which has no interaction between X_W and X_N. This assumption could be tested by fitting a more general model as explained in Section 5.4.3.

5.5 Exercises

1. The dataset `Chapter5_Framingham_exercises.dta` contains the observations used in Example 5.1 of Chapter 5 (4434 records, 4415 with BMI available) for illustrating NNE using risk factors for coronary heart disease (CHD). The available risk factors include:

   bmi3: a three-category variable for BMI: 1 (< 25), 2(>=25 and <=29.9), 3 (30+)

   obese: indicator for BMI >=30

   overwt_obese: indicator for BMI ≥ 25

   age: age in years

   age50plus: indicator for age >=50

   sex: 0=Male 1=Female

   (i) Use these data to obtain the adjusted OR and hence the adjusted NNE for both outcomes in the table in Example 5.1 (all other quantities in the table can be obtained from the 2-by-2 tables). Note that the ORs in the example were adjusted for sex, age (dichotomised at 50 years) and an interaction between these two.

   (ii) Validate that the adjusted ARI (and hence the NNE) in (i) is also obtained from the difference in the average probability of the outcome (predicted by the logistic model) for the exposed and unexposed individuals.

   (iii) Run a logistic regression analysis for CHD in males and find the adjusted NNE from the predicted probabilities and the adjusted OR. Verify that the predicted probabilities for males from the joint model give the same result as the male only model.

   (iv) Alternative approaches to obtaining the adjusted NNE use the logistic model to:

   (a) calculate the average change in risk from adding the exposure to the individuals who were unexposed

   (b) calculate the average change in risk by removing exposure from those who were exposed

Validate that the estimates from (a) and (b) are in good agreement with those from (i).

2. The summary dataset `neonatal_jaundice.dta` contains a summary of the infants analysed in Table 5.6 in Chapter 5, according to the event (diagnosis of jaundice), preterm delivery and a few other variables (mother aged 35 or older, BMI category, multiparity, sex of neonate).

   (i) Expand the data to one record per infant and calculate the crude RR and crude OR for the association between preterm delivery and jaundice.

   (ii) Run a logistic regression to obtain the OR for preterm, adjusted for maternal age, BMI, parity and sex of infant. Verify that your adjusted OR is close to the value reported in Table 5.6.

   (iii) Modify the dataset using the double-the-cases method. Tabulate exposure by outcome in the modified data, compare to the table from the original data and verify this agrees with Table 5.4.

   (iv) Run a logistic regression of the modified data to obtain the adjusted RR for preterm and compare to Table 5.6.

   (v) Select a 1:2 case-control sample from the cohort using simple random sampling of controls (use a random number), and compare the estimates of the adjusted OR from logistic regression and the adjusted RR from weighted logistic regression to the values obtained from the full cohort.

   (vi) Select a 1:2 case-control sample, frequency matched on mother's age and infant sex, by first identifying the number of cases in these four strata and then randomly selecting twice as many controls (using a random number).

   Double the cases and verify that an unweighted logistic regression provides a biased estimate of the adjusted RR, but a weighted logistic regression (weighted by the inverse of the sampling fractions) provides an unbiased estimate.

   (vii) Repeat the selection in part (vi) using a command in your software package for matched case-control sampling. Double the cases and re-run the logistic regression.

(viii) To obtain standard errors for the RR estimates from doubling the cases, further calculations are required. These are automatically provided if the data are analysed in R using the **DoublingOfCases** package available from https://github.com/nyilin/DoublingOfCases. If you have used Stata, comment on whether the invalid variance is too small or too large.

6

Estimates from Matched and Nested Designs

6.1 Matched Designs

In Chapter 2, we have seen examples of how confounding can be controlled at the design stage (by matching) or at the analysis stage (by adjusting). Here, matching will be introduced first for a cohort study setting where it is more easily understood intuitively, although it is more widely used in case-control studies. The purpose of matching on confounders in a cohort study is to ensure a similar distribution of the confounding factors in the exposed and unexposed individuals. If a confounder is very unbalanced, a random (i.e. unmatched) selection of subjects can result in difficulties adjusting for the confounder at the analysis stage due to sparse data in some strata. Selecting reasonable numbers of exposed and unexposed cohort members in the strata defined by the confounder(s) overcomes the imbalance, with the greatest gains in efficiency when the imbalance is large and the matching factor is strongly related to the outcome (i.e. is itself an important risk factor) [110].

There are two ways of drawing a matched sample from a cohort: **frequency matching** where the number of unexposed individuals selected in each stratum is equal to (or a multiple of) the number of exposed; or **individual matching** where one or more unexposed individuals are selected *for each exposed individual* from those that match on one or more characteristics. Where the matching factors define very specific characteristics of the case and their individually-matched control(s), thus representing a very fine stratification of the cohort, it is referred to as **fine matching**. Individual matching where the matching ratio is 1:1 is often referred to as **pair matching**. For a binary outcome, frequency-matched cohort data is analysed using unconditional logistic regression with the matching stratum variable included in the model, together with the exposure and other variables of interest. As with any regression model of data where records with specific values of a predictor variable have been preferentially selected, the effect of the matching factors on the outcome can be validly estimated. For individually-matched data, the effect of exposure on outcome within the matched strata is estimated from a conditional logistic regression model, where each exposed individual is compared to the unexposed subjects in their matched set. Since the model is fit within each stratum, the stratum effects are not estimated, as they are 'matched away'. Thus the matching variables are usually confounders that are not of interest in themselves, but for which the exposure effect needs to be adjusted. The conditional model can include additional terms to adjust for other potential confounders that were not considered in the matching. Matching is particularly useful when we wish to adjust for potential confounders that are difficult to measure, but for which the implementation of matching is straightforward. One of the early reviews of matched cohorts [42] presents a number of such examples from injury research. Other examples are matching on neighbourhood, which controls for a number of socio-economic and life-style factors, or matching on family, such as twin and sibling studies [188], which controls for genetic factors and the family environment. Pair-matching is an appealing method and commonly used, but such fine matching is not always useful. For example, if the categories of the matching variables are wide, such as 10-year age groups, the pairs generated by individual matching are artificial, since any unexposed person of the same age group (of which there will be many) could have been paired with a specific exposed individual. Conditional logistic regression of data with such 'random' matching will be inefficient since it is adjusting for an uninformative factor (the pair membership).

Whether using frequency matching or individual matching, the choice of which variables to consider as matching factors requires careful consideration to avoid **overmatching**. This occurs in a matched cohort when the matched sampling results in the exposed and unexposed persons being more similar with respect to the outcome and is often due to inadvertently including as a matching factor a variable that is a intermediary between exposure and outcome (i.e. a 'mediator'), or a variable that is strongly associated with the outcome but has little or no association with the exposure (i.e. is *not* a confounder). The first of these situations will result in dilution' (i.e. bias) of the estimate of the exposure effect, and the second in a less precise estimate (wider confidence interval). This loss of precision is referred to as lower **efficiency** and is expressed in terms of the relative magnitude of the variance compared to the variance of the reference design (in this case the unmatched sample), i.e.

$$\text{Efficiency} = \frac{\text{Var}(Reference)}{\text{Var}(Design)} \tag{6.1}$$

For example, if the variance from a random sample is twice as large as the variance from the full cohort, the sample has 50% efficiency, which can be understood as the sample extracting only half the information that is in the cohort.

As a general principle, the categories for matching should be based on just a few well-established confounders. Continuous variables (such as age) can be categorised to facilitate the matching: for example, it is very common practice in epidemiology to match on 5-year or 10-year age categories. An alternative is to use **caliper matching** where the unexposed individuals are chosen to be within ±5 or ±10 years of the exposed. A coarse categorisation of an important continuous variable may not completely adjust for its confounding effect, but if such **residual confounding** is suspected, the original continuous variable can included in the unconditional logistic regression model or, in the case of individual matching, added to the conditional logistic model.

6.1.1 Matched case-control studies

Matching is widely used in case-control studies to overcome imbalance in the confounding factors in cases and controls and thus improve efficiency. Unlike the matched cohort design, the matching in a case-control study depends on the outcome (i.e. the case status). However, only the relationship between the outcome and the matching factor is altered, and not the association between the exposure and outcome, which is of primary interest. This is illustrated with fictitious data in Table 6.1, where a random sample results in unbalanced samples in both strata, with 10 times more cases than controls in Stratum 1 and twice as many controls as cases in Stratum 2. The two tables in the bottom row present the numbers of observations that would be expected in each cell if the number of controls chosen in each stratum was equal to the number of cases, i.e. 10 times more controls in Stratum 1 and half as many in Stratum 2. Example 6.1 illustrates this with the Framingham data that was used to demonstrate interaction in Chapter 2 (Example 2.5), where a total of 57 males and 59 females had a diagnosis of diabetes. It is important to note that choosing a balanced sample does not alter the ability to investigate effect modification, and in fact provides more precise estimates of the separate odds ratios than the sparse data from a

TABLE 6.1: *2-by-2 tables of association between an exposure and outcome in two strata, where data are unbalanced (top row) and balanced (bottom row).*

Stratum1 — Case

	Yes	No	
Exposed	50	5	55
Unexposed	50	5	55
	100	10	110

OR = 1

Stratum 2 — Case

	Yes	No	
Exposed	25	20	45
Unexposed	25	80	105
	50	100	150

OR = 4

	Yes	No	
Exposed	50	50	100
Unexposed	50	50	100
	100	100	200

OR = 1

	Yes	No	
Exposed	25	10	35
Unexposed	25	40	65
	50	50	100

OR = 4

Example 6.1. *Balanced case-control sample of males (57 + 57) and females (59 + 59) from data in Example 2.5 (**top row**) and random samples of approximately the same size (**bottom row**). OR (95% C.I.) in bold face under each table.*

Male — Diabetes

	Yes	No	
HTN	25	20	45
No HTN	32	37	69
	57	57	114

1.44(.67, 3.1)

Female — Diabetes

	Yes	No	
HTN	42	22	64
No HTN	17	37	54
	59	59	118

4.1(1.9, 9.1)

	Yes	No	
HTN	2	39	41
No HTN	3	71	74
	5	110	115

1.21(.14, 8.5)

	Yes	No	
HTN	3	43	46
no HTN	2	72	74
	5	115	120

2.5(.36, 22)

very unbalanced sample. The balanced sample provides estimates of the stratum-specific ORs that are closer to the values from the full cohort (1.43 for males, 4.14 for females) than those from the random sample and with much narrower confidence intervals. The balance has also increased the power for detecting effect modification, with the Breslow-Day test of homogeneity having p-value .055 versus p=0.59 in the random sample.

Where there is confounding but no effect modification, a lack of balance can lead to either positive or negative confounding in the crude OR, and where there is no association in the strata (i.e. each stratum-specific OR=1), can result in a spurious association in the combined table. While balancing can help to reduce the bias, it does not completely remove it. In contrast to unbalanced data, which can result in positive or negative bias, the crude OR from a balanced sample will always have negative bias: the OR from the combined balanced data will be on the same side of 1 as the stratum-specific OR, but biased towards 1. This is illustrated in Example 6.2, where the crude OR =5.44 although the OR is 9 in each of the two strata.

Example 6.2. *Example of balanced strata for case control data with negative bias in crude OR.*

	Stratum 1			Stratum 2			Overall		
	Case			**Case**			**Case**		
	Yes	No		Yes	No		Yes	No	
Exposed	50	10	60	90	50	140	140	60	200
Unexposed	50	90	140	10	50	60	60	140	200
	100	100	200	100	100	200	200	200	400
	OR = 9			**OR = 9**			**OR = 5.44**		

As with cohort studies, frequency matching or individual matching can be used in a classical case-control study. One important limitation of a frequency matched case-control study, that is not shared by a matched cohort, is that the associations between the matching factors and disease cannot be estimated from the unconditional logistic regression model, since this relationship is a result of the matching, i.e the effect of those factors on disease has been 'matched away'.

Many applications of the individually matched case-control design use pair-matching, with each pair consisting of one case and one control. Twins discordant for a disease provide a case-control pair that is matched for genetic and environmental effects. Studies of paired organs also offer a 'twin' design that adjusts for the individual's genetic factors and environmental/behavioural effects such as smoking [174]. As for the matched cohort study, pairing on a 'random' factor will result in a loss of efficiency. This loss in efficiency is a simple function of the proportions of cases and controls that are exposed, p_1 and p_0 respectively. With the pooled (i.e. unpaired) design as reference, the efficiency of the randomly-paired design is the ratio of the variances:

$$\frac{p_1 q_1 + p_0 q_0}{p_1 q_0 + p_0 q_1} \tag{6.2}$$

where $q_i = 1 - p_i$, the proportion of cases ($i = 1$) or controls ($i = 0$) that are unexposed. From this it can be shown that when there is no association between exposure and disease (OR=1), there is no loss of efficiency from random pairing. It will be left as an exercise to show that the loss is small in other scenarios, except for extreme values of the OR.

While any number of controls can be selected for each case, the ratio is usually no more than 5:1, as there is little gain in efficiency from sampling more (see the $M/(M+1)$ 'rule of thumb' presented in Section 2.5.6). A nested case-control study is automatically an individually-matched design, since time-matched controls are chosen for each case. In a matched nested case-control study, the controls will also be selected to match their case on one or more confounder variables. This offers the increased efficiency of implementing a study of smaller size, as the HR can be estimated without following up the whole cohort (see Chapter 4). We will see in later chapters that this property of the nested case-control design is especially useful in simplifying the analysis of the effects of time-dependent covariates.

In choosing matching factors, the purpose of the matched design should be kept in mind, i.e. to ensure a reasonable balance of cases and controls in the different confounder strata. The same principles apply as outlined for matched cohorts above: matching should be based on just a few well-established confounders and matching on a variable that is intermediary' between exposure and outcome will lead to bias and should be avoided. Matching cases and controls for a factor that is strongly associated with the exposure but has little or no association with the outcome, will result in overmatching and a loss of efficiency. This can be understood intuitively in the context of paired case-control studies, where it will result in pairs being more likely concordant for exposure, and thus contributing no information to the analysis.

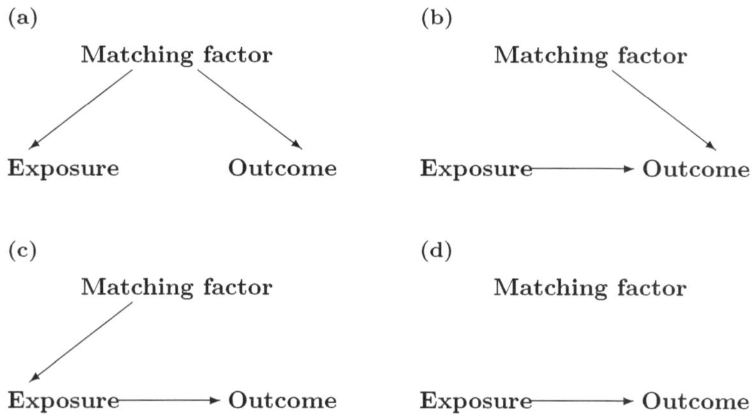

FIGURE 6.1: ***(a)*** *and* ***(c)*** *potentially useful matching factors for cohort studies;* ***(a)*** *and* ***(b)*** *potentially useful matching factors for case-control studies;* ***(b)*** *overmatching for cohort study;* ***(c)*** *overmatching for case-control study;* ***(d)*** *overmatching for both designs.*

Figure 6.1 uses DAGs to illustrate settings that can lead to overmatching in a cohort or case-control study: (a) displays a typical confounder (i.e. a factor associated with the exposure and outcome) that might be matched in a cohort or case-control study; (b) is a potentially useful matching factor in a case-control design but would lead to overmatching in a cohort design, while (c) is potentially useful in a cohort design but would lead to overmatching in a case-control design; factor (d) is not associated with either the exposure or outcome and so would result in overmatching in both designs.

The previous paragraphs have presented the similarities, and some subtle differences, between matching in case-control and cohort studies. A summary comparison is presented in Table 6.2 in the following pages. An essay in the European Journal of Epidemiology from 2018 presents a detailed discussion, with a focus on the misconceptions with regard to matching in case-control studies [141].

TABLE 6.2: *Comparison of matching in cohort and case-control designs.*

	Cohort	Case-control
Purpose	Balance confounders in exposed and unexposed	Balance confounders in cases and controls
Analysis		
Frequency matching	No need for matching strata if underlying continuous variable available	Keep matching factors
Fine Matching	Conditional logistic regression	
Advantages	Efficiency (sample size)	
	Can adjust for confounders that are difficult/impossible to measure: neighbourhood, family, genes (twins)	
	Reduces selection bias where no population register (e.g. geographic region, hospital)	
		Concurrent sampling: clearly defined 'exposure window', e.g. screening studies; biological specimens subject to same storage time and/or measured by same technology
Disadvantages		
Overmatching	Matching factor strongly related to *disease* but not exposure (reduced efficiency)	Matching factor strongly related to *exposure* but not disease (reduced efficiency)
Cost-efficiency	Time and effort to find a match (maybe none), cost and loss of many unsuitable 'candidates'	
Planning		For concurrent sampling, number of controls that will be needed in confounder categories is unpredictable
Choice of matching categories	Wide categories (e.g. of a continuous variable) may not sufficiently adjust for confounding (i.e. 'residual confounding' remains), so a more precise variable needs to be modelled	
	Fine matching can result in failure to find a match; relaxed matching (e.g. wider categories) may result in residual confounding	
Unnecessary matching	Matching on a weak/random factor will result in little or no bias, but loss of efficiency	
'Matched away' effects		Cannot estimate effects of the matching factors

6.2 Ignoring or Breaking the Matching

There is a good deal of confusion surrounding the question of whether and when matching can be ignored or 'broken' at the analysis stage. This is largely due to imprecise vocabulary, where it is often unclear whether it refers to the arrangement of the data, the method of analysis, the model, or some combination of these. Here we will distinguish between:

- Ignoring and breaking the matching,
- Pooled/marginal vs. stratified data
- Conditional vs. unconditional analysis
- Adjusting (or not) for matching variables

In particular, **ignoring the matching** will mean just that: the data are regarded in the same way as if they had arisen without matching, so that the matching variable is irrelevant and could be eliminated from the dataset to be analysed. In contrast, **breaking the matching** will refer to data that were acquired in a matched design and the matching is 'broken' prior to analysis, but the matching factor may play a role in the final analysis. Thus, breaking the matching is the first step in relaxing the constraints of a matched design, while the most crude second step is to completely ignore the matching. For data gathered in a matched design, assuming the primary interest is in estimating an adjusted OR, there are essentially only three approaches to the analysis, ranging from the most correct for the design to the most crude:

- Conduct a conditional/adjusted analysis, such as Mantel-Haenszel estimation or conditional logistic regression, that respects the design through conditioning on the matched sets
- Conduct an unconditional analysis, adjusting for the matching by including the matching variable(s) in the model
- Ignore (completely) the matching: in the simplest case, obtain an overall (crude) OR from a pooled analysis over all strata; where adjustment is to be made for confounders other than the matching factors, these can be included in an unconditional logistic regression

6.2.1 Ignoring the matching in cohort studies

The consequences of matching for the analysis of cohort or case-control data can be different, as already seen in Table 6.2. In particular, for matched case-control data, the matching factors generally cannot be ignored: whether analysis proceeds by conditional or unconditional regression, the matching factors will almost always need to be retained in the analysis. For a matched cohort study, standard epidemiology text books differ regarding whether the matching factor(s) can be ignored in the analysis. While Woodward's simple advice is to always take account of the matching in the analysis [235], several others (summarised in [195]) argue that since matching will result in the ratio of exposed and unexposed subjects in a matched cohort study being the same in all strata defined by the matching variable, this variable is independent of exposure in the matched dataset, and thus cannot be a confounder of the exposure-disease relationship. Except for studies with loss to follow-up or competing risks (where the balance may be disturbed), these authors conclude that the matching factor can be ignored. However, this is only true in the very limited setting where there are no other confounders. Even where another confounder has been measured and included in the analysis, failure to adjust for the matching will result in bias [195]. Conditional analysis automatically adjusts for the matching, but an unconditional analysis will need to include the matching factor. Thus, in one way or another, the simple statement of Woodward holds true as a general principle, that the matching must be accommodated in some way in the analysis.

6.2.2 Unconditional analysis of matched cohort data

A simple and familiar alternative to conditional logistic regression for matched data is to adjust for the matching factors by including them in an unconditional logistic regression model. Such a decision might be motivated by the loss of matched sets in the conditional analysis because they are concordant for the outcome (for example due to overmatching) or concordant on an important (unmatched) confounder that is rare in the population. Another situation where it could be useful to break the matching is where a matching factor was defined by creating categories from a continuous measure (e.g. 10-year age groups from age in years) but where there is evidence that some residual confounding by age after adjustment for the categorical variable. By including the continuous variable in the conditional analysis, adjustment for the residual confounding is achieved by modelling the effect of small increments in age within each age group. However, in many applications, it may be sufficient to fit an overall effect of (continuous) age which can be done in an unconditional analysis that includes this variable. In this case, the crude matching variable (e.g. age group) would not be included in the model but if other matching factors (e.g. sex) were used in the data collection, these must also be included in the unconditional model. A parallel situation arises where the matching was considered unnecessarily fine, such as age-matching within one year of age, while the risk would be expected to be stable over a larger interval. Breaking the matching in this case would allow for adjustment of the continuous age effect or a meaningful stratum effect (e.g. 5-year age groups), which approach could offer a gain in power over the conditional analysis.

6.2.3 Unconditional analysis of matched case-control data

The reasons presented in the previous paragraph for choosing to use an unconditional analysis are not unique to cohort studies, and any of these situations could arise in matched case-control data. However, there is a critical difference between matched case-control data and matched cohort data: the matching in a case-control design depends on the *outcome*. Analysis of matched case-control data using an unconditional logistic regression model with a stratum effect can be prone to bias. The magnitude of the bias depends on the exposure rate in controls, the size of the true odds ratio and the size of the strata. Where there are many small strata, the bias can be serious: in a 1:1 matched design, the estimate of the OR from the unconditional analysis is $(\frac{n_{10}}{n_{01}})^2$ [5] as opposed to the correct estimate from conditional analysis, $\frac{n_{10}}{n_{01}}$, that we saw in Chapter 2, where n_{10} and n_{01} are the numbers of discordant pairs with only the case or only the control exposed, respectively. While the bias is most severe for matched pairs, it is still present for larger sets. Figure 6.2 presents an extract from the numerical example in Breslow and Day's text book ([24], Table 7.1) illustrating the main pattern: a reduction in bias with the number of cases and number of controls per set, and more serious bias for larger odds ratios. The pattern is similar regardless of the prevalence of exposure. The main message is that conditional analysis should be used for matched case-control data, and if there are strong reasons for conducting an unconditional analysis that adjusts for matching strata, the strata should be reasonably large. A simple

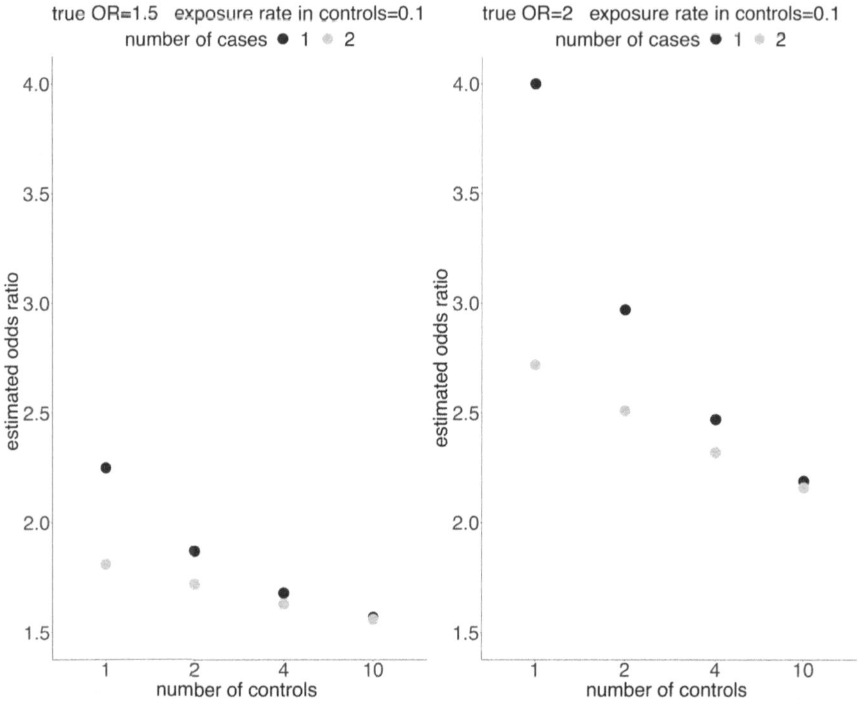

FIGURE 6.2: *Expected value of the estimated OR from unconditional logistic regression analysis of matched case-control data with 1 and 2 cases per set (from [24]).*

precaution against biased results from choosing an unconditional model for its better precision is suggested by Breslow and Day [24]: compare the estimates from the unconditional and conditional analysis, and if the difference in the estimates suggests bias, then report the estimates from the conditional analysis and accept the loss in precision.

6.2.4 Ignoring the matching in case-control analysis

The most crude approach to analysis of matched data is to disregard the matched sets, and in the analysis of the individuals, ignore the matching factors. As for the matched cohort discussed above, this pooled analysis will almost always result in bias. Prior to the adoption of conditional methods of analysis, it was widely accepted that data were only 'poolable' across strata if either of the following conditions held:

1. the stratification variables are conditionally independent of disease given the risk factors
2. the stratification variables are conditionally independent of the risk factors give the disease status

In either of these situations, the pooled and matched analysis yield the same asymptotic results. In matched case-control studies, the design will ensure that the matching variables are uncorrelated with disease in the overall sample, but this does not ensure a lack of correlation for groups defined by the risk factors, so that pooled analysis will often be biased. Similarly, overmatching on a factor that is associated only with exposure and not with disease can induce a bias in the selected data where none was present in the population, so that adjustment becomes necessary, resulting in a potential loss of efficiency. The only situation where there is no bias is where the matching is 'random'. In this setting, which is most unlikely to describe any real investigation, there is some loss of efficiency from breaking the unnecessary matching, but the loss is modest except for rather extreme odds ratios.

Where the matching factor is not random, i.e. it carries some information, the bias in a pooled estimate of the OR tends to be conservative, with the extent of the bias depending on the exposure probabilities of cases and controls in the different strata [7]. The pooled estimate will be unbiased only where there is equal probability of exposure for controls in all strata (the proof of this will be left as an exercise). But as mentioned above, an unconditional analysis of matched data, even if unbiased, can sacrifice efficiency. A pooled OR estimate can be especially biased when the strata are unbalanced, with either a positive or negative bias. Balanced case-control sampling can reduce, but not eliminate, the bias of the pooled estimate, but results in a conservative estimate, as discussed in Section 6.1.1. This is illustrated in Table 6.3, which compares an unbalanced and balanced case-control sample of size 200 in each of three strata. To reflect a situation where the samples are selected from the same underlying cohort, the odds of exposure in the cases and controls in each of the three strata are preserved.

To conclude, although a balanced design will overcome the loss in efficiency due to sparse data, and will mitigate the bias of the pooled OR due to imbalance, the main message remains as stated above: *a matched case-control design should be analysed with a conditional analysis.*

TABLE 6.3: *Unbalanced and balanced case-control samples of size 200 in three strata, with stratum-specific OR of approximately 2.0, illustrating the less biased pooled OR from balanced sampling.*

Unbalanced	Cases		Controls		
Strata	**Exposed**	**Unexposed**	**Exposed**	**Unexposed**	**OR**
1	107	13	64	16	2.06
2	54	26	60	60	2.08
3	49	97	11	43	1.97
All	210	136	135	119	**1.36**
Balanced Strata					
1	89	11	80	20	2.02
2	67	33	50	50	2.03
3	33	67	20	80	1.97
All	189	111	150	150	**1.70**

6.3 Breaking the Time Matching

Unconditional logistic regression analysis is routinely used for frequency-matched case-control data, but as concluded in the previous section, it will generally lead to a loss of efficiency in finely-matched data. However, there are several reasons why one might wish to conduct an unconditional analysis: to obtain estimates of the effects of the matching factors (not available from conditional analysis); to overcome the loss of concordant sets from the conditional analysis; or make use of the controls from the matched set of a case who is missing a variable necessary for analysis. Missing values for a control in a 1:1 case-control study will also result in a case that would be lost from conditional analysis but could be recovered by breaking the matching. The loss of cases from conditional analysis is less likely for 1:m matching, as the set can still be analysed provided at least one control has complete data. In Chapter 3 we saw that a case-control sample can be regarded as the second stage of a two-stage study, where the 'first stage' is the underlying cohort. Where matching has been used in a classic case-control design, the available data is simply a stratified random sample within the strata defined by the outcome and matching factors. Provided these sampling fractions are known or can be estimated, valid estimates of population parameters can be obtained from a weighted analysis where the weights are the inverse of the sampling fractions.

The data collected in a nested case-control study cannot simply be regarded as a finely-matched two-stage design, as now the available controls are individually matched to the cases *on time*, and perhaps other matching factors. But what if the matching is broken? Is there some way to calculate the sampling probabilities for the individuals who were in the case-control sample, so that valid estimates of population parameters can be obtained from an unconditional weighted analysis?

In Chapter 4, we saw that the Cox model estimates the HR for a cohort using a likelihood where the component at each event time is the ratio of the hazard of the case to the total hazard of the individuals in the risk set at that time. This 'full risk set' consists of the case and all non-cases in the cohort at the time of the case's event. However it is not necessary to have all non-cases, as the HR can also be estimated from data sampled in a case-cohort design: at each event time, the total hazard in the full risk set can be estimated from the individuals in the case-cohort sample who are still at risk, by weighting them to represent the background cohort. In contrast, for the nested case-control design, the conditional likelihood compares the hazard of each case to the total hazard in the *sampled* risk set at that event time.

This (conditional) likelihood for nested case-control data differs from the full cohort and case-cohort Cox models (see Table 4.10 in Chapter 4), in that it does not attempt to represent the full risk set in the cohort at each event time, but instead uses a conditional likelihood, with the component at each event time expressing the probability that the event happened to the case individual, given that that one event occurred in the case-control set at that time. However, if the nested case-control data has been sampled from a well-defined cohort, it should be possible to break the matching and use information from the cases and all sampled controls whenever they are at risk to 'reconstruct' the cohort experience as done for the case-cohort design.

If for each individual in a nested case-control dataset, the probability of being selected into the sample during the study period can be calculated/estimated, then the inverse of these probabilites can be used to weight the study subjects to represent the background study base. If all cases in the cohort are selected into the nested case-control study, the weight for cases will be 1, as for the case-cohort design. The probabilities for the non-cases will be more complex than for a case-cohort sample, which is unsurprising when we consider that an individual may be selected as a control for more than one case, and in order to have a non-zero probability of being selected for any specific case, needs to survive free of disease up to that event time. However, the probability of *not being sampled* in the nested case-control study (i.e. not selected as a control at any of the event times) is quite straightforward and can be understood from a simple example. Figure 6.3 presents a toy cohort of just 15 individuals followed from time 0 to 15 years, with 7 cases occurring during that time, for each of whom one control is selected from those available.

The probability the first control was sampled is 1/12 (probability 11/12 of not being sampled), as this individual is only available at the first event time, being censored shortly afterwards. The control who was selected for the second case, at time 5, had the opportunity to be selected at event times 3, 5 and 6. Thus the probability that this individual (number 7) was *not* selected at all into the study, i.e. was not selected at any of the times they were available:

$$P(\text{individual 7 not selected}) = \frac{11}{12} \times \frac{9}{10} \times \frac{8}{9}$$

so that their probability of being selected is 0.266. For the final control (individual 15), the probability of not being selected is the product $(\frac{11}{12})(\frac{9}{10})(\frac{8}{9})(\frac{5}{6})(\frac{4}{5})(\frac{3}{4})(\frac{1}{2})$ as this control had the opportunity to be sampled at every event time in the study. Note that individual 14, who was selected as the control for the second last event has the same weight: although they were actually sampled at $t = 11$, they still had the opportunity to be sampled at $t = 13$.

From this simple example it should be clear that once we can identify the event times when an individual was available to be selected, and the number of control candidates at those times, a simple product provides the probability of not being selected at all into the study, and hence the probability of being selected. Thus for any individual control, their weight can be calculated from the risk set sizes at each event time when they were in follow-up, i.e. the events prior to the control being censored, if individuals enter follow-up at $t = 0$ as in the simple cohort above. Where there is staggered entry, the weight for a specific control is calculated from the risk sets for the events between their entry and exit times.

6.3.1 Kaplan-Meier type weights

In the previous section, we have seen that time plays a key role in the probability that an individual is sampled as a control in a nested case-control study. The probability of being selected as a control for a specific case depends on the number of 'candidate' controls available at that event time, i.e. the number of non-cases in the risk-set. This probability also depends on the number of controls to be matched to each case, which in the simple example above was 1. An individual's overall probability

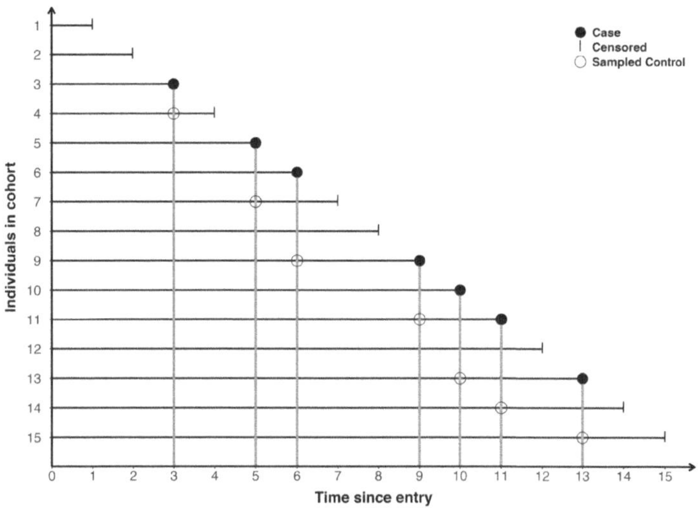

(a) *Illustration of a nested case-control study in a cohort of 15 individuals, with 7 incident cases and one time-matched control per case*

Event Time t	3	5	6	...	13
Probability not selected:					
at time t	$\frac{11}{12}$	$\frac{9}{10}$	$\frac{8}{9}$	...	$\frac{1}{2}$
by time t	$\frac{11}{12}$	$(\frac{11}{12})(\frac{9}{10})$	$(\frac{11}{12})(\frac{9}{10})(\frac{8}{9})$	...	$(\frac{11}{12})(\frac{9}{10})\dots(\frac{1}{2})$

(b) *Probability of not being selected by event time t for controls who are still in follow-up*

FIGURE 6.3: *Line plot of a nested case-control study in a cohort of 15 individuals, illustrating the calculation of the probability of being selected into the study.*

of being selected at some time into the study will depend on the cases that occur during the time period when they are available (i.e. 'at risk'), and they may be selected as a control for more than one case during this period. If the entry and exit times of the control individuals are available, then together with the event times and corresponding risk set sizes, the probability that individual i was not sampled into the study is the product of not being sampled at any of the event times (labelled j):

$$1 - p_i = \prod_j (1 - \frac{m}{R_j - 1}) \quad (6.3)$$

where m is the number of controls per case, R_j denotes the full risk set (including the case) at the time of event j and the product is taken over all events j that occurred during the period for which individual i was available as a potential control. Here we are assuming unique event times, but where there are ties, the number of tied events at time j will replace the 1 in the denominator, $R_j - 1$, since the m controls are then selected from the remaining observations at that time. By using the inverse of the probability in Equation 6.3 to upweight the controls from a nested case-control study, it was shown by Samuelsen [185] that the weighted Cox regression provides a valid estimate of the HR. Statistical analysis that weights observations by the inverse of their selection probability is commonly referred to as **inverse probability weighting**. The weights computed by inverting the p_i from Equation 6.3 are sometimes referred to as 'Kaplan-Meier type weights', as the risk sets necessary for the calculation are readily obtained from a simple Kaplan-Meier analysis of the cohort (see Figure 4.4 in Chapter 4).

Stratified weights

As for the classic case-control design discussed in Chapter 3, the nested case-control design will often include matching on additional characteristics that are known confounders, not only on time. The controls at each event time are selected from the individuals still at risk and who match the case on these additional characteristics. Since the available data is a *stratified random sample* within the strata defined by the matching factors, the probability of not being sampled in Equation 6.3 generalises to:

$$1 - p_i = \prod_j (1 - \frac{m}{R_j - 1}) I[U_i = U_j] \tag{6.4}$$

where U_j denotes the matching stratum to which case j belongs, and I[ ] is the indicator function, equal to 1 when true (i.e. individual i matches the case), and zero when false (i.e. when individual i does not match the case). This means that the only events of relevance for the sampling probability (and thus the weight) of a control are the events in cases with the same matching variables. Thus the weights for a matched design need to be calculated separately for each stratum, so that they reconstruct the cohort by faithfully reconstructing the strata.

6.3.2 Data necessary for reweighting

There are two practical considerations worth mentioning concerning the data that are necessary to enable a nested case-control study to be up-weighted to represent the background cohort. Firstly, the entry and exit times of each control that are essential for the weight calculation are not routinely collected: since controls are matched on time with their cases, and the matched sets analysed by a conditional logistic regression, the entry time of a control or their fate after the sampling time are irrelevant. Even if a 'skeleton' of the cohort is available that contains the entry and exit times of all individuals and the event times of any cases, as well as any matching factors, this may not enable the individual controls to be identified. It will however enable the risk sets at each event time to be readily found from a Kaplan-Meier analysis, but this risk set information needs to be combined with the at-risk time of each control to obtain their weight. Thus, if data collected in a nested case-control design are to be potentially useful for additional unconditional analysis, it is important that the critical dates of each study subject are recorded. With these dates available, even a deidentified skeleton cohort is sufficient for the computation of the risk sets, so that weights can be obtained.

Where individual-level (skeleton) data are not available for the cohort from which the nested case-control sample was drawn, it may be possible to estimate the risk sets from available population counts. For example, the population counts by age and sex over calendar years are published by the government statistics office in many countries. Such statistics would be reasonable estimates of the risk set sizes, provided the selection of the case-control study subjects from the population was well-defined and the cases under study constituted only a small proportion of the population (i.e. the 'rare disease assumption').

6.3.3 Illustration of weighted risk sets

Using the same set-up as in [49], a cohort of N=5000 subjects was generated, with each assigned male/female sex S with 50% probability, an event time t that was associated with an exposure X_e, another continuous independent risk factor X_c and a binary factor Z that is common in the cohort (prevalence 30%). To generate confounding, the exposure was assigned with probability 0.8 to males and 0.5 to females and the effect was modified by Z using the following (log-)hazard function to generate the time-to-event

$$\ln h(t) = \ln h_0(t) + \beta_e X_e + \beta_c X_c + \beta_s S + \beta_Z Z + \beta_{ef} Z * X_e \qquad (6.5)$$

with a constant baseline hazard $h_0 = 0.0005$. The coefficients and corresponding hazard ratios used to generate the simulated cohort are presented in Table 6.4. All individuals entered the cohort at time $t = 0$ and were followed until the event of interest or a censoring time (generated from an exponential distribution with a rate of 0.05) with a maximum follow-up time of 25 years. These settings generate an event rate of approximately 2.5%.

The cohort of size 5000 was generated five hundred times, and for each cohort a nested case-control sample was drawn, with each case matched to 2 controls selected randomly from those still at risk at the case's event time. The average sample size of the nested case-control sample over the 500 simulations was 399. For each of the simulation cycles,

TABLE 6.4: *Coefficients (and corresponding hazard hazard ratios) used to generate a time-to-event outcome according to the hazard function in Equation 6.5 for a simulated cohort.*

Variable		Coefficient	Hazard Ratio
X_e	Exposure	0.405	1.5
X_c	Continuous risk factor	0.020	1.02
S	Sex (confounder)	0.095	1.1
Z	Binary effect modifier	1.386	4
$Z * X_e$	Interaction between Z and X_e	0.69	2

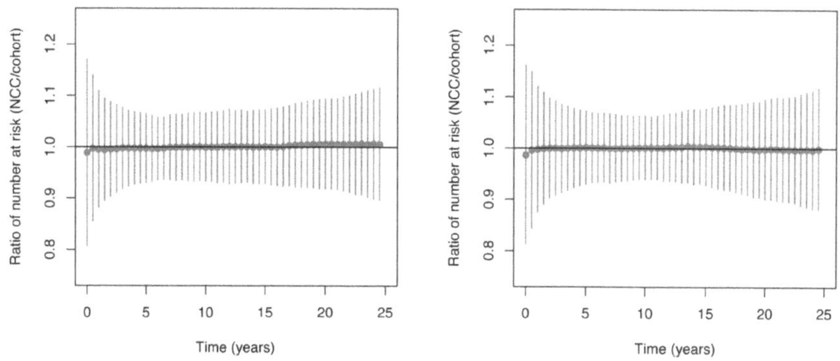

(a) *Controls sampled randomly* **(b)** *Controls matched on sex*

FIGURE 6.4: *Recovered risk set sizes from weighted nested case-control data, compared to actual risk set sizes in the cohort, presented as the average ratio (with two standard deviations) over 500 simulation cycles.*

the Kaplan-Meier weights were used to estimate the number of subjects at risk in the cohort from the case-control data. The performance of the weighting in recovering the person time experience of the cohort is summarised in Figure 6.4(a) which presents the mean ratio over the five hundred simulations (with two standard deviations) of the numbers of individuals at risk over time recovered from the nested case-control data compared to the actual numbers of individuals in the cohort. The recovered risk set sizes are unbiased and have good precision. The estimates are slightly more variable at the beginning of follow-up where information is limited due to short observation time and few events, with a gradual increase in variability as time elapses and the number of individuals in follow-up is depleted. Figure 6.4(b) presents a similar summary for a matched design, where controls were matched to cases on the binary variable for sex.

6.4 Weighted Cox Likelihood

In Chapter 4, Table 4.10 presents the likelihoods that are solved for estimating the HR from cohort, nested case-control and case-cohort designs. The full cohort Cox likelihood compares the case to all non-cases at each event time, whereas a case-cohort or case-control study estimates the HR in the underlying cohort when only a representative sample of each risk set is available. Since the sub-cohort in a case-cohort design is a random sample from the full cohort, a weighted Cox regression that reweights by the inverse of the sampling fraction provides an unbiased estimate of the HR. In contrast, the traditional analysis of nested case-control data uses conditional logistic regression to estimate the HR from the time-matched case-control sets, so that the controls simply act as a comparison group for their own case. However, we have seen in the previous section that if there is sufficient basic information for the controls, they can be reweighted to represent the full cohort from which they were drawn. Thus, with reweighting, a nested case-control sample can be used in a weighted Cox regression in much the same way as a case-cohort sample. Figure 6.5 illustrates a cohort where bold lines represent the individuals sampled in a nested case-control study and dashed lines are those not sampled. The full cohort likelihood uses the full risk set R_i at each event time t_i, whereas the nested case-control data only contains some of these individuals, which we refer to as the **sampled risk set**, $R_i^{\#}$. Unlike the ith sampled risk set of Chapter 4, this sampled risk set consists of any individuals in the nested case-control sample (including future cases) who are at risk at that event time. Thus the case-control sample functions like a 'mini-cohort', and if these individuals are up-weighted appropriately, a weighted Cox regression will provide valid HR estimates and a conservative confidence interval is obtained from the robust standard error. If all cases have been included in the case-control sample, then they are assigned a weight of 1 and each control will be weighted as described in the previous section. Note that it is the *individuals* in the sample that are used to represent the larger cohort, so that the 'mini-cohort' should only contain unique individuals: controls sampled more than once should have just one record retained in the weighted data and controls sampled later as cases should retain only their case record (with weight 1).

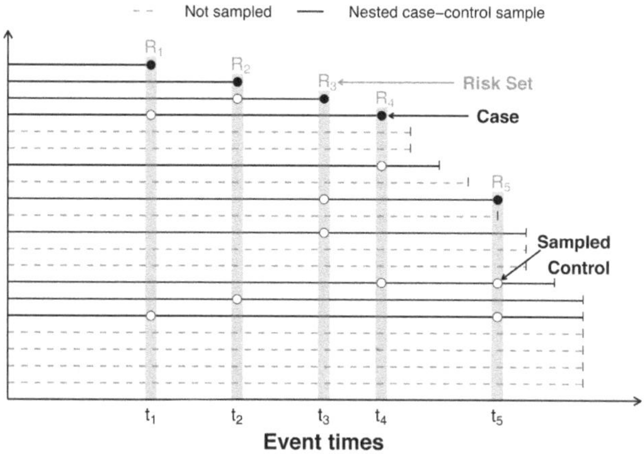

(a) *1:2 case-control study*

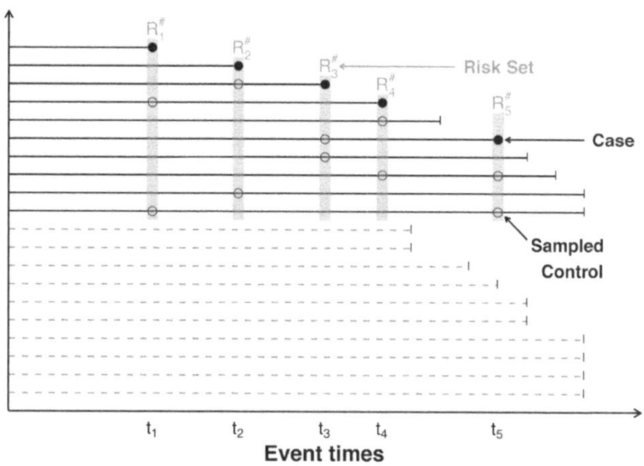

(b) *Rearrangement of (a) to clarify individuals sampled and not sampled*

Cohort likelihood	**Weighted likelihood**
$\prod_{t_i} \frac{e^{\beta X_i}}{\sum_{k \epsilon R_i} e^{\beta X_k}}$	$\prod_{t_i} \frac{e^{\beta X_i}}{\sum_{k \epsilon R_i^{\#}} w_k e^{\beta X_k}}$

where $R_i^{\#}$ all cases and controls at risk at t_i

$w_k = 1$ for cases and $\frac{1}{p_k}$ for controls

FIGURE 6.5: ***(a)*** *Cohort with a 1:2 nested case-control sample;* ***(b)*** *rearrangement of (a) to separate the individuals sampled and not sampled; the full likelihood for the cohort and weighted likelihood using only those sampled.*

6.5 Illustration of Weighted Analysis of Nested Case-control Data

In this section, two real data examples are used to illustrate the feasibility of breaking the matching on time in a nested case-control sample and conducting a weighted Cox regression of the individuals. In these examples, the whole cohort is available for computing the Kaplan-Meier weights for the sampled controls. However, as pointed out previously, where the cohort information is not available, weights can be estimated from the number of individuals in the background population from which the nested case-control study was drawn, or in the case of matching (e.g. on age and/or sex), the numbers in the matching strata. Commands are available in Stata and in R for computing the weights in each of these settings, i.e. from the full (or skeleton) cohort or from summary information on risk set sizes in the background cohort.

6.5.1 Estimation of HR from nested case-control data

To illustrate the estimation of a HR from a weighted Cox regression of the individuals in a nested case-control sample, we return to the study presented in Table 4.9 of Chapter 4, investigating the association of postpartum VTE with preeclampsia and other factors. In the full cohort of 970,778 pregnancies, there were 1163 cases of VTE within one year of delivery. Selecting 2 time-matched controls per case resulted in a sample of size 3489, which was first analysed by conditional logistic regression of the matched sets. The time-matching was then broken and the information in the cohort used to calculate the Kaplan-Meier weights for the 3481 unique individuals in the sample: two cases had been sampled earlier as controls and six controls were selected twice. The results of the conditional logistic regression and weighted Cox regression are presented in Table 6.5, where the Cox regression of the full cohort is included for comparison.

While the estimates are similar from the two methods of analysis of the case-control sample, many have better precision (narrower confidence intervals) from the weighted Cox regression: for the conditional logistic regression analysis, 1006 of the 3489 risk sets were dropped due to the case and their matched controls being concordant for the main exposure of interest (preeclampsia). This type of situation can occur when there is a rare exposure or confounder, as in this example where a very small

TABLE 6.5: *Adjusted hazard ratio estimates (with 95% confidence intervals) of the effect of various risk factors on postpartum VTE, using the full cohort, a nested case-control sample with 2 controls per case and a case-cohort sample with a subcohort of twice as many individuals as the number of cases.*

	Full Cohort	**NCC(1:2) CLR**	**NCC (1:2) IPW**	**CCH IPW**
PE*	1.83(1.43,2.33)	1.59(1.10,2.30)	1.79(1.41,2.28)	1.54(1.20,1.98)
Age	1.02(1.01,1.04)	1.03(1.01,1.04)	1.03(1.01,1.04)	1.03(1.01,1.04)
BMI				
Overwt	1.60(1.39,1.83)	1.63(1.36,1.95)	1.57(1.37,1.80)	1.43(1.25,1,65)
Obese	2.16(1.84,2.53)	2.14(1.72,2.65)	2.02(1.72,2.37)	1.97(1.68,2,32)
C-Section	1.75(1.53,2.01)	1.62(1.34,1.96)	1.67(1.46,1.92)	1.85(1.61,2.12)
First birth	1.13(1.00,1.29)	1.19(1.00,1.41)	1.16(1.02,1.32)	1.05(0.92,1.19)
Smoker	1.62(1.35,1.95)	1.87(1.43,2.46)	1.76(1.46,2.12)	1.53(1.27,1.85)
Transfus	2.68(2.10,3.41)	2.83(1.89,4.25)	2.75(2.16,3.51)	2.63(2.06,3.37)

* Preeclampsia (PE)
NCC: Nested case-control; CCH: Case-cohort
CLR: Conditional logistic regression; IPW: Inverse probability weighting

proportion of the pregnancies (2.8%) had a diagnosis of preeclampsia. The final column of the table presents the results from analysis of a case-cohort sample with a subcohort of 2326 (i.e. twice as many individuals as the number cases). This subcohort is less than 1% of the cohort, and so most of the 1163 cases will occur outside the subcohort, yielding a case-cohort sample of comparable size to the nested case-control study. Thus the precision of the estimates is similar to that of the weighed Cox regression that uses all of the sampled individuals in the nested case-control sample. Some variation in the estimates from the different designs is to be expected, as this illustration uses just a single nested case-control sample and a single case-cohort sample from the cohort. Although all cases are selected by design, the selected controls will be subject to sampling variability.

6.5.2 Estimation of absolute risk from case-control data

This illustration uses a cohort of 75,856 individuals who are children or siblings of non-Hodgkins lymphoma (NHL) patients[181]. Follow-up begins at the time of diagnosis of the first NHL in a parent or sibling (referred to as the index case or proband) and the children and siblings are followed from their age at this time until their age at diagnosis of NHL or censoring due to death, emigration, or end of follow-up. The risk of NHL is assumed to follow a Cox proportional hazards model, and in addition to age, sex and birth cohort, which are important factors in cancer epidemiology, the model includes the relationship with the proband (whether child or sibling) and sex of proband. These additional factors have been found to have strong effects for some cancers, such as leukemia [177].

There were 293 cases of NHL diagnosed in the relatives of patients during follow-up. To simulate the performance of the case-control design in estimating the cancer-free survival experience of the cohort of relatives, five hundred nested case-control samples were drawn from the cohort, each with 2 controls for each of the 293 cases, matched only on time. A further 500 nested case-control samples were drawn in a matched design, where controls were sampled from the risk set members whose index family member was the same sex as that of the case: (i.e. sex of the proband was used as a matching factor). For each of the 500 case-control samples, following computation and assignment of the Kaplan-Meier weights for controls (cases were given a weight of 1 since all were included), a weighted Cox regression analysis provided the estimates of the baseline hazard and hazard ratios from which the absolute risk could be calculated for any subgroup of interest.

For sons of male NHL patients, the average absolute risk at different ages is presented in Figure 6.6 for those with average birth year 1954. The grey whiskers extend to the upper and lower 2.5% of the estimates and lie within the 95% confidence interval of the absolute risk computed from the full cohort and marked by dashed lines. Panel (a) of the figure presents the results from the unmatched design, while for panel (b) controls were sampled from relatives with an affected father or brother (i.e. matched on sex of proband). The weighted estimates from the nested case-control data are in very good agreement with the absolute risk estimated from the full cohort.

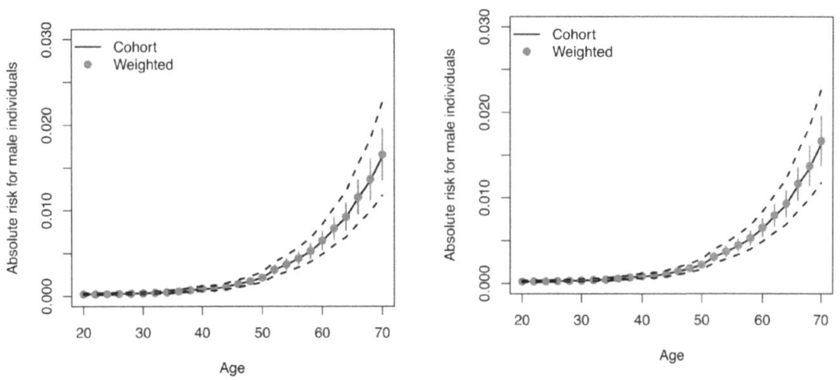

(a) *Controls sampled randomly*

(b) *Controls sampled from relatives of male patients*

FIGURE 6.6: *Average absolute risk for men with average birth year (1954) whose father was the first NHL patient in the family, estimated from weighted Cox regression of 500 nested case-control samples from a cohort of all children and siblings of NHL patients. The grey whiskers extend to 2 standard deviations each side of the average risk (grey points) and the dashed lines indicate the 95% CI of the absolute risk computed from the full cohort.*

Alternative estimate of absolute risk

A method of estimating the absolute risk from nested case-control data was proposed as early as 1997 by Langholz and Borgan [113]. The method involves first conducting the conditional logistic regression of the matched sets to obtain the hazard ratio estimates for the exposure variable X and other variable(s) Z in the hazard function

$$h(t|X) = h_0(t)e^{\beta X + \gamma Z}$$

These estimates, $\hat{\beta}$ and $\hat{\gamma}$, are then used in the following estimator of the absolute risk (i.e. cumulative hazard) up to any time-point t:

$$\hat{H}_0(t) = \sum_{i=1}^{n_c} \frac{I_{[t_i \leq t}}{\sum_{k \in R_i^*} w(t_i) e^{\hat{\beta} X_k + \hat{\gamma} Z_k}} \qquad (6.6)$$

where I is the indicator function, n_c is the number of cases, t_i is the time of the ith case and R_i^* denotes the matched set at time t_i. The weight $w_i = \frac{R_i}{m+1}$ where R_i is the full risk set at time t_i (including the case) and

m is the number of controls per case. The purpose of the weights is to inflate the sampled matched risk set at any event time to represent the full risk set size at that time. Thus the weights apply to a *time point*, not an individual as for the Kaplan-Meier weights above, and an individual sampled more than once as a control will have different weights at the different sampling times. When there is no matching except for time, this estimator and the Kaplan-Meier/Samuelsen estimator have very similar performance, but the Samuelsen estimator has somewhat better precision when a matched design is used [181]. The Langholz-Borgan estimator is also more prone to bias when fine matching results in the baseline hazard being estimated in strata with small numbers of cases. The Samuelsen estimator avoids this problem as the baseline hazard is estimated from all the individuals in the case-control sample.

6.6 Advantages of Breaking the Matching

Now that we have seen *how* to upweight a nested case-control sample to represent the whole cohort, let us return to *why* we might wish to do this. This methodology, first developed by Samuelsen [185], provides a very powerful tool for epidemiological analysis, as any parameters that could have been estimated from a Cox regression of the full cohort can also be obtained from a weighted Cox regression of the nested case-control sample. For example, one shortcoming of nested case-control data that is commonly cited is that, unlike cohort or case-cohort data, the absolute risk (cumulative hazard) cannot be estimated. However, breaking the matching yields estimates of absolute risk, as illustrated in the previous section.

Where risk sets have been lost from the conditional logistic regression due to missing data or concordant exposure or confounders, the weighted Cox regression can also provide hazard ratio estimates with much better precision than those from a conditional (matched) analysis. This was apparent in the illustration in section 6.5.1 where approximately one-third of the matched sets were lost from the conditional analysis due to concordance. The weighted Cox regression is of course less efficient than the full cohort analysis, due to the smaller sample size, but as with conditional logistic regression, the loss in efficiency is surprisingly little provided there are at least 3 controls per case.

Section 6.1 introduced the problem of overmatching. In a case-control study, this results from matching cases and controls on a factor that is associated with exposure but not associated, or only weakly associated, with outcome. Thus in the matched sets, there may be very little variation in exposure, resulting in a loss of efficiency. Where the exposure is binary or categorical, the case and their matched controls may have the same value, and so be lost from the analysis. But even where the exposure is continuous and the set is not lost due to concordance, the narrowing of the range of exposure will also reduce the information content of the data and result in reduced efficiency. Such a situation arose in a nested case-control study of subsequent lung cancer in a cohort of patients diagnosed with breast cancer in Sweden between 1958 and 2001 [47]. Cases of lung cancer were matched to breast cancer patients from the same region, who were diagnosed at the same age and in the same 10-year period, and were free of lung cancer at the time of diagnosis of the case. The purpose of the study was to investigate the effect of exposure to radiation (from radiotherapy for the breast cancer) on the woman's subsequent risk of lung cancer, and whether this was modified by smoking. The ability to address these questions was hampered by the unfortunate overmatching on calendar time. Figure 6.7 illustrates that from 1958 until approximately 1975, a large majority of patients received radiotherapy for their breast cancer and after 1975, the exposure to radiotherapy was still common. Thus a conditional logistic regression analysing the effect of any radiotherapy versus none will lose many risk sets due to concordance: during 1958–1974, 76% of patients in Stockholm and 85% in the rest of Sweden shared the same treatment; during 1975–1994, 51% of patients in both regions shared the same treatment.

To mitigate this problem of overmatching, the radiation dose (in Gray) that was collected in the study might have been used in the logistic model . However, this dose was estimated for 9 different technologies in use over the study period, so that it too was strongly associated with calendar time (see Table 2 of [174]), so that it was overmatched in the chosen design. Faced with this difficulty, the researchers conducted an analysis of only the cases in a 'twin design' of the woman's two lungs [174], since the radiation dose to each breast was recorded. By comparing the lung affected by cancer to the contralateral lung, the effect of exposure to radiotherapy could be estimated and its modification by smoking investigated in a stratified analysis. The authors found an increased risk of lung cancer on the irradiated side in smokers (OR 3.17;

95% CI: 1.66 to 6.06) but not in non-smokers (OR= 0.9; 95% CI: 0.37 to 2.22). They also reported evidence of a dose response trend in smokers.

6.6.1 Illustration of breaking the (over)matching

In the cohort of Swedish breast cancer patients described in [47] and summarised above, there were 900 with a subsequent lung cancer. For 726 of these, a matched control was identified and 4 cases had no match. Restricting to the 565 cases diagnosed more than 5 years after breast cancer (since the effect of radiation will not be acute), there were 565 case-control pairs and 4 unmatched cases. The information on treatment was available for 509 of these pairs, and for a further 29 cases and 16 controls. After breaking the matching, all of these 1063 records can contribute to the weighted analysis, provided they are from unique individuals. However, four of the cases had been a control at a previous time (so their control record was dropped) and eight controls were sampled twice (so only one record was retained). The number of unique individuals in the final weighted analysis was 1051: 538 cases and 513 controls. The cases were assigned a weight of 1, since all lung cancers were included, and for the 513 controls, the weights were calculated from the numbers of breast cancer patients at risk of lung cancer at each event time from when the control entered the cohort to when they were censored.

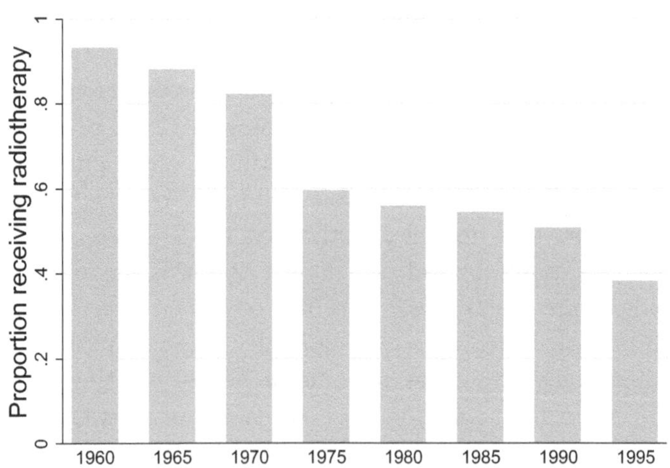

FIGURE 6.7: *Proportion of Swedish breast cancer patients receiving radiotherapy in 5-year intervals from 1958 to 2001.*

The adjusted estimates of the HRs for radiotherapy and smoking are presented in Table 6.6. The conditional logistic regression used the 509 matched case-control pairs, whereas the weighted Cox regression used all 1051 women and adjusted for the matching factors in the model. The estimates from the two analyses were similar, with the weighted Cox regression having better precision, and most importantly, revealing a significant interaction between smoking and radiotherapy.

The modification of the effect of radiotherapy by smoking noted in Table 6.6 could be explored in detail by a weighted Cox regression with lung as the unit of analysis, as the radiation dose was recorded for both the ipsi-lateral lung (on the same side as the treated breast cancer) and the contralateral lung. The 2102 lungs of the 1051 women in Table 6.6 were analysed using weighted Cox regression, with the dependence in these paired measurements accommodated by a cluster term for woman. The effects of smoking and radiotherapy dose (adjusted for age as a linear term) are presented in Table 6.7, demonstrating a large increase in the risk of radiation-associated lung cancer in smokers, with evidence of a dose-response (p-value for trend .026).

Breaking the matching also enables absolute risk to be estimated. Figure 6.8 presents the absolute risk profile between 5 and 25 years after breast cancer diagnosis (and treatment) for the lung of a 54-year old woman. Figure 6.8 reflects the same pattern as Table 6.7, with strong evidence of increasing risk of lung cancer in smokers associated with larger doses of radiation.

Breaking the matching and conducting a weighted analysis of this nested case-control study offered many advantages: a formal test for the

TABLE 6.6: *Adjusted hazard ratios (95% confidence intervals) for the associations of smoking and radiotherapy with a subsequent lung cancer diagnosis in breast cancer patients, estimated from conditional logistic regression (CLR) and inverse probability weighted Cox regression (IPW Cox).*

Exposure	CLR	IPW Cox[a]
Radiotherapy only	0.997 (0.56, 1.76)	0.77 (0.47, 1.26)
Smoking only	3.97 (2.13, 7.41)	3.96 (2.25, 6.97)
Radiotherapy and smoking	1.71 (0.80, 3.65)	2.19 (1.12, 4.30)

[a] *Adjusted for matching variables used in sampling: age (continuous), decade of diagnosis, region.*

TABLE 6.7: *Age-adjusted hazard ratios and 95% confidence intervals from a weighted Cox regression analysis of the 2102 lungs of 1051 breast cancer patients.*

Radiotherapy	Non-smoker	Smoker
None	Ref	4.09 (2.31, 7.24)
< 5 Gy	0.74 (0.42, 1.3)	5.42 (3.06, 9.60)
5 –13 Gy	0.92 (0.49, 1.75)	7.15 (3.60, 14.20)
13+ Gy	0.77 (0.43, 1.38)	8.63 (5.04, 14.79)

interaction between radiotherapy and smoking; increased power from inclusion of all individuals in the analysis; the ability to conduct analysis with lung as the unit of analysis in Cox regression, using the individual identifier as a cluster term to accommodate the dependence within woman; estimation of the absolute risk of lung cancer over time following

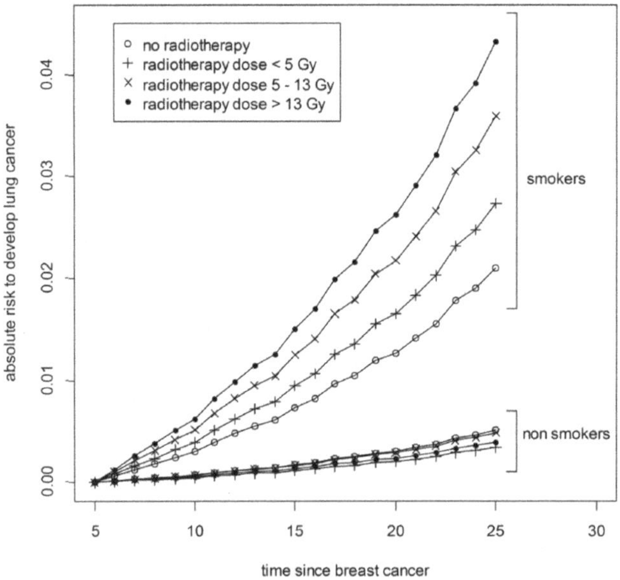

FIGURE 6.8: *Estimates of absolute risk of cancer in a lung exposed to different doses of radiation, from weighted Cox regression of 2102 lungs from 1051 breast cancer patients, stratified by smoking status (reproduced from [47] with permission).*

therapy; presentation of how the absolute risk changes with radiotherapy dose, an important treatment-safety question.

6.6.2 Further uses of reweighted case-control data

One strength of a case-cohort study is that the subcohort can be used to provide the reference group for more than one outcome. In cancer epidemiology, this has obvious potential for studies of cancers at different sites where controls are cancer-free, but even when the outcomes are different diseases and/or cover a wide age range, a judicious choice of subcohort by researchers working with the same cohort can be very cost-efficient.

Since a reweighted a case-control sample is representative of the cohort, it is also possible to reuse the data to address a research question about a new outcome in the same cohort. For example, individuals in the nested case-control data could be used as the reference group for a case-series identified in the same cohort, eliminating the time and cost needed to gather new controls. Where the available nested case-control data is insufficient, due to a small control:case ratio or controls being 'less informative' for the new outcome, these existing data could be used to supplement newly-selected controls, again leading to cost-efficiency. These settings will be presented in detail in Chapter 7.

6.7 Exercises

1. The following questions concern the paper *Preeclampsia and COVID-19: results from the INTERCOVID prospective longitudinal study* in the American Journal of Obstetrics and Gynecology in Sept 2021 (PMC8233533).

   (i) Is this a cross-sectional, cohort, or case-control study?

   (ii) Comment on the matching scheme, which the authors refer to as 'unmatched'. Is there potential for bias?

   (iii) Are the reported estimates "risk ratios" as claimed? Why/why not?

2. This exercise investigates the role of balance using the following cohort of 10,000, from Table I in the paper *Ignoring the matching variables in cohort studies - when is it valid and why?* by Sjölander and Greenland, in Stat in Med 2013 (PMID: 23761197), which is provided as a summary dataset **sjolander.dta**.

	Men		Women	
	Exposed	Unexposed	Exposed	Unexposed
Cases	4972	7154	7843	2756
Total	16256	70895	8788	4061

   (i) Expand the data to one record per person and verify that the crude OR is 6.88, but the common OR for men and women is 3.92

   (ii) Implement each of the following sampling strategies to select 1000 individuals (M=Male, F=female, E=exposed, U=unexposed) and complete the table with the estimates of the crude OR, sex-adjusted OR (with 95% C.I.) and the OR for the sex effect, from unconditional logistic regression.

	Crude OR	Adjusted OR (95% CI)	Sex OR
Full cohort			
Samples			
Random 1000			
500 M, 500 F			
500 E, 500 U			
250 E+250U M 250 E+250 U F			
500 cases, 500 controls			
M: 250 Cases+250 controls F: 250 Cases+250 controls			

(iii) Comment on the bias in the crude OR from the different samples.

(iv) Compare the estimates of the effect of sex from each of the samples to the 'true' effect in the full cohort. Comment.

(v) Re-weight the final sample to get the valid estimate for sex.

3. The dataset **Example 2.5 Framingham.dta** contains the aggregated data from Example 2.5 in Chapter 2.

   (i) Expand the data to one record per person and verify that you can reproduce the ORs in Example 2.5.

   (ii) Create a dataset with five times as many individuals, but with the same distribution of sex, exposure and outcome. Verify that you can again reproduce the ORs. Save this data for the following steps.

   (iii) Use the logistic model with an interaction term to obtain the ORs (with 95% confidence intervals) for males and females, by using either males or females as the reference group and a suitable post-estimation command to get the OR for the other sex.

(iv) Select a random sample of 1000 individuals and estimate the male and female ORs.

(v) Repeat the random sampling with several different seeds to verify that the OR for males can be biased in either direction due to the imbalance.

(vi) Record your results from (iii)-(v) on the table below and continue with the other sampling strategies to complete the table (M=Male, F=female, E=exposed, U=unexposed).

	Male **OR(95% CI)**	**Female** **OR(95% CI)**
Full cohort		
Samples		
Random 1000 from (v) **seed=** **seed=** **seed=**		
500 M, 500 F		
500 E, 500 U		
250 E+250U M 250 E+250 U F		
500 cases, 500 controls		
M: 250 Cases+250 controls F: 250 Cases+250 controls		

4. A cancer research group is planning to study whether a specific gene, or gene signature, is associated with the risk of a patient with Adenoid Cystic Carcinoma (ACC) having a recurrence. The study is to be conducted in a cohort of ACC patients, some of whom have experienced a recurrence (cases)

while others have not yet had a recurrence (controls). The original suggestion discussed by the group was to match cases and controls 1:1 according to treatment, tumor origin (i.e. gland), presence of lymph node metastases, in addition to age and gender.

(i) One investigator in the group proposes that it is essential to include time-matching. Do you agree? Why/why not?

(ii) Another investigator proposes that a matched cohort design should be used in order to ensure that the modification of gene effects by matching factors could be estimated. Do you agree? Why/why not?

(iii) What regression model would be used to analyse the data from the proposed matched design in (i), and what main effects and interactions are, and are not, available from such analysis?

(iv) For the effects not estimable in (ii), is it reasonable to assume that these are not of interest?

(v) If the regression model for the matched case-control data has no term representing modification of the effect of gene signature by any of the matching factors, what is the assumption concerning the OR for the gene effects. Is this reasonable?

(vi) Might the matching strategies result in sets where the exposures of interest or an unmatched confounder is the same for the case and control?

(vii) Could some of the proposed matching factors be potential mediators (i.e. in the pathway from gene to recurrence)? If so, what are the consequences?

(viii) Could some of these matching factors be strongly associated with exposure (the gene) but weakly, or not at all, associated with recurrence? If so, what are the consequences?

(ix) How would you advise the group regarding the design of this study?

5. The odds ratio for an exposure can be written in terms of the exposure rate in cases (p_1) and in controls (p_0). In Chapter 6,

the expression for the efficiency from random pairing (Equation 6.2) depends only on p_1 and p_0.

(i) Show that when the true OR=1, there is no loss of efficiency.

(ii) Rewrite the expression for an OR to provide a formula for p_1 in terms of p_0 and the OR.

(iii) Use the formula from (ii) to express the efficiency of random pairing in terms of p_0 and the OR.

(iv) Use the efficiency expression from (iii) in an Excel sheet or statistical software program to calculate the efficiency of random pairing for a range of ORs from 1 to 12, assuming a p_0 of 0.9

(v) Repeat the calculations in (iv) for p_0 values of 0.7, 0.5, 0.3 and plot the efficiency vs. the ln(OR) for each of the four curves on the same axis.

(vi) From your plot in (v), comment on if/when there is a serious loss in efficiency from random pairing.

6. This and the following four exercises need purpose-written commands for computing weights for nested case-control data provided with the datasets, which you should first install in your statistical software package.

   The variables ID, t, and 'event' in the dataset `tiny_cohort.dta` describe a cohort that is similar (but not identical) to the cohort in Figure 6.3 in Chapter 6. Use these data to:

   (i) sketch a line-plot similar to Figure 6.3 using the frame provided on the left below, marking on your plot the individuals identified by the indicator variable 'chosen' in the dataset (i.e. one potential 1:1 nested case-control sample).

   (ii) For each of the event times, complete the shaded boxes at the bottom of the plot on the next page with the following quantities:

   p: probability a potential control is sampled at this event time

   q: probability a potential control is *not* sampled at this event time

   Q: probability a potential control is not sampled for this or any prior event

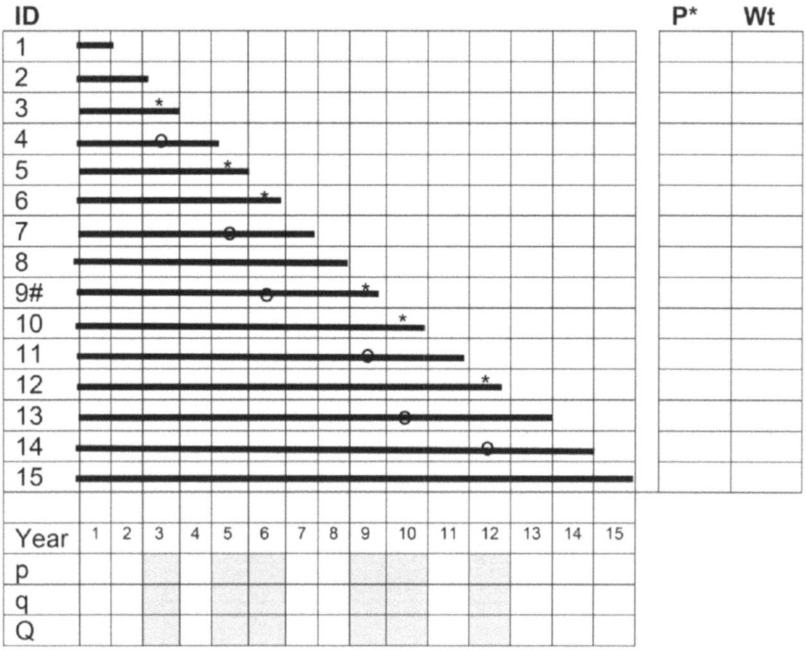

(iii) Use the quantities from (ii) to calculate the probability for each control being sampled for the study and hence their inverse probability weight. Enter these in the columns P^* and Wt to the right of the plot.

(iv) Compare your weights in (iii) to the weights obtained from a purpose-built command in your statistical package.

7. Repeat steps (i) to (iii) of the previous exercise to complete the weights in the following figure for the dataset `tiny_cohort2.dta`, which is similar to `tiny_cohort.dta` but has two shared event times.

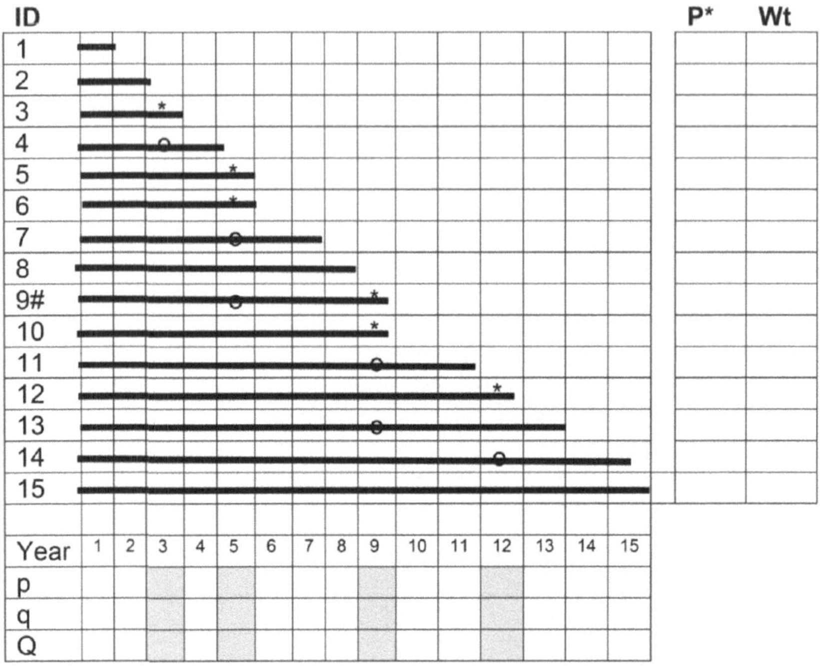

8. For the `tiny_cohort` data in Exercise 6:

   (i) Use the survival analysis commands in your statistical software to create a file with the risk sets and number of failures, and save this as a temporary dataset.

   (ii) Open the `tiny_cohort.dta` dataset and select just the case and control individuals that were 'chosen' as a nested case-control sample.

   (iii) Use the external risk set information you saved in (i), together with an appropriate purpose-built command in your software package, to obtain the weights for the individuals in this nested case-control sample.

   (iv) Compare the results from (iii) to what you obtained in Exercise 6.

9. Repeat the steps in Exercise 8 for the `tiny_cohort2.dta`, taking care with the repeated event times (*the risk set information must only have one observation for each time point*).

10. If data are available with time measured in calendar years (integer values), how would you weight a control if they were censored in the same year as they were selected? Modify one of the tiny cohorts above to include one such control and check that your weights agree with those from the purpose-built commands.

11. The dataset `tiny_cohort_strata` is similar to `tiny_cohort`, except that individuals now belong to two strata, and the 'chosen' individuals represent a *matched* nested case-control study.

    (i) Sketch a line plot of the cohort, showing the two strata and marking the selected nested case-control sample.

    (ii) Calculate the weights from the full cohort `tiny_cohort_strata` using the purpose-built command in your statistical software and specifying the stratum variable.

    (iii) Use the survival analysis commands in your software to prepare a dataset with the risk set information from `tiny_cohort_strata`, saving a temporary dataset.

    (iv) Open `tiny_cohort_strata`, select the 'chosen' nested case-control sample and obtain the weights using the appropriate purpose-built command in your software, with the stratification option and the external risk set information from (iii).

    (v) Compare the results obtained with the summary risk sets information in (iv) to those obtained from the full cohort in (ii).

12. Returning to the `full_cohort.dta` data example from Chapter 4, and using the same 10-year age categories as in Exercise 4.1, draw a 1:1 nested case-control sample that is matched on sex and age category. Examine your dataset and note the variable `_set` which identifies the matched sets, each of which will have 2 individuals (1 case and 1 control).

    (i) Fit the same full model as in part (iii) of Exercise 4.1 and compare the OR from conditional logistic regression (using `_set` as the conditioning variable) to the HR in the full cohort.

(ii) Create a variable called **selection time** containing the event time for the case and the selection time for their control. Round this variable to the nearest year. Now suppose that researchers have saved these data with the rounded selection time, the case-control identifier at that time, and the covariates, but have forgotten to keep the matched set variable that identifies the control that 'belongs' to each case. To mimic this situation, save the dataset containing just this information before proceeding.

(iii) If the only data available is the information on cases and controls from part (ii), can an unconditional analysis of this data provide valid estimates of the underlying OR or HR? Why/why not?

(iv) For the data saved in part (ii), the rounding of the time means that for each case there may be many individuals that might have been their matched control (check for any covariate pattern that there are as many controls as cases, due to the 1:1 sampling design). Assign controls randomly to appropriate cases and conduct a conditional logistic regression, using your new matched sets. Compare your results to those from the 'intentional' matched design.

(v) Repeat parts (i)-(iv) with a 1:3 case-control sampling design.

13. The purpose of this exercise is to illustrate how reweighting nested case-control data can provide estimates of hazard ratios and a Kaplan-Meier curve representing the population.The exercise uses the dataset `full_cohort` from Exercise 1 in Chapter 4, which contains information on outcome (coronary heart disease) and covariates for 50,000 individuals. The variables and coding used in this exercise are as follows:

t time (in years) from enrolment to coronary heart disease(CHD)

censored event indicator (0=CHD, 1=censored)

Age age in years

Gender 1=Male, 0=Female

Chol cholesterol in mg/dL

HDL high-density lipoprotein in mg/dL

SBP systolic blood pressure in mmHg

Treat antihypertensive treatment (1=Yes, 0=No)

Smoke smoking status (1=Yes, 0=No)

(i) Create a new variable from each of the continuous covariates age, cholesterol, HDL, and SBP, by centering them at their mean values (i.e. subtract the mean from each value). Then run a Cox regression with these new variables and the remaining binary variables (gender: 1=Male, 0=Female, Treat: 1=Yes, 0=No, Smoke: 1=Yes, 0=No).

(ii) Estimate the survival at each 5-year point from the start of follow-up to 20 years for one simple comparison of interest (e.g. smoking vs non-smoking females not on treatment, or male vs. female non-smokers not on treatment, female non-smokers who are on vs. off treatment). Save these survival estimates.

(iii) Draw a nested case-control sample using simple random sampling.

(iv)For the sampled controls, calculate the probability of inclusion in the nested case-control study using Kaplan-Meier type weights.

(v) Run a weighted Cox regression to obtain the estimates of the coefficients and the baseline hazard.

(vi) Calculate the survival at 5-year time points for the same two groups you compared in (ii).

(vii) Draw a plot to compare the survival curves obtained from the whole cohort and from the nested case-control sample.

14. This exercise illustrates how external population counts can be used to conduct a weighted analysis of nested case-control data. For this illustration we will use real population counts from the Swedish female population and a constructed dataset representing cervical screening in Sweden in the 10 years from 2002 to 2011 inclusive. The constructed dataset has been constructed from a real case-control dataset used for the audit

Cervical cancer case-control audit: Results from routine evaluation of a nationwide cervical screening program reported by Wang et al in Int Jour Cancer 2020 (doi: 10.1002/ijc.32416). From these data, women in their 30s, 40s and 50s were extracted together with 10 of their 30 controls, all dates where replaced by a random day during that calendar year and all ages were randomly perturbed in a 3-year window. The only variables in the dataset provided for this exercise are these fictitious dates and ages together with a categorical variable describing the attendance at the two previous screening rounds and the matched-set identifier. These fictitious matched nested case-control data are available as a Stata dataset (`chap6_cxcaNCC10_age30-60.dta`) and the population counts of women in Sweden during the study period are available as an Excel file (`tidy_risksets_23to100.xls`) or can be downloaded from the population database at Statistics Sweden (www.scb.se).

(i) The population counts required are the numbers of women in Sweden of each one year of age (starting from age 23) in the 10 years from 2002-2011.

(a) Rearrange the wide data in the Excel sheet (or the downloaded data) as a long dataset with three columns (age, year, count), containing the number of women of each age in each of the ten calendar years.
(b) Add a new variable to the dataset with the age in 2002.
(c) Extract from these data the counts for each one year of age for women who were aged 30-60 in 2002, and arrange these in a dataset with just four columns: age in 2002 , current year, age in current year, total number. Save this dataset before proceeding.

(ii) Use the nested case-control dataset with a conditional logistic regression analysis to find the hazard ratios for the different levels of screening, using the women screened in both periods before 2002 as the reference group. Note that your results will differ somewhat from the published paper since you only have women aged 30 to 60 and the dates and ages have been randomly altered.

(iii) Prepare a dataset containing all unique individuals from the case-control dataset where any case who was previously a control keeps their case record, and any control selected more than once keeps only one record (outline the steps and counts on a flowchart). Before saving this dataset, generate a variable for the follow-up time in days from 1st January 2002 to the date of the event for cases and censoring date for controls (this will be used in part(v) below).

(iv) Compute the number of events in each year for each age, by aggregating the cases from the dataset in (iii) to count the number of events at each diagnosis date for each year of age. Assuming that the population remains the same for every day of the year, merge this dataset to the data from part(i) using year of diagnosis and age, to get the external riskset information. Before saving, generate a variable for the age in 2002 and time in days from 1st January 2002 to the date of event (for using in part(v) below).

(v) Assign weights to the unique individuals from (iii), using a purpose-built command in your software package, with time in days as the time variable and the age in 2002 as the matching factor. Check that all cases received a weight of 1 and that controls with the smallest and largest weights can be explained in terms of their follow-up time and/or the size of population they represent.

(vi) Estimate the crude hazard ratio for the screening variable using a weighted Cox regression. Repeat the analysis adjusting for age in 10-year categories and compare with the results from conditional logistic regression in part(ii).

(vii) Use the weighted data to examine the crude Kaplan-Meier or cumulative hazard curve, and the curve stratified by (a) screening status and (b) 10-year age categories.

7

Reusing Case-Control Data

7.1 Using Classic Case-control Data for new Outcomes

7.1.1 Explanatory variable as outcome

Case-control studies that are not matched on time will be referred to as 'classic' in the following, to discriminate them from the time-matched nested case-control design. Classic case-control data collected for a previous study may contain all the variables that are needed to address a new research question concerning an 'outcome' that was the exposure or a confounder in the original study. An example of this was provided in Chapter 3, where the explanatory variables collected in a case-control study of cot death included infant immunisation and mother's marital status, and the association between the infant immunisation outcome and mother's marital status in the population was of interest. A naive application of a logistic regression model to the available case-control data will not provide a valid estimate for the new association of interest, as the available data are not representative of the population. In addition to being enriched with cases (50% in a simple unmatched 1:1 case-control dataset), available case-control data may also be matched. However, if the case-control design has been reported clearly, and if there is sufficient information to calculate the sampling fractions of cases and controls (within matching strata if the study was matched), then the data can be simply viewed as a two-stage design, where the first stage is the cohort. Thus, as illustrated in Chapter 3, a weighted regression, using the inverse of the sampling fractions as weights, provides valid estimates of the association of interest in the cohort.

7.1.2 Reusing controls for a new outcome

For a classic case-control study (i.e. non-nested), if the controls were sampled randomly from the study population, then it is often reasonable to reuse them as the reference group for a new case series from the same population or cohort in which the case-control study was conducted. Controls will often be selected from individuals that are not only free of the disease that defines the 'case', but also free of other (perhaps related) diseases: hence the expression 'healthy controls'. In studies of expensive genetic markers, it is not uncommon for investigators to gather information only on cases and then compare these to controls that are already available from another study in the same population, or even in a different population.

If the prior case-control study was matched, it may be possible to 're-match' the available controls to cases of another disease in the same population, assuming the matching factors are also considered as confounders for the new association of interest. In this case, a conditional analysis of the new matched sets will provide the estimate of interest. But what if one or more of the matching factors in the original study are of interest as risk factors for the new outcome? Provided the sampling fractions in the strata defined by the matching factors are known, a weighted analysis can correct for the biased sampling that led to the available data and a valid adjusted estimate obtained for the association of interest. Where the original case-control study, and the cases for the new study, have both been sampled from a well-defined cohort, the sampling fractions (and thus the weights) can be derived from the cohort provided the size of the risk sets (the counts of individuals in the cohort) are available at each event time. If the original case-control data was matched, these counts must be available for the strata defined by the matching factors.

Where the matching is coarse, for example involving demographic variables such as sex, age group and calendar period, the sampling fractions can often be computed from official statistics for the population that yielded the original case-control sample. But if matching in the original study involved variables not routinely collected in population registers, then the sampling fractions may not be available.

7.2 Reusing Nested Case-control Data

Where data have been gathered in a nested case-control design, the time matching makes it most unlikely that these individuals could be 're-matched' to another outcome in the same cohort to enable a conditional logistic regression analysis. However, we have seen in Chapter 6 that if the sampling probabilites can be calculated for nested case-control sample, these individuals can be reweighted to represent the person-time experience of the cohort. The illustrations presented were both concerned with the same outcome as the original case-control study, but since the reweighted data are representative of the cohort, they can also be used in the study of a new outcome.

In Figure 7.1, a cohort of 20 individuals is used to illustrate a prior nested case-control study (solid circles for cases and open circles for controls). The triangles represent cases of a new outcome of interest, for whom controls are *not* selected, but instead the prior case-control study subjects are to be used to represent the background cohort. There were 5 events in the prior study during the follow-up time, and for each of these, 2 time-matched controls were selected. A conditional logistic regression of the 15 observations in these 5 matched sets would provide an estimate of the HR, but as we saw in Chapter 6, the HR could also be estimated from a weighted unconditional Cox regression of the 10 unique individuals (numbered 11 to 20), with a weight of 1 assigned to the cases (numbered 15, 17, 18, 19, 20) and Kaplan-Meier weights for the controls.

On deciding to study the new outcome, we would identify three cases in the existing data (individuals 12, 14 and 16) and three more cases in the cohort who had not been sampled into the prior case-control study (individuals 6, 7 and 9), so that the combined data available for investigating the new outcome consists of 10+3=13 unique individuals from the cohort. The study base for the new outcome, i.e. the cohort, can be represented by these individuals if they are weighted by the inverse of the probability that they are available in this (non-random) sample of 13. The probability of being in the sample is clearly =1 for all cases of the new outcome, so these have weight 1. But cases of the original outcome were all selected for the prior study (with probability 1) so these also have a weight of 1. The sampling probabilities (and thus weights) for the remaining individuals can be computed from the risk-set information as already presented in detail in Chapter 6. In this example there are only two subjects whose weight will be > 1 (number 11 and 13) and these will have the same weight, as they are both available for selection at all the same event times!

In the weighted Cox regression, the new cases will be defined as events and the other individuals as censored. Thus the cases in the prior

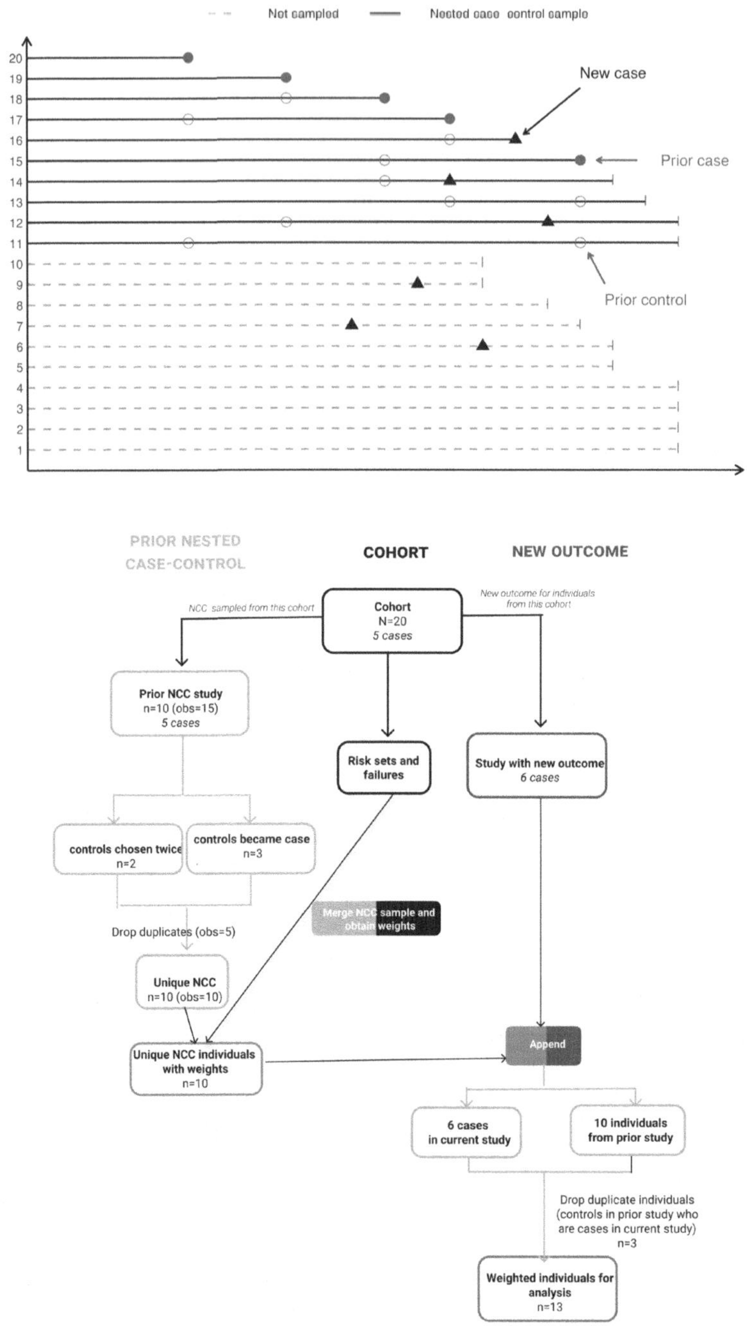

FIGURE 7.1: ***(a)*** *Line plot of a nested case-control sample (circles) and a new outcome (triangles) ascertained for the same cohort.* ***(b)*** *Steps to prepare a dataset of unique individuals from the prior data and the new events.*

study will be defined as censored at the time of their diagnosis. Note that this assumes the same censoring would have been considered appropriate if the new outcome had been investigated in the full cohort. This would be reasonable if the two outcomes are thought to be independent or are rare: for example, in cancer epidemiology, it is common to censor individuals with a cancer other than the one under investigation. While the two outcomes in Figure 7.1 might be independent (at least they never occur in the same individual), they are certainly not rare, but for a more realistic situation, we can imagine that the cohort is much larger and that the great majority are non-sampled individuals who have neither disease. Where outcomes with risk factors in common are not rare, the non-independent censoring (**informative censoring**) will bias the effect of these risk factors. In such instances, competing risk analysis or multi-state modelling would be more appropriate than simple Cox regression.

7.2.1 Illustration in a realistic cohort

The 'prior' study

This illustration uses a simulated cohort which was generated to be similar to the actual Singapore Chinese Health Study [77], including a nested case-control study of coronary heart disease (CHD). As described in detail previously [181], the following demographic characteristics and CHD-related factors were first generated to reflect the values and their correlations in the actual cohort: sex, age (in years), smoking status, anti-hypertensive treatment (yes/no), systolic blood pressure, cholesterol and high density lipoprotein. To generate a time to CHD onset, a proportional hazards model was used with each of these variables having the coefficient that was estimated from the real data. Random censoring times were also generatedand the outcome for any individual set to the event time or censoring time, whichever occurred first. A cohort of 50,000 individuals was generated, with the follow-up set to a maximum of 25 years, during which time the cumulative incidence of CHD was approximately 4%. For each of these cases, two time-matched controls were selected, and the analysis of this 1:2 nested case-control sample gave HR estimates in good agreement with the full cohort analysis, as expected. In the next paragraph, this case-control sample will be used to analyse cases of a new outcome in the same cohort.

The 'new' outcome

To mimic a study of stroke in Singapore [214] that reported a number of risk factors in elderly Singaporeans, a time to stroke was generated for individuals older than 60 years, using age group (60–74, 75–84, 85+), sex, smoking status and hypertension:

$$h(t) = h_0(t)e^{1.2*\text{Age1}+0.8*\text{Age2}+0.8*\text{sex}+1.5*\text{smoker}+2.5*\text{HT}}$$

where $Age1$ and $Age2$ are the 75–84 and 85+ age groups, and sex, smoker and HT (hypertension) are indicator variables. All events occurring before a random censoring time and within the 25 years follow-up (8.8% of subjects aged 60 or older) constitute the cases to be analysed. Instead of sampling controls from the cohort, the prior nested case-control sample from the CHD study is to be used to analyse the stroke outcome.

Preparing the sample for analysis

The preparation of the data for analysis follows the same steps as in the very simple example in section 7.2 above, i.e.

1. break the matching and keep unique individuals: the case record for any case who was previously a control, and just one record for any control sampled more than once
2. ensure that data contains the entry time, and the event or censoring time, of all individuals
3. compute the weights for these individuals: weight=1 for cases if all have been selected, and Kaplan-Meier weights for controls
4. append the new cases and drop any of their prior records
5. assign weight=1 to the new cases (assuming all were sampled) and define prior cases as censored

These steps were executed for the 1:2 nested case-control study sampled from the full cohort that was analysed in Section 7.2.1 and the flowchart in Figure 7.2 used to check the numbers of observations at each step. The alert reader will note one additional feature in this flowchart that was not in the simpler Figure 7.1(b): the unique individuals from the prior study who represent the background study base for the new outcome are at least 60 years old, so only these individuals are retained for analysis. On appending these to the (new) stroke cases, any stroke case who was in the prior nested case-control data has their prior record

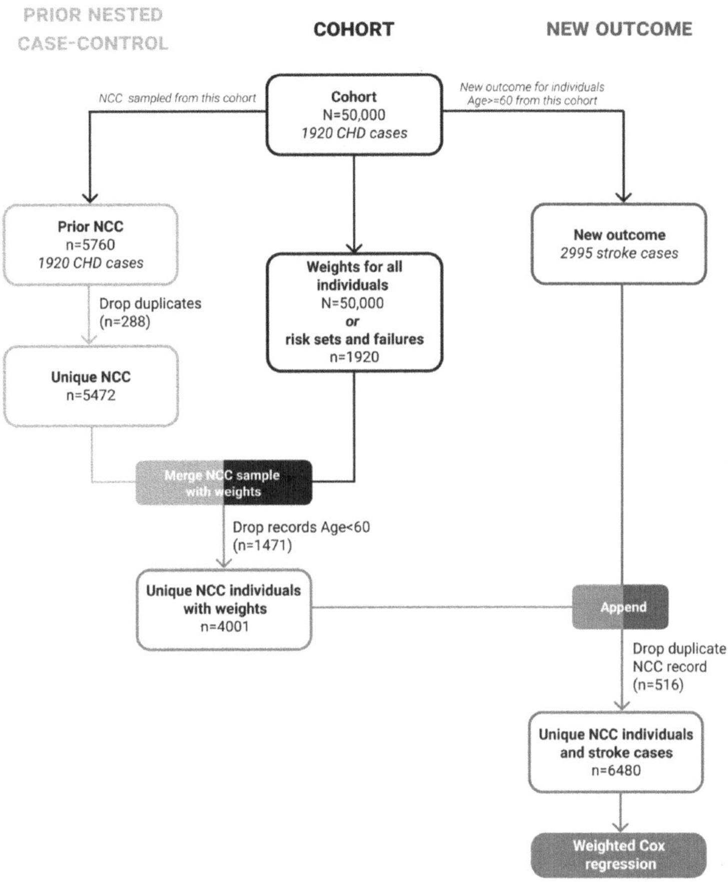

FIGURE 7.2: *Flowchart of the data preparation to reuse a nested case-control sample to analyse a new outcome in the same cohort.*

dropped: for example a new case who was a control in the prior study of CHD will have their control record(s) dropped, and a new case who was also diagnosed with the prior outcome will have only the new outcome retained [184]. All new cases are assigned a weight=1 and defined as having the binary outcome of interest, while all prior records are defined as censored.

Results from weighted Cox regression

The first column of Table 7.1 presents the results from the analysis of the full simulated cohort of individuals who were younger than 60 years

TABLE 7.1: *Weighted Cox regression analysis of stroke cases and reused data from a prior nested case-control study of CHD in the same cohort (the simulated Singapore Chinese Health Study [181]).*

	Full Cohort	**Reuse NCC of CHD**	**Reuse NCC controls only**
Age 75–84	1.17 (1.05,1.30)	1.18 (0.99,1.40)	1.20 (1.00,1.44)
Age 85+	0.65 (0.38,1.12)	0.82 (0.38,1.80)	0.92 (0.39,2.12)
Sex	0.80 (0.74,0.86)	0.85 (0.76,0.95)	0.87 (0.77,0.97)
Smoker	1.38 (1.26,1.50)	1.30 (1.13,1.50)	1.33 (1.15,1.53)
Hypertension	4.64 (4.25,5.08)	4.70 (4.18,5.27)	4.77 (4.24,5.36)

at baseline ($N = 34,116$), among whom there where 2995 stroke cases during follow-up. The coefficient estimates agree closely with the 'true' values used to simulate the data, as expected for such a large cohort. The estimates in the second column are from the analysis of the stroke cases by reusing the data from the prior nested case-control study of CHD, i.e. the 6480 unique individuals described in the flowchart in Figure 7.2. Reusing only the prior controls provided very similar results (third column of Table 7.1). This is to be expected, as the 1920 CHD cases in the prior sample of 5760 were weighted by a factor of 1 when reused, while the 3840 controls will generally be upweighted by large factors to represent the cohort of size 34,116.

The above illustration overlooks a number of issues that would require more careful attention to the study design and data management in a real epidemiological investigation. For example, it is likely that if a nested case-control study of CHD was conducted in a cohort such as the Singapore Chinese Health Study, the controls would be selected from those who were not only free of CHD but also free of other cardiovascular diseases (such as stroke). The cases of interest might also be those without such a history. Likewise, in a nested case-control study of incident stroke, controls might be sampled from individuals without stroke or other cardiovascular disease. These complications have been ignored above, but will be explored further in some of the exercises related to this chapter.

It was assumed in the illustration above that controls were sampled randomly, although it is common for nested case-control sampling to match controls on one or more confounders, such as sex and age group.

This does not generate any additional difficulty, as it simply requires the sampling weights for individuals from a prior matched study to be calculated within the matching strata (see section 6.3.1 of Chapter 6) to properly reflect the cohort. If the new outcome is only of interest in some of these strata (for example in females) then the relevant individuals from the prior study can be used with their weights. Other valid subset analyses are discussed in Section 7.4 below.

7.2.2 New outcome in restricted follow-up time

In all the examples so far, it has been assumed that the prior outcome and new outcome have been obtained during the same observation period. This results in a simpler calculation of the weights for the prior individuals: remembering that the purpose of the weights is to reconstruct the background study base in which the new outcome occurred, this is straightforward when the new study base is the same as for the prior study. When the new study base is a subset of the cohort, defined by baseline characteristics such as age (60 and older) in our illustration above, this is also trivial to accommodate. However, if the new study base covers a different period of observation, then the weights for each of the prior individuals, which depend on their observation time, will need to reflect this. Subsequent to conducting a nested case-control study in a cohort of individuals followed up from T_0 to T (line A in Figure 7.3), a likely scenario is that a new case series is to be identified in the same

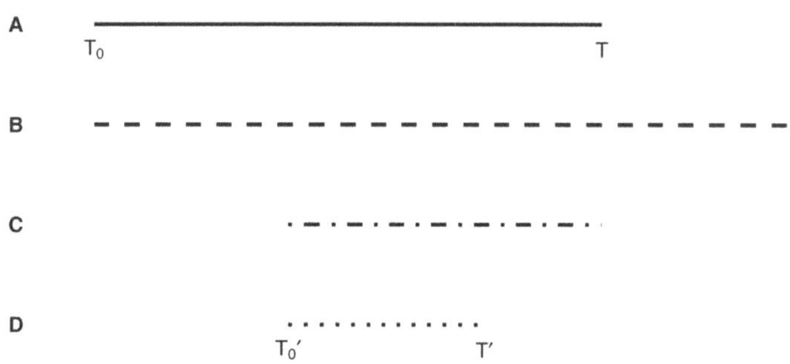

FIGURE 7.3: *For a nested case-control study conducted by following up a well-defined cohort from T_0 to T (A), the broken lines B, C and D represent three follow-up protocols for identifying a new outcome that could be studied in an overlapping study base by reusing the existing controls from A.*

cohort of individuals that has been updated to a later time (line B). Clearly the available prior data can be used to analyse all new cases up to T but not those that occurred between T and the end of the extended follow-up, as there are no individuals available to represent that part of the cohort's experience. It is also possible that the new study is more focused on recent time and has excluded cases in the earliest part of the observation period (line C in Figure 7.3). In this situation, the available prior data needs to be reweighted to represent the cohort's experience from the later starting time (T_0') to T, i.e., the **overlapping study base** for the new and prior outcomes. Cases whose prior event time was before the starting time of the new study will have weight 0, and the weight for any control must reflect their (inverse) probability of being sampled from the study base relevant to the new outcome, which will exclude any individuals censored before the starting time of the new study.

Where the follow-up time for the new study starts later and finishes earlier (line D in Figure 7.3), the weight for any prior case whose event has not occurred by this earlier finishing time will be > 1, as their probability of being selected (as a control) in the new study period is < 1. This weight, like the weights for other controls, will be calculated from the probabilities of being sampled (as a control) for events in the restricted study period (T_0' to T').

Whether the new outcome is recorded during a shortened or extended follow-up time, from the same starting time T_0 or a delayed starting time T_0', reusing the prior data involves identifying the overlapping study base and representing it by appropriate weighting of the available data. A new outcome that is recorded during a restricted follow-up period with both left truncation and right censoring (line D in Figure 7.3), will be used in the next paragraph to illustrate how restriction can be accommodated appropriately when re-weighting nested case-control data for use in the study of a new outcome.

Figure 7.4(a) presents a simple line plot of new cases (denoted by triangles) identified in a cohort. In contrast to the previous illustrations of this small cohort, here the new cases have only been identified during a limited follow-up period, from T_0' to T', shaded grey in the figure. The individuals denoted by circles represent a prior case-control study that enrolled subjects over the entire follow-up. Assuming that the outcome, exposure and confounders of interest for the analysis of the new cases are also available in the prior case-control dataset, the objective now is to use those data to estimate the HR describing the association between the new outcome and an exposure of interest. This involves

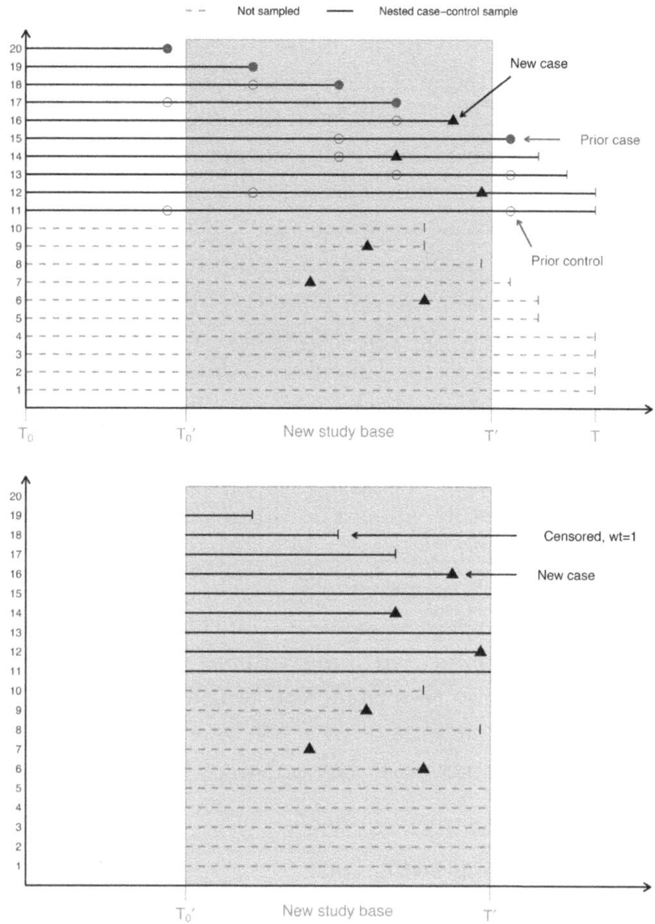

FIGURE 7.4: *(a) Schematic drawing of a nested case-control sample from a cohort of 20 individuals: sampled individuals are denoted by solid lines, cases by closed circles and time-matched controls (2 per case) by open circles; cohort members not selected are denoted by dashed lines; triangles denote a new outcome of interest in the cohort during the shaded follow-up period.* ***(b)*** *the individuals who will contribute to the analysis of the new outcome (solid lines and triangles) and the study base they represent (shaded grey).*

re-weighting the available individuals so that they correctly represent the study base *from which the cases were obtained.* The study base that is relevant to the new outcome consists of the cohort observed during the restricted period (Figure 7.4(b)) and excludes individual 20. Individual 11 is not in the nested case-control sample selected from *this study base*, and individual 15 would have been observed only until T' and so would not have been identified as a case. Eight of the 10 individuals from the prior case-control study (with the exception of number 11 and number 20 as explained), together with the 3 additional new cases (numbered 6, 7 and 9) are members of the appropriate study base, i.e. the 'overlapping study base' of the prior study and the new cases. These individuals can be used to reconstruct the study base by weighting them by the inverse of the probability that they are available in our sample. The sampling probability is 1 for any prior case (except number 15) or new case, and the probabilites (and thus weights) for the prior controls can be computed from the relevant risk sets in the time period from T_0' to T'.

As before, the illustration is simplistic, as there are no individuals with both outcomes, and the question arises as to how such comorbidity might be accommodated in practice. For example, if the cases (and thus the controls) for the new study should not have had the prior event, such as a study of cardiovascular disease in individuals who do not have diabetes (studied earlier in the same cohort), then the case-control dataset from the diabetes study needs to contain the second outcome (cardiovascular disease) to determine which individuals are eligible for the new study. Although the precise reconstruction of the correct study base in such a setting requires the modified risk set sizes, it will be demonstrated later that the weighted analysis is not sensitive to imperfection in the weighting.

Illustration of overlapping study base

Using the same simulated cohort as in Section 7.2.1, we identify cases of stroke that occurred in a 10-year interval, between year 5 and year 15 of the full follow-up. Instead of sampling time-matched controls for these cases, we propose to reuse the nested case-control sample from the previous CHD study, consisting of cases and their matched controls during the whole 25 years of follow-up. The preparation of the data for analysis is outlined in the flowchart in Figure 7.5 using one randomly selected nested case-control sample.

Of the available 5760 records in the prior nested case-control study, only 3391 (from 2369 unique individuals) were retained in the new study: 809 of these individuals experienced the event during the study period. For those who were sampled only as controls during the restricted study period, but were cases at a later time in the full follow-up, it is important that their outcome status is reset to censored at the new end of follow-up

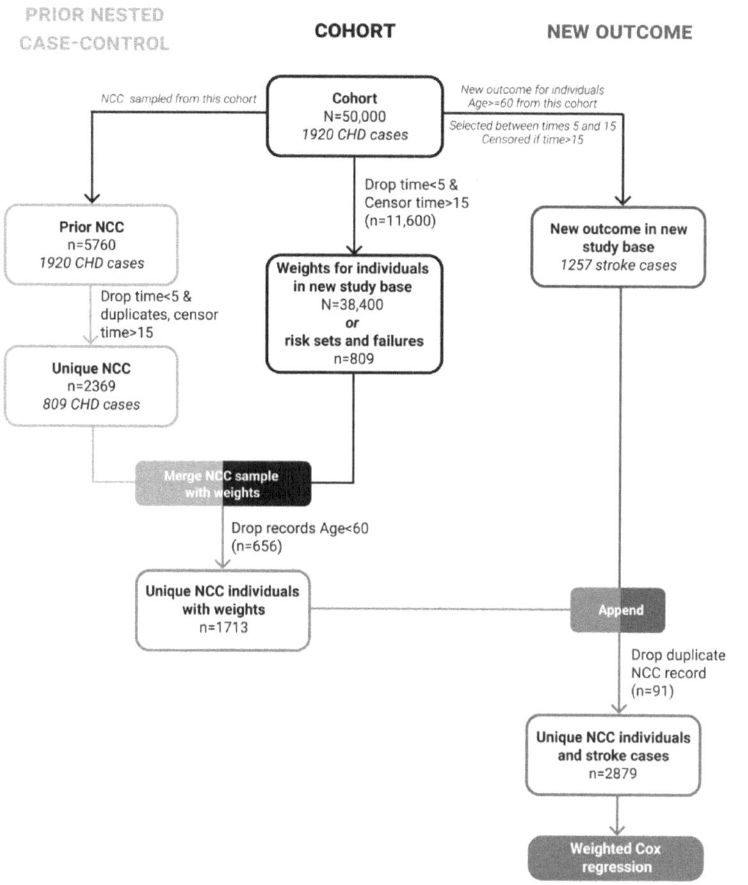

FIGURE 7.5: *Flowchart depicting the preparation of data for weighted Cox regression of new cases selected during a restricted follow-up time of the full cohort, from which prior nested case-control data are to be used as controls.*

($T = 15$). To represent the study base from which the 2369 individuals were sampled, it is clear that any individuals censored before $t = 5$ are excluded. While individuals who had a diagnosis of CHD before $t = 5$ could in principle still be followed up, we will also exclude them so that the study base is consistent with the prior nested case-control study of (incident) CHD. The new study base has 38,400 individuals, among whom there were 809 CHD cases in $t \in [5, 15]$ and as before, any cases that occurred at $t > 15$ are censored at $t = 15$. This study base (or a summary of the 809 event times with their risk sets and tied failures) can be used to assign weights to the data to be reused. Note, as before, that individuals younger than 60 are excluded, as the stroke outcome was studied only in those 60 years and older. This exclusion, which can be done either before or after merging with the study base to get the weights, simply selects the relevant records from the prior data. Note that the exclusion based on age is *not* applied to the study base, as there was no age restriction on the controls who were sampled for the CHD study! It will be left as an exercise to explore the reuse of prior data from a study where cases and controls were sampled from a restricted age group.

Following the steps in the previous paragraph, there were 1713 unique individuals available from the prior case-control sample of CHD who could be reused to study the stroke outcome. Of the 2995 total stroke cases in the full cohort, 1257 were diagnosed during the time period $t \in [5, 15]$. Appending these to the 1713 prior records and keeping only the new case record for any individual who was duplicated in the prior data, 2879 records were used in the weighted Cox regression analysis.

Results from weighted Cox regression

The first column of Table 7.2 presents the results from the analysis of incident stroke in the 'full cohort' of 25,315 individuals 60 years or older who were under observation from year 5 to year 15. During this follow-up time, there were 1257 stroke events: any earlier events are truncated and any later events are censored at year 15. The second column in the Table presents the results from a weighted Cox regression analysis of the 2879 individuals described above: the 1257 stroke cases and the additional individuals representing a nested case-control study of CHD in the same study base. The estimates from the weighted analysis are similar to those from the full cohort, but with wider confidence intervals, due to the much smaller sample size. Even if the available prior dataset size was equivalent to a 1:2 or 1:3 nested case-control study, it cannot be assumed that the 'old' controls in the reused data carry the same information as (new) controls that are explicitly sampled for the stroke cases. We will return to this point in Section 7.3.

7.2.3 Application to study of breast cancer

The various issues introduced above were encountered in a study that compared incident cases of contralateral breast cancer to controls from a nested case-control study of metastases [48]. The cases of contralateral breast cancer (CBC) were identified in a cohort of breast cancer patients

TABLE 7.2: *Weighted Cox regression analysis of stroke cases and reused data from a prior nested case-control (NCC) study of CHD. The overlapping study base represents individuals 60 years and older who were in follow-up during a restricted time period in the simulated Singapore Chinese Health Study[181].*

	Full Cohort (n=25,315)	**Reuse NCC of CHD (n=2879)**
Age 75–84	1.07 (0.90,1.27)	0.95 (0.71,1.25)
Age 85+	0.83 (0.39,1.74)	1.25 (0.39,4.03)
Sex	0.78 (0.70,0.87)	0.80 (0.67,0.96)
Smoker	1.43 (1.25,1.64)	1.31 (1.05,1.64)
Hypertension	4.92 (4.28,5.65)	4.70 (3.92,5.65)

whose diagnosis was recorded in the Stockholm-Gotland cancer register from 1976 to 2005. The researchers wished to investigate multi-focality of the initial breast cancer as a risk factor for CBC, and parity as a protective factor. For the 853 cases identified, this information, together with other variables, was retrieved from the medical charts. Prior to identifying controls and abstracting their medical records, investigators were aware of a nested case-control study of metastases in the breast cancer patients in the same register who were diagnosed between 1997 and 2005, i.e. an overlapping cohort. In addition to time since their initial breast cancer diagnosis, the controls for that study had been matched to the metastases cases on the calendar period of diagnosis (1997–2000, 2001–2005), age group (<45, 45–54, >54 years) and intended treatment (chemotherapy, hormonal therapy or a combination). The variables that had been abstracted for the CBC cases were also available in the nested case-control dataset for the metastases study.

Although the new cases of CBC and the prior study of metastases were both sampled from the same register, the common study base is not simply the overlapping cohort of breast cancer patients registered between 1997 and 2005. A contralateral breast cancer was defined as a cancer diagnosed in the opposite breast at least three months after the initial cancer diagnosis, so the study base represented by the CBC cases must reflect this condition. The metastases study had no minimum follow-up but had inclusion criteria concerning age (at most 75 years) and intended treatment (must include chemotherapy or hormone therapy). Thus the metastases study base differs from that of the CBC cases.

The first task is to identify the restricted (common) study base from which a subset of individuals in both the metastasis study and CBC study were sampled: this subset will be CBC patients in the overlapping calendar period (1997–2005) who meet metastases study criteria, and metastases patients who meet CBC study criteria (see Figure 7.6). The common study base (double-bordered rectangle) and the corresponding subsets of CBC cases and metastases study subjects (dashed circles) are referred to as the 'aligned' datasets, and once these are defined, weights can be correctly assigned to the records to be reused.

Of the total 6867 patients in the common study base, 106 had a diagnosis of CBC, and 528 (148 cases and 380 controls) were in the metastases study. Stratified Kaplan-Meier weights were calculated for the controls to reflect the matched sampling. A weighted Cox regression was conducted using the unique individuals in the combined data.

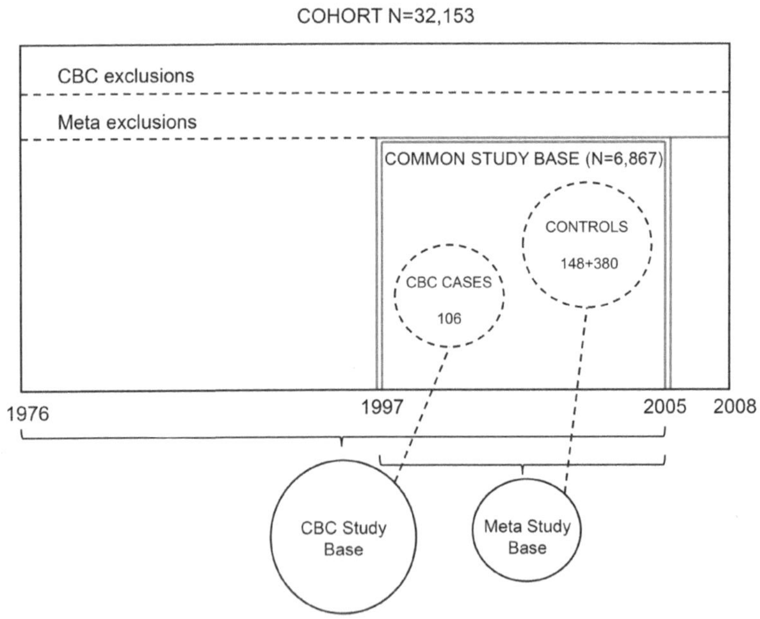

FIGURE 7.6: *Alignment of contralateral breast cancer (CBC) cases (1976–2005) with a matched nested case-control study of metastases (1997–2005). CBC cases were diagnosed at least 3 months after the initial cancer diagnosis and the metastases study had several inclusion criteria in addition to the matching.*

The first column of results in Table 7.3 presents some of the published estimates of the adjusted hazard ratios.

This analysis enabled the authors to conclude that a multifocal first tumor was a risk factor for CBC and that parity was negatively associated with the risk, after adjustment for known factors such as histology and family history. In the published results, similar estimates were obtained from an analysis that reused only controls. Prior cases will usually contribute only a small increase in efficiency as observed here, since they only have a weight of 1, while control weights may be large, especially for a large study base and rare outcome.

It is important to note that the weighted analysis provides a valid estimate of the association with treatment, although this was a matching factor (together with age group) in the data available. An interesting observation was that there was little or no change in the estimates if the weights were calculated from an 'imperfect' study base: the second column of results in Table 7.3 presents the estimates from using the study base from which the metastases study sample was drawn, rather than the (correct) common study base. When the study base is large, and consequently the risk sets are large throughout follow-up, then the imperfections in the exact risk set sizes will not exert much influence on the product in the Kaplan-Meier weights. This might often be of practical importance, as an investigator will usually have skeleton information

TABLE 7.3: *Weighted Cox regression analysis of contralateral breast cancer and reused data from a nested case-control study of metastases (from [48]).*

	Weighted Cox HR (95% C.I)	
Risk Factors	**Common Study Base**	**Metastases Study Base**
Multifocal tumor	1.99 (1.07, 3.70)	1.98 (1.07, 3.70)
Multiparous	0.40 (0.18, 0.89)	0.39 (0.18, 0.86)
Non-ductal histology	2.09 (1.21, 3.59)	2.11 (1.22, 3.66)
Positive family history	1.91 (1.11, 3.28)	1.92 (1.12, 3.32)
Treatment:		
Chemo (Ref)	1	1
Hormonal	0.71 (0.39, 1.26)	0.65 (0.36, 1.16)
Chemo + Hormonal	0.57 (0.30, 1.07)	0.57 (0.30, 1.07)

about the study base from which the cases arose, but is less likely to have such details for the study base of a prior investigation. However, for study bases that are small, highly stratified, or grow 'thin' over follow-up, it becomes more important to use the correct study base for weighting.

7.2.4 Supplementing controls

In the illustration in Figure 7.5 on page 275, the 5760 records in the prior nested case-control study of CHD only provided 1713 individuals that could contribute to the analysis of the 1257 stroke cases: only 1622 actually contributed data, as 91 of the 1713 were already present among the stroke cases. This resulted in a control to case ratio just a little over the minimum that would be considered in practice, i.e. a 1:1 nested case-control study. Where prior data are available, but not sufficient, investigators can use those data to supplement controls that have been explicitly sampled for the new cases. Using **supplementary control data** could result in significant cost savings, as fewer 'new' controls would be required to achieve the same statistical power as from implementing a standard nested case-control study of the new outcome.

In addition to identifying the overlapping study base, combining prior data with a new nested case-control sample also requires the data from these sources to be weighted appropriately. In the final dataset of individuals to be analysed by weighted Cox regression, the weight must be the inverse of the probability that an individual *is in the sample.* Since an individual might enter the sample from either study, the probabilities of being sampled in the two studies both need to enter the calculation. As before, it is simplest to calculate the probability that an individual is *not* sampled and subtract from 1. Denoting the prior study as A and the new study as B, then from Equation 6.4 of Chapter 6, the probabilities that an individual i is selected for a specific study is:

$$p_{iA} = 1 - \prod_j (1 - \frac{m_A}{R_{jA} - 1}) I[U_i = U_{jA}] \tag{7.1}$$

$$p_{iB} = 1 - \prod_j (1 - \frac{m_B}{R_{jB} - 1}) I[U_i = U_{jB}] \tag{7.2}$$

where the product is taken over all events j of type A in the first equation and of type B in the second, m_A and m_B are the ratios of controls to cases in the two studies, and U_{jA} and U_{jB} denote any matching factors. The probability that an individual is not selected for either study is:

$$(1 - p_i) = (1 - p_{iA})(1 - p_{iB}) \tag{7.3}$$

If Study A individuals had been analysed by IPW, the sampling weights would be the inverse of p_{iA}, and likewise for Study B individuals if the matching was broken. Thus, if the weights appropriate to just Study A and just Study B are known, the combined weight can be computed as follows:

$$\begin{aligned}(1 - p_i) &= (1 - p_{iA})(1 - p_{iB}) \\ &= (1 - \frac{1}{w_A})(1 - \frac{1}{w_B}) \\ \implies p_i &= 1 - (1 - \frac{1}{w_A})(1 - \frac{1}{w_B}) \qquad (7.4) \\ w_{AB} &= \frac{1}{1 - (1 - \frac{1}{w_A})(1 - \frac{1}{w_B})} \qquad (7.5)\end{aligned}$$

where w_{AB} denotes the combined weight. The procedure is the same as previously, with just one record being retained for each individual in the final dataset for analysis. Note that any individual selected as a case in either study (and thus assigned a weight of 1 in that study) will have a weight of 1 in the combined analysis.

A flowchart outlining the data preparation for a combined analysis of a nested case-control study supplemented with prior controls is presented in Figure 7.7. For a new outcome of interest (Outcome B), the nested case-control sample is represented on the right. On breaking the matching, the unique individuals can be combined with the unique controls from a prior nested case-control study of outcome A (on the left) in the same study base. Using information from the study base, the individuals from these two sources can be weighted to reflect the probabilities of being sampled *in each study* (i.e. not only the study where they were actually sampled). On combining the two datasets, only one record is retained for each individual: for individuals who appear as a control in both datasets, the information is duplicated, so one record is dropped; for a case (of outcome B) who was also a prior control, the case record is retained.

As a practical example, a 1:1 case-control sample was selected for the 2995 stroke cases in Figure 7.2 on page 269. The conditional logistic regression of the matched sets is less efficient than the weighted Cox

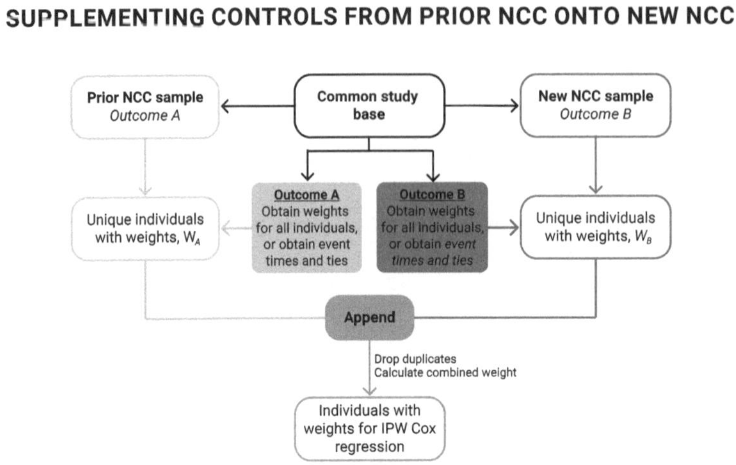

FIGURE 7.7: *flowchart illustrating the steps required to combine and weight data from two nested case-control studies. The combined weight is expressed in terms of the two separate weights in Equation 7.5.*

regression of the 5648 unique individuals (first and second column of Table 7.4). When these data records were supplemented with unique controls sampled for a 1:2 nested case-control study of CHD in the same cohort, the resulting dataset had 7486 unique individuals. The estimates from the weighted Cox regression are presented in the third column of results in Table 7.4. There is a further gain in efficiency from using the prior controls, although the ratio of controls to cases in the analysed sample of 7486 is only approximately 1.5.

TABLE 7.4: *Results from analysis of stroke in a 1:1 nested case-control sample from the simulated Singapore Chinese Health Study cohort, before and after supplementing the data with controls from a nested case-control sample of CHD in the same cohort.*

	Conditional logistic n=5990	**IPW 1:1 NCC n=5648**	**IPW 1:1 NCC Supplemented n=7486**
Age 75–84	1.21 (1.01, 1.46)	1.21 (1.02, 1.43)	1.20 (1.04, 1.39)
Age 85+	1.27 (0.49, 3.31)	1.18 (0.50, 2.74)	1.18 (0.58, 2.41)
Sex	0.83 (0.74, 0.94)	0.79 (0.71, 0.88)	0.84 (0.76, 0.92)
Smoker	1.40 (1.21, 1.62)	1.39 (1.21, 1.59)	1.36 (1.21, 1.53)
Hypertension	4.31 (3.79, 4.89)	4.38 (3.92, 4.90)	4.58 (4.13, 5.07)

The ability to break the matching of nested case-control data and conduct weighted Cox regression, enables a small nested case-control study to be supplemented with controls from a prior study. This results in improved cost efficiency due to the reduced data collection and the increased statistical efficiency from using a weighted Cox regression rather than conditional logistic regression.

7.2.5 Combining two nested case-control studies

In the examples above, only the controls from a prior nested case-control study were used as supplementary data in the study of a new outcome. However, a valid analysis can also be conducted using all prior records from a nested case-control study to supplement another nested-case control study, i.e. data from two case-control studies are combined and analysed. The paper that provided the explicit expressions for computing the probability of (not) being sampled in either of two studies (Equations 7.1– 7.3), provides an application of the methodology to the analysis of risk factors for anorexia using data from a study of schizophrenia [182]. The cases of anorexia were 781 girls born in Sweden between 1978 and 1984, who were diagnosed between the age of 10 and 21 years. Five controls were selected per case, from girls born in the same calendar year, in the same hospital, and the study investigated the association between anorexia nervosa and several factors measured at birth[33]. Here we focus on two of the risk factors: gestational age and birth trauma, both coded as binary variables.

For the purpose of illustration, only one randomly selected control is retained for each of the anorexia cases, to emphasise the boost in the efficiency of this small study when combined with data from an earlier nested case–control study. The earlier study with data available was a study of schizophrenia and other psychosis in 657 children born in Sweden between 1973 and 1979 [89]. For this study, 5 controls per case had been sampled from the risk sets at each event time, matched on sex, year of birth and hospital. The cases from this study included 274 girls, who together with their 5 controls (matched on year and hospital of birth) provide data for reuse in the analysis of anorexia. However, the prior study did not include information on whether or when the subjects were diagnosed with anorexia, so this information had to first be obtained by linking them to the Swedish hospital discharge register, using their unique national identifier.

TABLE 7.5: *Weighted likelihood analysis of anorexia data with one control per case combined with 1644 data records from a 1:5 case-control study of schizophrenia in an overlapping cohort (results derived from [182]).*

	Gestational age < 33 weeks		Birth Trauma	
	HR	**95% C.I.**	**HR**	**95% C.I.**
Exponential baseline	2.20	(1.06, 4.55)	1.66	(1.10, 2.51)
Weibull baseline	2.16	(1.03, 4.51)	1.59	(1.04, 2.42)
Cox prop. hazards	2.17		1.59	

On breaking the matching of both studies, the individuals need to be weighted by the inverse of the probability that they were sampled into either study. The sampling probabilites in the two studies (Equations 7.1 and 7.2) were first computed using the numbers of girls born in each year and hospital (available from the national birth register). These probabilities were inverted to give the separate weights, which were then combined (Equation 7.5). The original publication that reused these data [182] reported the coefficients from weighted Cox regression and also from weighted likelihood analyses that did not assume proportional hazards. These are presented as hazard ratios in Table 7.5. The HRs from weighted Cox regression reported in the publication were similar to the estimates from both of the weighted likelihood analyses, and almost identical to the results using a Weibull baseline hazard. In practice, the data analyst can check the proportional hazards assumption before reporting the results from a Cox regression, by inspecting the Schoenfield residuals that are provided with the output from the regression model: in this application, there was no evidence against the proportional hazards assumption.

There was a marked increase in power from combining the 1:1 anorexia data with the prior schizophrenia data, reflected in the much narrower confidence intervals: the 95% confidence intervals for the HR for premature birth and birth trauma from analysis of the schizophrenia data alone were (1.16, 10.84) and (1.13, 3.42) respectively.

7.3 Value of Reused Data

The previous sections illustrated the feasibility of reusing nested case-control data in the analysis of a new outcome in the same study base. One possibility is to gather no controls for the new cases and instead rely on the available records (or just the controls) from a previous study. If the available prior data is insufficient, then some controls can also be sampled for the new cases and combined with the prior data for analysis. These decisions regarding the study design depend on the statistical power. Power calculation for a standard nested case-control study is straightforward, but if data from a prior study are to be appended to the case-control sample, one needs to also estimate the additional information in this sample of individuals who were *not* selected as controls for the outcome now being studied. Clearly, these reused records will be less informative if they are very different to the control records that would have been selected for the new cases: for example, if the prior and new events tend to occur in a different age range.

The value of reused data was examined in a simulation study [184] in order to provide some practical guidelines on the potential gain in power from reusing prior data. Two time-to-event outcomes were generated in a simulated cohort of 5,000 individuals, where the hazard ratios (for age, gender and a binary exposure that depended on age and gender) differed for the two outcomes. For each of the simulated cohorts, a matched nested case-control study was sampled for each of the two outcomes, using different control to case ratios, with cases matched to controls of the same gender and age category. For the event representing the 'new' outcome, a ratio of 0 (i.e. a sample consisting of cases only) was also considered.

For 500 repetitions of the simulation followed by sampling, the 'new' outcome was analysed by standard conditional logistic regression, and weighted Cox regression was used to analyse the combined data from both outcomes. The efficiency of the combined study relative to the new study was expressed as the ratio of the estimated variance of the exposure coefficient, β (i.e. the ln(HR), from the two analyses. The reduction in variance from the combined analysis depends on the magnitude of the exposure effect, β, the number m of controls sampled per case of the new outcome, as well as the number of prior data records available relative to the number of new cases to be analysed. If the size of the prior dataset is m_p times the number of cases of the new outcome, it is clear that the combined data from an $m : 1$ case-control study and the records from a prior study is equivalent to a newly sampled $m' : 1$ case-control study where $m < m' < m + m_p$ since the reused records are not as informative as those selected explicitly for the new outcome. Thus we would expect that combining a new 1:3 case-control study with a prior dataset of any size will not lead to large gains in efficiency, as a 1:3 case-control ratio already captures a large proportion of the information in the whole cohort (the $M/(M+1)$ rule). Greater gains are possible where fewer controls are sampled for the new cases: an example of a 1:1 nested case-control study combined with prior data on three times as many subjects as the cases [184] had a relative efficiency of 0.7, which means a reduction of 30% in the variance.

Figure 7.8(a) presents the average of the variances for a HR=1.2, from the analysis of only prior control data and analysis using a standard nested case-control sample. From this plot it can be seen that a new 1:2 case-control study (the solid line) has the same variance as a reused dataset that has four times as many records as the number of cases of the new outcome: one can say that with the reused data records, the **effective number of controls** per case is 2. Expressing any combination of the prior records and controls per case in this way leads to Figure 7.8(c). When the cases of study A and study B differ with respect to their covariate profile (in particular, the matching factors), the reused controls will be less 'effective'. An example of this can be seen in Figure 7.8(b) and (d), which are the results from a simulation where there was less overlap in the covariates of the individuals with the two outcomes: compared to plot (c), where 4 reused controls were as effective as 2 newly-sampled controls, the plot in (d) indicates that 4 reused controls are not even as effective as one new control.

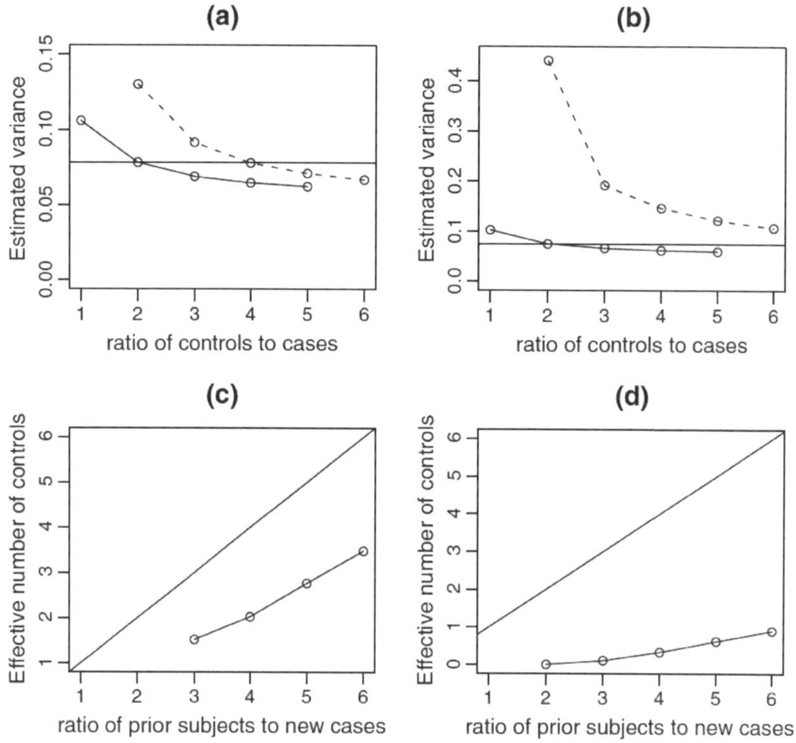

FIGURE 7.8: ***(a)****Average over 500 simulations of the variances of an exposure coefficient of 0.18 (HR = 1.2), using only prior control data (dashed line) and a nested case-control sample (solid line).* ***(c)*** *Transformation of (a) to express the number of reused subjects equivalent to (fewer) new controls. For plots* ***(b)*** *and* ***(d)****, the covariate profiles of the prior cases and new cases were less similar (plot reproduced from [184] with permission).*

7.4 Analysis of Subgroups from Nested Case-control Data

There are many published examples of data from a case-control study being used to investigate an exposure in greater detail for a subgroup of interest. This investigation may involve only the data collected in the original study, with the analysis using more complex models, for example including interactions that are important only in the subgroup. Such subgroup analysis may be presented as supplementary results with the main findings of the case-control study, or could be undertaken as stand-alone analysis at a later time when the hypothesis of interest arises. However, there are also situations where the research question concerning the subgroup involves additional data collection, such as laboratory assays of specimens that had been collected and stored at the time of enrolment into the original study.

If the original study was a nested case-control design, perhaps with additional matching on a confounder, then the traditional approach to analysis is conditional logistic regression of the matched sets. This is also be a valid approach to the analysis of the subgroup, although it could be highly inefficient. If the subgroup is defined by a characteristic that is rare in the study population, then the conditional analysis includes only the risk sets where cases and controls have this characteristic. In the situation where the characteristic was a matching factor, any case belonging to the subgroup enters the analysis together with their matched controls, provided they are not concordant for exposure. For example, if the nested case-control study had been matched on age group and sex, analysis of only males (or females) or of a specific age group would include all cases in the group of interest and all their matched controls. However, if the subgroup is defined by some other risk factor, or an unmatched confounder or effect modifier, then a matched set can only enter the analysis if the case and at least one control belong to the subgroup.

In the simple example of matching on age and sex, analysis of only individuals with a specific level of education will include cases who belong to that group and any of their controls who have the same education level. Thus the loss of risk sets from the analysis will depend not only on the proportion of the population that belongs to the subgroup of interest, but on how the characteristic defining the subgroup is correlated with the outcome and matching factor(s) of the original study. The loss of risk sets will be further exasperated by a rare exposure, as seen in Section 6.5.1 of Chapter 6, where 1006 of the 3489 risk sets were dropped due to the case and their matched controls being concordant for the main exposure of interest (preeclampsia).

It is clear from these considerations, that breaking the matching and conducting a weighted Cox regression offers the potential for more efficient subgroup analysis. The performance of the weighted analysis in estimating an exposure effect in subgroups was examined in a simulation study [49] where the subgroups were defined by various variables in a nested case-control study: a matching factor, another unmatched confounder, an effect modifier, or an independent risk factor. Using the sampling weights (stratified if the study was matched) not only enabled the cohort to be reconstructed as seen in Figure 6.4 of Chapter 6, but also recovered the numbers of individuals in the various subgroups [49]. The weighted analysis offered valid estimates that were more efficient than those from conditional logistic regression, and in many instances similar to the full cohort analysis (see Figure 7.9). The authors found the weighted estimates to have good accuracy and precision, Even in an extreme setting and when using the unstratified weights despite stratified sampling.

Returning to the illustration in section 6.5.2 in Chapter 6, the cohort of 15,727 siblings of the NHL patients were analysed by Cox regression to estimate the hazard ratio for siblings of a female patient compared to siblings of a male patient [49]. The time scale was the age of the sibling. In addition to the main exposure of interest (sex of patient), the model included the calendar year of birth as an independent risk factor, and to accommodate potential effect modification, an interaction

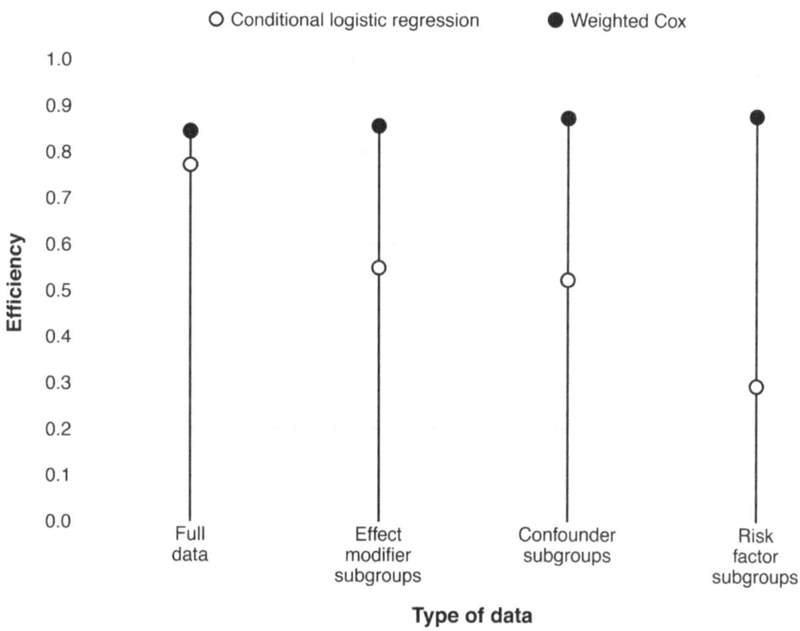

FIGURE 7.9: *Efficiency (relative to a full cohort analysis) of the HR estimates from nested case-control data, for subgroups defined by different variables, from a simulation study [49]. The nested case-control data was analysed using conditional logistic regression and weighted Cox regression.*

between the sex of the patient and sex of their sibling. Thus in the analysis of the full cohort of siblings with male sex as reference, the coefficient of patient sex in the model estimates the ln(HR) for brothers of female patients (compared to brothers of male patients) and the sum of the coefficients for patient sex and the interaction term provides an estimate of the ln(HR) for sisters of female patients compared to sisters of male patients. The same estimates can be obtained from a separate analysis of each of the two subcohorts (brothers and sisters of patients) using the simpler model with no interaction term. These 'full cohort' estimates of the hazard ratios in the two subgroups were compared to the average estimates obtained from fitting the same models to one hundred unmatched 1:2 nested case-control samples.

From the results presented in Figure 7.10, the risk of NHL in brothers of patients has little or no association with the sex of the patient, while for sisters of patients, the hazard when the patient is female is more than twice as high as when the patient is male ($HR = e^{0.979} = 2.66$). The weighted Cox regression was more efficient than conditional logistic regression for the subgroup analysis. The authors also reported unbiased results for nested case-control sampling matched on the sex of the sibling (i.e. the effect modifier).

7.4.1 Subgroups defined by outcome

Following a nested case-control study, it may be of interest to analyse a subgroup defined by the outcome. For example, cancer epidemiologists are often interested to conduct analysis of one or more subtypes. If conditional logistic regression is used for analysis of a given subtype, then only the controls selected for those specific cases (i.e. the selected risk sets) are included. However, all controls in the larger study will be cancer-free at their selection time, and thus constitute an appropriate comparison group for any site-specific cancer. For example, in a nested case-control study investigating high sensitivity C reactive protein as a risk factor for lung cancer [155], the authors conducted analyses of the five histological subtypes (large cell, small cell, squamous cell, adenocarcinoma and other). The study was a 1:1 nested case-control design, so that all the conditional logistic regression analyses were based on case-control pairs, resulting in small sample size for the rarer subtypes. For example, there were only 173 cases of large cell carcinoma, and in all analyses, the confidence interval for the HR was wide and included 1. If the information for re-weighting is available for the underlying cohort, the matching could be broken and any control records used in a weighted Cox regression of a specific subtype. In particular, this might be a better use of the 1186 controls for whom the corresponding case's subtype was unknown. It would also make fuller use of the results from the biochemical analysis of the frozen plasma or serum samples that had been obtained from cohort members at baseline.

Another situation that may arise is in the study of a **subsequent event**, where a second (rare) event may occur at some time after a first event, such as cancer-specific death (second event) following cancer diagnosis (first event). Such data may accrue following a nested case-control study of incident disease, when vital status and cause of death of the original study participants becomes available from more recent health or population records. A conditional logistic regression analysis to estimate the association between exposure and the second event (cancer-specific death) would make use of only those cases and their matched controls (who have not had the second event). However, if the matching is broken, much more information is available from the data, as any control who has not had the second event can contribute to a weighted analysis. This was illustrated in an analysis of the association between vitamin D

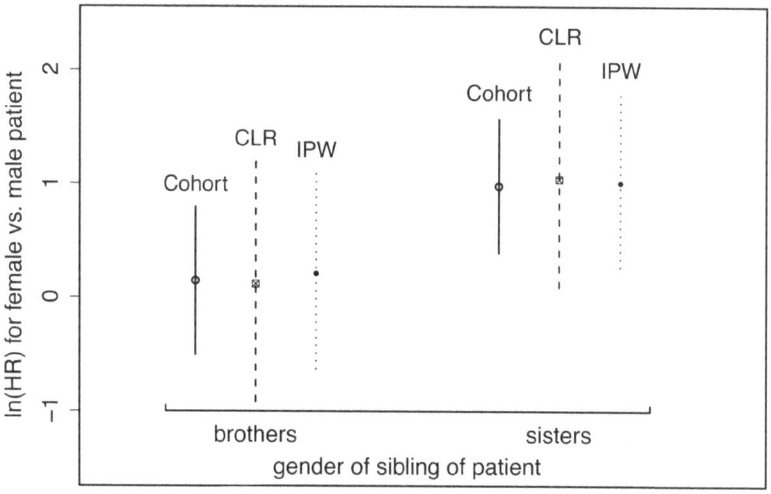

FIGURE 7.10: *Estimates and 95% confidence intervals for the ln(HR) of NHL in siblings of female vs. male patients, obtained from combined and stratified analysis of the full cohort data, compared to the average estimates from 100 nested case-control samples analysed by conditional logistic regression (CLR) and weighted Cox regression (IPW).*

and lethal prostate cancer (death from prostate cancer) using the data from a nested case-control study of vitamin D and prostate cancer incidence [205]. The setting was based on a real cohort of 15949 Norwegian men with blood samples taken at their enrolment into a health survey, who were followed up for approximately 20 years. During this time, 698 were diagnosed with prostate cancer, among whom 162 subsequently died from prostate cancer. The results from 1000 simulations mimicking the real data illustrated a large gain in efficiency for the analysis of prostate cancer death from breaking the matching and using all the control information in a weighted analysis: a standard error only 16% larger than that obtained from the whole cohort, whereas the standard error from the conditional analysis was almost 50% larger.

7.5 Conclusion

It will be clear from the many examples presented in this chapter, that where a population or large cohort has basic information for all members, this **skeleton cohort** [185] makes it possible to reuse nested case-control data in various ways: to estimate absolute risk in the underlying cohort, to conduct analysis of a subgroup, to supplement controls in the study of a new outcome, or where the available nested case-control data is sufficient, to dispense with the need to sample any controls for the new cases. The ability to obtain valid estimates from reused data can result in significant savings. Where subjects in a case-control study have been identified from national registers, the basic information in the registers can be viewed as the 'skeleton cohort' from which the subsample of selected individuals are studied in more depth. Thus studies sampled using national registers result in data that, provided ethical approval is obtained, can easily be reused for addressing other research questions using the same variables, or providing or supplementing controls in a new investigation.

7.6 Exercises

1. Referring to Figure 7.1 of Chapter 7 (provided below), if individual 15 had not been sampled as a control prior to becoming a case, would their contribution to the weighted analysis change? Explain.

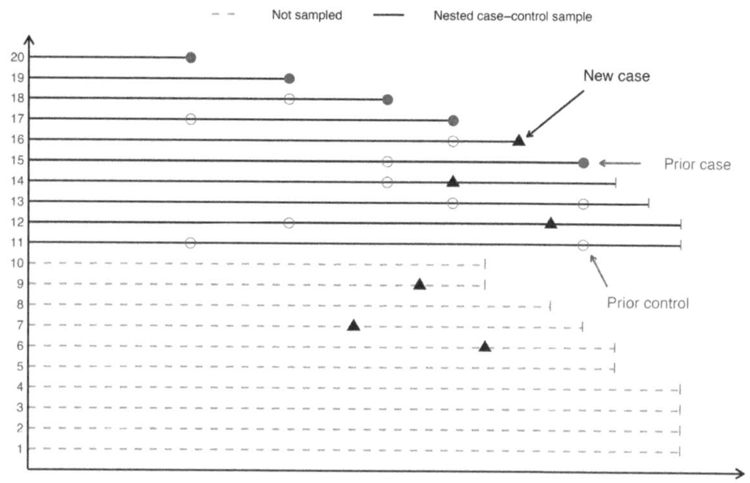

2. Table 7.1 in Chapter 7 presents results from weighted analyses of prior nested case-control data using all individuals and using only control individuals. Explain why these results are very similar.

3. For the illustration in Section 7.2.1 on reusing CHD controls for stroke cases:

   (i) If the nested case-control study of CHD had investigated only individuals aged 60 years or older, would the weights used for the stroke analysis be the same? Why/why not?

   (ii) If the study of CHD was a *matched* nested case-control study, and stroke was subsequently studied within one (or a subset) of the matching strata, would the weights be the same or different than for the original study? Explain.

   (iii) The the simulated dataset `full_cohort_new` is the same as the dataset (`full_cohort.dta`) used in the exercises in Chapters 4 and 6, but in addition to the CHD outcome (with indicator and time `event` and `t`) there are also variables for a stroke outcome (`event_stroke` and `t_stroke`). The dataset `ncc_absrisk_sample.dta` is a 1:2 nested case-control sample of CHD from the cohort.

Select a 1:2 nested case-control study of individuals aged 60 years and older from the cohort, compute the weights for these controls, and compare to the weights for the sample `ncc_absrisk_sample.dta` to verify your conclusion in (i).

(iv) Repeat the sampling in (iii) for a study matched on sex to verify your conclusion in (ii)

(v) Imagine if instead of selecting a new sample from individuals over 60, you had to use the original nested case-control sample, dropping every body under 60.

(a) What is the disadvantage of this compared to part (iii)?
(b) What weights would be used?
(c) If you were to analyse the data with conditional logistic regression, compare the sample size available to the sample available from part (iii).

Implement the sampling and weighted analysis of the data described in (v) with the simulated cohort and compare your results with part (iii).

4. For the illustration in Section 7.2.1 of Chapter 7, re-draw Figure 7.2 as far as the **merge** and **append** steps to outline the datasets, describing who is included and how many would be analysed in each of the following situations:

(a) If the cases in the original nested case-control study of CHD should have no history of stroke
(b) If in the study of stroke, the cases of stroke should have no history of CHD.

How would the computation of weights change in these two analyses compared to the situation where there are no restrictions (as in the illustration in Section 7.2)?

5. For the lung cancer subtype analysis in *Circulating high sensitivity C reactive protein concentrations and risk of lung cancer: nested case-control study within Lung Cancer Cohort Consortium* by Muller et al in BMJ 2019 (DOI: 10.1136/bmj.k4981):

    (i) What skeleton data would be required to conduct an IPW analysis?

    (ii) Suggest some difficulties that could be encountered with access to such data.

    (iii) Consider an imperfect weighting scheme using readily-available data that would be accessible and consider how one could still obtain valid estimates by referring to *Inverse probability weighting in nested case-control studies with additional matching–a simulation study* by Stoer and Samuelsen in Stat Med 2013.

    (iv) Suggest any other way of obtaining the probabilities for the IPW analysis.

8

More Complex Designs

8.1 Case-cohort Design as a Two-stage Study

Chapter 3 introduced 'two-stage' studies of a binary outcome and illustrated how to analyse the data using weighted logistic regression. However, as seen in the subsequent chapters, many cohort studies investigate a time-to-event outcome that is analysed using Cox regression. The case-cohort design introduced in Chapter 4 is an example of such two-stage design, where the subcohort and any additional cases are the 'second-stage' observations for which all exposure information is available, while the remaining members of the cohort will only have their event/censoring status, and perhaps some easily-obtained explanatory variables. The case-cohort study was introduced in Chapter 4 as a design that was implemented for a prospective cohort study. Thus the subcohort was selected at baseline to have all details gathered and be followed up for the study period, during which time any cases occurring outside the subcohort also had their details recorded. For the remaining cohort members, it is only necessary to record the event/censoring time.

A case-cohort study may also be conducted retrospectively within an existing cohort. In this setting, the investigator would choose all cases that occurred during follow-up and a randomly sampled proportion p of non-cases. The reader will recognise that this is simply a two-stage design, with sampling fraction 1 (for cases) and $1/p$ for non-cases. These data can be validly analysed by specifying the sampling probabilities in a weighted Cox regression, or using custom-written software commands for case-cohort analysis.

8.1.1 Stratified case-cohort

The motivation for a case-cohort study is to enable efficient estimation of an exposure effect from information collected only from a fraction of the whole cohort (called the subcohort) and from all the cases. In the simplest case-cohort design described above, and illustrated in Figure 4.13 in Chapter 4, the subcohort is a random sample of the whole cohort at the start of follow-up. However, this efficiency can be further improved in situations where there is a variable known for all members of the cohort that is correlated with the exposure of interest that is to be measured in the case-cohort study. An example of such a variable is a 'surrogate' of the exposure, such as a crude classification of exposure as low, medium and high. The stratified case-cohort design, first proposed in 2001 [15], selects a sample that is stratified on this surrogate, rather than a completely random sample. This ensures a better range of exposure values, which in turn can lead to better precision. For example, if BMI is to be measured as a continuous variable in a case-cohort study, where a three-level surrogate of BMI (underweight, normal, overweight) is available for the whole cohort, then stratified sampling can be beneficial. In our example of a case-cohort study of postpartum VTE in Chapter 4, maternal age was classified with a binary indicator for 'advanced maternal age' (35 years or older). This could be used to conduct a stratified case-cohort study where the effect of age (in years) was of interest.

In general, the stratum variable has levels 1,2, ... L, and Figure 8.1 presents a simple illustration of a stratified case-cohort study for $L = 2$, i.e. where the subcohort is selected by stratified random sampling from two strata. Denoting the number of individuals in the cohort that belong to a specific stratum l by N^l and the number of these that are selected into the subcohort as n^l, then the sampling fraction in stratum l is

$$p_l = \frac{n^l}{N^l}$$

Likewise, if a case-cohort study is conducted retrospectively by selecting all cases and a subsample of non-cases from an existing cohort, the sampling fraction of non-cases in stratum l is $p_l = \frac{n_0^l}{N_0^l}$, where the suffix 0 denotes a non-case. By using the inverse of these sampling fractions as weights for the non-cases, and a weight of 1 for cases, the same likelihood structure as in Equation 4.23 in Chapter 4 provides the estimate of the HR (see Equation 8.1). Thus the only modification to the random subcohort likelihood in Chapter 4 is that the weights for the controls now differ by stratum to reflect the sampling.

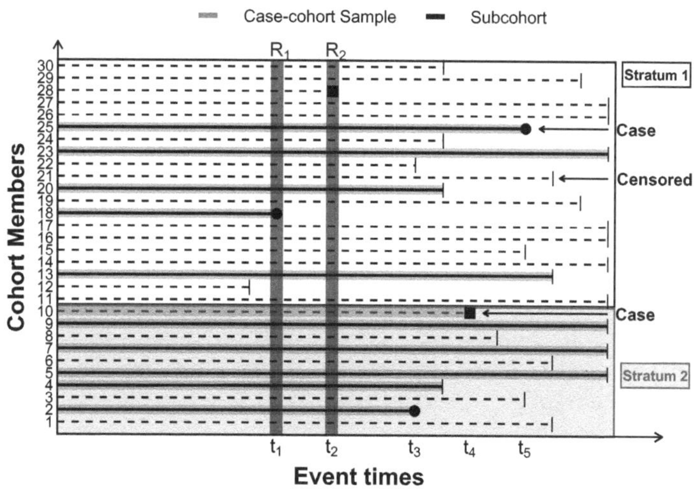

Hazard for case i $\quad h_0(t)e^{\beta X_i}$

Hazard for sub-cohort at t_i $\quad \sum_{l=1,2}\sum_{j\in S_i^l} h_0(t)e^{\beta X_j}$

S_i^l sub-cohort in stratum l at risk at t_i

Likelihood (IPW) $\quad \prod_i \frac{e^{\beta X_i}}{\sum_{l=1,2}\sum_{k\epsilon S_i^{l\#}} w_l e^{\beta X_k}}$

$S_i^{l\#}$ sub-cohort and cases in stratum l at risk at t_i

$w_l = 1$ for cases and $\frac{1}{p_l}$ for controls

FIGURE 8.1: *Stratified case-cohort sample (highlighting the risk sets R_1 and R_2 at the first two events), where S_i^l denotes subcohort members in stratum l who are at risk at time t_i, and $S_i^{l\#}$ denotes this subcohort supplemented with all cases in stratum l who are at risk at time t_i.*

$$\textbf{Likelihood (IPW)} = \prod_{t_i} \frac{e^{\beta X_i}}{\sum_{l=1}^{l=L}\sum_{k\epsilon S_i^{l\#}}[e^{\beta X_k} w_k]} \tag{8.1}$$

where $w_k = 1$ if individual k is a case

$$w_k = \frac{1}{p_l}\text{for a control in stratum } \ell$$

The likelihoods for random and stratified sampling are compared in Table 8.1. Since all controls in the same stratum will have the same weight, it is a simple data management task to assign the weights before running the weighted Cox regression. However, the robust variance can be much too conservative. A few simple R commands for computing the variance estimate have been available since 2007 (Figure 1 in [186]) and an R package **cchs** for stratified case-cohort studies is available since 2018. Alternatively, any standard software that allows weighting can use the IPW approach, which has been shown to perform well [186].

TABLE 8.1: *Comparison of risk sets and weights for case-cohort and stratified case-cohort design.*

Design	Likelihood	Risk Set
Case-cohort	$\prod_{t_i} \frac{e^{\beta X_i + \gamma Z_i}}{\sum_{k \epsilon \boldsymbol{S}_i^{\#}} \boldsymbol{w_k} e^{\beta X_k + \gamma Z_k}}$	$\mathbf{S_i}^{\#}$: All members of the subcohort and cases outside the subcohort who are at risk t_i. $\mathbf{w_k}$: the weight assigned to individual k. Assuming the case-cohort sample consists of all cases in the full cohort and a fraction p of non-cases: $\mathbf{w_k}$ =1 if individual k is a case $\mathbf{w_k} = \frac{1}{p}$ if individual k is a control
Stratified case-cohort	$\prod_{t_i} \frac{e^{\beta X_i + \gamma Z_i}}{\sum_{k \epsilon \boldsymbol{S_i}^{\ell\#}} \boldsymbol{w_k} e^{\beta X_k + \gamma Z_k}}$	$\mathbf{S_i}^{\ell\#}$: All members of the subcohort and all cases outside the subcohort who are in stratum l (l=1,2 ...L) and are at risk at time t_i. For non-cases, the sampling fraction depends on the stratum. $\mathbf{w_k}$ =1 if individual k is a case $\mathbf{w_k} = \frac{1}{p_l}$ for controls in stratum ℓ

8.1.2 Post-stratification

Further efficiency gains are possible in a case-cohort study conducted within a cohort where the censoring time is known for all members [30]. The procedure includes the information contained in the censoring times as follows:

- Conduct a case-cohort study, with random or stratified sampling
- group the censoring times into intervals
- obtain the frequency distribution of the censoring intervals in the cohort
- conduct the analysis with the censoring interval as a stratification variable

The grouping of censoring times should be chosen to have a reasonable number of censored subcohort members in each interval, since their proportion relative to all cohort members censored in the same time interval is used (i.e. inverted) to obtain the weights for analysis.

The term **post**-stratification (also called 'local averaging') refers to the fact that the study sample is assigned to these strata after they have been sampled, in contrast to stratified sampling of a subcohort of individuals selected at random from pre-defined strata. The gain in efficiency from such after-the-fact classification can be understood intuitively by considering that some of the reasons for censoring may be due to characteristics of the study subjects that have not been measured, so that the censoring time can capture information additional to what is available in the collected data. As a simple example, if cohort members in a few cities or geographic locations had been censored at specific times following (local) public criticism of the cohort study, then the censoring variable carries demographic information. Censoring due to death from causes unrelated to the outcome under study would carry information about comorbidity or frailty that could contribute to more precise estimation of the effects of the exposures of interest.

8.2 Optimal Two-stage Designs for Binary Outcome

Chapter 3 introduced 'two-stage' studies of a binary outcome and illustrated how to analyse the data using weighted logistic regression. Such data might arise from a planned two-stage study, where investigators gather some information only for a subset of the study subjects. These data will often be expensive or difficult to obtain, such as dietary factors or biochemical and genetic markers. Thus the objective of the two-stage design is a practical one, to reduce the time and/or cost of the study by collecting the more difficult/expensive information for a subsample of subjects. This 'second-stage sample' may be selected by simple random sampling, or by stratified random sampling within strata defined by the 'first stage' information that is available for all subjects: for example the strata defined by the binary outcome and one or more confounders or surrogates of exposure. Two-stage data collection may also arise in situations that were not planned in advance. For example, investigators may realise during the study that there are insufficient resources to gather an expensive variable for all study participants, or may become aware of an important variable that has been overlooked in the data collection so far.

For the study of post-menopausal breast cancer described in Chapter 3 [55] the description of the sampling suggests that there were several revisions of the remaining budget that led to the inclusion of additional laboratory analyses. The resulting design, where women with more exposure to HRT are over-sampled for genetic analysis, is thus a consequence of efforts to optimise resources, by sampling the women that investigators perceived to be more informative. In the study of chlamydia and ectopic pregnancy [194] introduced in Chapter 3, both an overlooked variable and insufficient resources contributed to the final design. When investigators became aware of the importance of chlamydia antibody testing, they did not make plans to collect serum samples from all (remaining) study participants, but from all cases and a subsample of controls, with over-sampling of black women. Another example presented in Chapter 3 was a cross-sectional study of H. Pylori in schoolchildren in Stockholm [106], where investigators determined the H.pylori infection status of the family members of all children from 4 of the 11 schools and just the infected children from the other 7 schools. These families were thought to be more 'informative', as they would ensure better representation of children with immigrant background and lower socioeconomic status

(SES), both of which were demonstrated risk factors for H. Pylori infection.

In all of the studies described in the previous paragraph, the investigators were faced with two questions regarding the subsample of individuals from whom to collect laboratory measurements:

- how many individuals to sample?
- which individuals?

Presumably the number sampled was dictated by simple considerations of time and cost, and in the breast cancer study [55], it appears that there were several revisions/recalculations of the affordable sample size. The choice of which individuals to sample may be somewhat ad hoc, but it is clear from all three studies that investigators had prior evidence, or at least intuition, regarding which individuals they considered most 'informative' for their research question.

In these examples and others in Chapter 3, the data had already been gathered and the focus was on how to analyse it efficiently using weighted logistic regression. But what if investigators wish to *plan* a two-stage study from the beginning? How can they design an 'efficient' two-stage study, that makes the best use of available resources to collect data that will be adequate to address the research question of interest? This is not a new problem. Optimal sampling has long concerned medical investigators, particularly in case-control studies. Common designs have equal numbers of cases and controls, overall or within strata, and we have already encountered these 'balanced' designs in Chapter 6. However, a simple balance of numbers is not necessarily optimum when there are different costs associated with collecting data from different individuals, for example from a case versus a control or from individuals in certain strata such as categories of age or occupation (e.g. schoolchildren or adults in the workplace). Another important consideration is whether the 'information' contributed by an individual is different across strata, as perceived by the investigators in the studies described in the previous paragraph.

Since the 1960s, methods for designing more efficient studies have been published in the statistical and epidemiological literature, with many researchers addressing the important consideration of cost. The early work in survey sampling [34] and in medical applications [159] showed that if a fixed budget is available for a study where the cost for each study subject is C_1 for a case (or treated) individual and C_0 for a control, then the optimal ratio of controls to cases (for maximum power to test the hypothesis of no effect) is the square root of the ratio of the cost per case to the cost per control, i.e. the case and control sample sizes are in inverse proportion to the (square root) of the costs.

$$\frac{n_0}{n_1} = \sqrt{\frac{C_1}{C_0}} \tag{8.2}$$

A later paper [160] extended these findings to matched case-control studies, where the cost per case C_1 was fixed, but the cost per control varied between strata. Unlike the earlier work [159], the fixed total cost C was now the budget available for sampling controls, as it was assumed that all case information was already available. The authors derived an expression for the control to case ratio in each of the strata that would result in the estimate of the common odds ratio having greatest efficiency (i.e. minimum variance). These sampling fractions depend on the true adjusted odds ratio, so an external estimate, or range of estimates, is needed. The design was shown to maximise the power of Cochran's test of an association when the true adjusted odds ratio is 1 [159]. Equal numbers of cases and controls is optimal when $C_0 = C_1$ *and* the exposure rate is the same in all strata. This is consistent with a presentation a couple of years previously, of the 'balanced design' as an efficient approach for sampling the cases and non-cases at the second stage of a two-stage study of a binary outcome [28].

8.2.1 Optimal sampling

The concept of **optimal design** in the previous paragraph referred to the choice of the ratio of controls to cases that maximises power or efficiency. However, in the practical examples of two-stage studies introduced in Chapter 3 and summarised earlier in this chapter, investigators were faced with the decision regarding how many and/or whom, to sample at the second stage for the most 'efficient' study. The 'balanced sample' [28] provides a simple suggestion, but does not consider costs. The work that does consider costs ([159], [160]), refers only to a case-control design, and not to other first-stage designs, nor to optimal second-stage sampling. In addition, the differential cost of a case and control that is considered in that work, is not the issue in the illustrative examples, nor in most practical applications, where it is the (high) cost of an exposure that results is this information only being gathered for a subsample. Although the first-stage sample size was already decided in all the applications presented earlier, it is reasonable to ask whether that too might be part of an optimal design that is derived before embarking on the study.

Here we will outline how one can derive optimal sampling designs for two-stage studies for the following three scenarios:

- Where first stage data is already available and a specified number of observations are to be sampled at the second stage: an example of this situation is where basic data is available from an existing database or registry, and additional information is to be gathered from some subjects in order to address a specific research question

- Where a coefficient of interest is to be estimated with a specified precision: the optimal design to be determined is the total first stage sample size and the numbers of second stage observations that will achieve the required precision for minimum cost

- Where a fixed budget is available and a study (first and second stage sample sizes) is to be designed to estimate the effect of an exposure with the maximum possible precision (i.e. minimum variance)

Section 3.2.1 of Chapter 3 introduced the weighted likelihood for two-stage data, where a binary outcome Y and other categorical variables, Z, are available for all (Stage 1) observations, and an exposure X (categorical or continuous) is available only for a subsample of Stage 2 observations. Estimates of the coefficients of interest are obtained by maximising the weighted likelihood, where the weights are the inverse of the sampling fractions, or equivalently by solving the corresponding (weighted) score equation. The first stage variable(s) Z, will typically include confounders, Z_c and perhaps an auxiliary/surrogate measure of X, Z_a. The second-stage sample is selected from the strata defined by the outcome and some components of Z, which we denote as Z_s, which may include confounders, auxiliary exposure or other covariates. The weighted score equation corresponding to that in Chapter 3 is:

$$\sum_{i \in 2^{nd} stage} \frac{N_{Z_{si}Y_i}}{n_{Z_{si}Y_i}} S_\beta(Y_i|X_i, Z_i') \tag{8.3}$$

where Z' includes variables of interest in the model, and excludes Z_a since the auxiliary variable for X no longer contributes to the model when the true X becomes available. Here the N and n used to weight each second-stage individual are the total number of subjects in the same sampling stratum, i.e. with $Z_s = Z_{si}$ and $Y = Y_i$. Thus the weights are the reciprocals of the sampling fractions, and this was our first encounter with inverse probability weighting. It was pointed out in Chapter 3, and for all the weighted regression analyses introduced in subsequent chapters, that a **robust standard error** should be used for the (weighted) estimate of the exposure coefficient.

The mathematical equations for computing the standard errors are beyond the scope of this book, but it is helpful to know that the computation depends on (i) the proportions of the total observations in the sample that are in each of the Z, Y strata, and (ii) the proportion of each Z, Y stratum that is selected for measuring X at the second stage. The first set of proportions will depend on the design chosen for the first stage of the study, for example whether cross-sectional or case-control, stratified or unstratified. However, for a given first-stage design, different choices of sampling fractions at the second-stage will result in different standard errors, so a good choice of sampling fractions is one that results in the smallest standard error!

Expressions for calculating these 'optimal' sampling fractions were derived [179] for the situation where a sample of first stage data (Y and Z) of size n are already available, and n_2 of these are to be sampled at the second stage. This is referred to as the **fixed sample size** scenario, as the sample sizes, both first and second stage, are already decided and the task is simply to distribute the agreed number of second stage subjects across the strata in the 'best' way. The formula for the optimal numbers to choose from each of the strata depends on the statistical 'information' in the strata about the exposure coefficient of interest and the proportion of the first-stage observations in each of the strata (the concept of statistical information is closely related to variance). Thus in addition to the estimated or observed proportions of observations in each of the first-stage strata, another ingredient is needed in order to estimate the information/variance components in the calculation of the optimal sampling fractions: some **pilot** second-stage data, i.e. a small number of observations selected at random from each of the strata.

Illustration using ectopic pregnancy data

To illustrate the optimal selection of a fixed number of second-stage subjects, consider again the ectopic pregnancy example from Section 3.1.1 of

Chapter 3. The total sample size was 979, among whom there were 264 cases of ectopic pregnancy and 715 controls. The variable that was only available for a subsample (of 327 women) was the result of a chlamydia antibody test. This second-stage sample was not selected randomly, but depended on case-control status and a number of other factors that investigators believed would enrich the sample. The data is provided with the Stata **meanscor** command and the analysis presented in the help file assumes the second-stage sampling depended on case/control status, history of gonorrhoea, use of contraceptives and multiple sexual partners. It will be left as an exercise for the reader to show that it is reasonable to assume that sampling had little or no dependence on history of gonorrhoea, and here we will assume that the women selected in each of the eight strata defined by case/control status, contraceptive use and multiple sexual partners, can be considered as representative of the stratum. Table 8.2 presents the total numbers of women in each of these eight strata together with the number (and %) sampled at the second stage. The second stage sample represents an overall proportion of 135/264=51% of cases and 192/715=27% of controls in the study.

As outlined in Chapter 3 and explained in the original publication [194], the selection of the 327 women for antibody testing was based on

TABLE 8.2: *Number of observations, N, in each of the strata defined by case/control status, contraceptive use and multiple sexual partners, in a case-control study of ectopic pregnancy [179], and number n and percent of each stratum with chlamydia antibody results available.*

Stratum	Case/ Control	Contraceptive Use	Multiple Sexual Partners	N	n (%)
1	0	No	No	56	13 (23%)
2	0	No	Yes	138	41 (30%)
3	0	Yes	No	146	36 (25%)
4	0	Yes	Yes	375	102 (27%)
5	1	No	No	26	11 (42%)
6	1	No	Yes	189	97 (51%)
7	1	Yes	No	9	5 (56%)
8	1	Yes	Yes	40	22 (55%)

criteria that would include as many cases as possible (all cases from when testing began) and some other assumptions regarding which women might be more informative. The question now is whether the resulting sampling fractions are 'optimal' or whether the 327 could have been selected in a way that would improve the precision of the OR for the association between chlamydia and ectopic pregnancy, adjusted for other factors.

Using the available sample of 327 as 'pilot' information, the optimal sample sizes were computed using the Stata command **optfixn** and the resulting optimal sampling fractions are provided in column 6 of Table 8.3. Although the sample is the same size in the actual study (n=327), choosing these 327 women in different strata could have given a more efficient design: in particular, the optimal design suggests that there was more information to be gained from sampling more intensely from strata 2, 7 and 8, and less intensely from stratum 3. If the researchers had some pilot data in the 8 strata, then they could have planned in advance to collect chlamydia antibody results from more (or all) of the cases who were contraceptive users and from a higher proportion of controls with multiple sexual partners who were not contraceptive users. The estimated variance of the adjusted coefficient for chlamydia from a sample of 327 using the optimal design is .067. A weighted logistic regression of the actual data provides an adjusted OR (with 95 % confidence interval) for chlamydia of 2.43 (1.32, 4.51), and the coefficient for chlamydia in the logistic model has a variance of .0998. Thus the actual design is only 67% as efficient as the design that optimally chooses how to sample the 327 second-stage subjects.

Minimising cost or maximising precision

The subsampling of subjects in a two-stage study will usually be driven by cost considerations. While the basic information for a large number of first-stage individuals may be easily accessible and affordable (for example, demographic variables and other data from health registers), many important exposures, such as those involving collection of biological specimens and/or the conduct of laboratory analysis, can involve considerable expense. Thus, the total study budget, B, for data collection is:

$$B = N * C_1 + n * C_2$$

where N and n are the first and second stage sample sizes, and C_1 and C_2 are the costs per observation at the first and second stage respectively.

TABLE 8.3: *The numbers in column 5 are the actual sampling fractions in each of the strata defined by the indicator variables Y (case status), cont (contraceptive use) and sexp (multiple sexual partners) in a case-control study of ectopic pregnancy [179] and these are compared to three optimal designs.*

				Actual	**Optimal designs**		
					(a) n	**(b) precision**	**(c) budget**
					n = 327	$C_1 = 5$	$C_1 = 5$
Stratum	Y	Cont	Sexp	n = 327		$C_2 = 50$	$C_2 = 10$
1	0	No	No	.23	.34	.56	.81
2	0	No	Yes	.30	.71	1	1
3	0	Yes	No	.25	.05	.08	.12
4	0	Yes	Yes	.27	.14	.22	.32
5	1	No	No	.42	.59	.97	1
6	1	No	Yes	.51	.47	.77	1
7	1	Yes	No	.56	1	1	1
8	1	Yes	Yes	.55	.97	1	1
				N = 979	N = 979	N_{opt}= 672	N_{opt}= 1812
Variance of β for chlamydia				.0998	.067	.067	.02

(a) optimal sampling fractions if a fixed sample size of 327 second stage subjects were selected to maximise efficiency; (b) first and second-stage sample sizes to achieve the same precision as (a) for minimum budget if costs are $C_1 = 5$ and $C_2 = 50$; (c) the maximum precision achievable for the same budget as (b) if costs are $C_1 = 5$ and $C_2 = 10$.

The objective of the optimal sampling presented above was to select a *fixed number* of study participants for whom an exposure is measured at the second stage in order to achieve the best precision of a coefficient of interest. However, studies are usually designed to achieve a specified precision and this is the objective of the power and sample size calculations that are routinely done when a study is being planned. Thus if a two-stage design is being considered, a natural 'sample size' question to ask is whether it is possible to determine the total (first-stage) sample size and the sampling fractions at the second stage, that will yield the desired efficiency. Where the first- and second-stage costs are known, the

optprec command in Stata provides the optimal total study size, N_{opt} and the sampling fractions within the strata, to achieve a specified precision at minimum cost [179]. The expression for the optimal sampling fractions, like those for fixed sample size, depend on the prevalences and 'information' of the strata in the first-stage data. For the fixed sample size situation in the previous section, the expression for the optimal sampling fractions is of the form:

$$\frac{n_s}{N_S} = \frac{n}{N}(\text{function of prevalence and pilot data}) \qquad (8.4)$$

where the 's' subscript denotes the stratum, while for specified costs C_1 and C_2 at the first and second stage, the optimal sampling fractions are:

$$\frac{n_s}{N_S} = \sqrt{\frac{C_1}{C_2}}(\text{function of prevalence and pilot data}) \qquad (8.5)$$

The reader will notice the similarity with Equation 8.2 where the optimal case:control ratio was inversely related to the relative costs of case and control observations.

As an illustration, assume the chlamydia antibody laboratory test in the example above had cost \$50 per specimen and the cost of collection of all the other variables was \$5 per individual, then the total cost of the study would have been:

$$B = 979 \times 5 + 327 \times 50 = \$21,245$$

In the actual study, this would have been the total cost of sampling 327 individuals from a total of 979. If the 327 were sampled optimally, the exposure coefficient would have an estimated variance of.067. But could this variance be achieved by a different design at less cost? The results from the Stata **optprec** command with the variance specified to be .067, and with first- and second-stage costs of 5 and 50, are presented in optimal design (b) in Table 8.3. The design with minimum cost has a smaller total sample size (N=672) but with a larger proportion of all strata selected into the second stage, including all individuals in strata 2, 7 and 8, and most of those in stratum 5. The cost of this design would be \$19910, resulting in some small savings compared to the design with N=979 and n=327.

Finally, it may be of interest to determine the maximum precision that can be achieved for a given budget with alternative costs. Expressions and a Stata command **optbud** have been developed that provide the total study size, N_{opt}, and the sampling fractions within the strata, that result in maximum precision for a specified total budget, B. The optimal sampling fractions for this situation are of the form:

$$\frac{n_s}{N_s} = \frac{[B - N_{opt} * C_1]/C_2}{N_{opt}} \text{(function of prevalence and pilot data)} \quad (8.6)$$

The full expression, not shown here, is in fact identical to that for the fixed second-stage sample size in Equation 8.4, except the specified second-stage sample size, n_2, is now replaced by $\frac{B - N_{opt} * C_1}{C_2}$ which is the *affordable* second stage sample size!

If in the ectopic pregnancy study in Table 8.3 above, the chlamydia antibody laboratory test cost \$10 per specimen instead of \$50, then the budget for study (b) could have achieved much better precision (optimal design (c) in Table 8.3). Comparing designs (b) and (c) in the table, it can be seen that with cheaper second-stage data, the optimal design for the same budget is a larger study (N=1812), with chlamydia assays conducted on all women in 5 of the 8 strata and a large majority in one other stratum (81% in stratum 1): two other strata, consisting of controls who are contraceptive users, have a smaller proportion of subjects in the second-stage sample.

What pilot data is needed?

In addition to information on costs and/or precision, the computations for the optimal designs above require the user to have a random sample of subjects in each of the sampling strata. These strata will usually be defined by the outcome variable and one or more of the covariates available at the first-stage. A covariate that defines the sampling strata will often be of interest in the logistic regression analysis of the two-stage data, but this is not essential. An example of such an **auxiliary variable** is age group: one might sample within strata defined by outcome and age group, but use the actual age in the regression model.

The pilot dataset must have a small number of observations in each of the strata in order to compute the 'information' components in the optimal sampling fractions. Computation of the optimal design is possible even with very small numbers in some strata, provided the observations in a stratum are not identical (i.e. that they do not have the same outcome and explanatory variables in the logistic model). However, the optimal sample sizes calculated from a small pilot sample will be subject to greater uncertainty, and a larger pilot sample enables more precise estimation of the optimal design. This raises the question as to how one should allocate the budget to collecting the pilot data (usually by balanced sampling) and the main study data (by optimal sampling). We will return to this in the next paragraph, but assuming for now that users of the optimal sampling methods have some pilot data available, Table 8.4 summarises what else is needed as input for computation of the different optimal designs. Since the purpose of optimal sampling

TABLE 8.4: *Requirements for computation of sampling fractions for two-stage studies of a binary outcome that optimise precision or cost, where n denotes the total second stage sample size, N_s the first-stage sample sizes in the strata, and N_{opt} the total (optimal) study size.*

Fixed:	**n**	**Variance**	**Budget**
to optimise:	**precision**	**cost**	**precision**
INPUT	pilot data n, N_s	pilot data budget, B costs C_1, C_2	pilot data precision, v costs C_1, C_2
OUTPUT	2nd stage sampling fractions	N_{opt} 2nd stage sampling fractions	N_{opt} 2nd stage sampling fractions

is usually to accommodate an expensive exposure variable, such as a biomarker, the pilot data will also be expensive to obtain, and the cost of this step may need to be considered in relation to the gain in efficiency of the overall study. For the setting where a second-stage sample of fixed size n is to be selected, this sample can be considered as consisting of two parts: n_a observations (the pilot data) sampled at Stage IIa and n_b sampled optimally at Stage IIb using the information in the pilot data. This design has been explored through simulation studies [143] that compared the efficiency of a two-stage **adaptive** design with various choices of n_b to a balanced design (the same number of second-stage observations from each stratum) and a proportional design (the same proportion of observations from each stratum).

The simulation study also investigated a **fully adaptive** sampling design, where, starting with a small sample, the initial optimal sampling fractions guide the selection of the next second-stage observation, after which the sampling fractions are re-computed and the next individual selected, with these steps repeated until the n second-stage observations are sampled. This fully adaptive design is the most extreme, as the sampling fractions are re-estimated after the selection of every individual in the second-stage sample! Thus, although it is the most efficient, it would not be practical for use in a real research study. In contrast, the two-stage adaptive design would be straightforward to implement, and achieved close to the theoretical optimal efficiency in many settings, outperforming the balanced sampling supported by the work of Breslow and others [22], [23], which in turn was more efficient than proportional sampling. To implement the adaptive second-stage sample of size n, the investigator still needs to decide on the best split between the n_a pilot observations and n_b optimally-sampled observations, as there will be a trade-off between a larger n_a, with more precise estimates of the sampling fractions, and the increased precision resulting from a larger n_b chosen optimally. The general recommendation of the authors was an equal split, as the simulation studies indicated that two-stage adaptive designs with $n_a \approx n_b$ resulted in sampling fractions that were close to optimal.

8.3 Efficient Sampling for a Time-to-event Outcome

The hazard ratio represents the effect of a prognostic factor on a time-to-event outcome in a cohort. As seen in Chapter 4, it is not necessary to have data on the whole cohort, as the HR can be estimated more efficiently from a subsample of the cohort selected in a nested case-control or case-cohort design. Matching is often used in case-control designs to further improve the efficiency. The corresponding strategy for case-cohort designs is the stratified sampling discussed earlier in this chapter. The data from either of these designs can be analysed using weighted Cox regression, where the weights reflect the sampling fractions: data from a nested case-control study uses the Kaplan-Meier weights illustrated in Chapters 6 and 7; for a case-cohort study, cases are weighted by the inverse of the (stratum-specific) sampling fraction (often = 1) and controls are usually weighted by the (stratum-specific) subcohort sampling fraction or fraction of non-cases, although there are other choices.

Provided sufficient information is available to compute the sampling fractions, it is clear that a HR can be estimated from a subsample of time-to-event data where cases and non-cases are sampled in various designs. If the cases and non-cases are sampled from strata defined by confounders or other categorical variables, then the sampled cases and non-cases are a second stage sample, which together with the information available for all first-stage observations, constitute a two-stage design. The two-stage studies introduced so far for binary outcomes used one or more confounders to define the sampling strata, but it is also possible to use strata defined by other variables, such as a surrogate/auxiliary variable for the exposure [179] or an independent risk factor. The performance of two-stage designs for estimating a HR using these different sampling strategies has been compared to simple random sampling and proportional random sampling in a simulation study [71] that also investigated the efficiency relative to the full cohort analysis. The authors concluded that exclusive case-control sampling stratified on a surrogate of the exposure and nested case-control sampling can both provide HR estimates and power similar to what is achieved from the whole cohort but with a much reduced sample size.

8.3.1 Optimal selection to improve efficiency

The optimal designs in Section 8.2 are all concerned with a binary outcome, where the objective of the two-stage analysis is the efficient estimation of an OR from a logistic regression model. While there have been no explicit algorithms developed to date for optimal sampling for time-to-event outcomes, the methods for binary outcomes can also be used to improve efficiency of the estimation of HR in such studies. By first considering the simple binary outcome for whether or not the event occurred during the follow-up time, the optimal sampling fractions for estimation of the OR from logistic regression can be obtained as outlined in Section 8.2.1 above. Using the inverse of these sampling fractions, a weighted Cox regression then provides a valid estimate of the HR of interest. This was the 'novel design' used in a study of prognostic genetic factors for relapse in acute lymphoblastic leukemia (ALL) [68], which is described in detail in the following paragraph.

In the cohort of 1999 patients, there were 306 who relapsed, 92 of whom had been classified as high risk, 186 as medium risk and 28 as standard risk. A pilot sample of 164 individuals were genotyped, and these data used to estimate the sampling fractions in the six strata defined by case status (i.e. relapse) and risk group that would maximise the precision of the estimate of genotype effect from a logistic regression model. For the size of the second stage sample, the researchers chose a sample size equivalent to a case-control study where the ratio of controls to cases was 1.5 (i.e 765 individuals). The optimal second-stage sampling fractions for a second-stage sample of this size were 100% of cases in each of the three risk groups, and 64%, 26% and 13% of the 460 non-cases (non-relapsed patients) in the high, medium and low risk groups respectively, which yielded a total of 766 patients (see Table 8.5). The optimal number of controls was randomly selected from each of the three risk strata, and together with the cases, had their ID numbers passed to the laboratory. However, for some of these patients, there was no stored DNA available for conducting the genotyping, so that the total available sample size was 614. The authors assumed that these individuals were representative of the full strata to which they belonged, and used the inverse of these 'effective' sampling fractions for the weighted Cox regression. It is important to note that this results in a weight greater than 1 for cases: for example, the 22 relapsed cases in the low-risk group are weighted by $1/0.786 = 1.272$. The weighted Cox regression revealed some significant findings from the combined analysis of genetic details for approximately one-third of the cohort and the outcome and clinical information for all individuals. In the simulation study referred to above [68], this design was more efficient than any of the case-control designs investigated. Thus the availability of pilot data on 164 individuals was very valuable.

In this example, the authors selected a stratified case-control sample, but at the analysis step, the data are handled as a stratified case-cohort study. This emphasises the close relationship between the case-control and case-cohort designs, which are just different ways of sampling from a cohort. Provided the sampling strategy is known, the parameters of interest in the cohort (e.g. the HR above) can be estimated by appropriate weighting.

TABLE 8.5: *Optimal and available sampling fractions and sample sizes in the strata defined by relapse status and a three-category risk assessment of the ALL patients in a study of prognostic genetic factors [68].*

		Optimal		Available	
Stratum	**N**	**Fraction**	**n**	**Fraction**	**n**
Case-high	92	1	92	0.870	80
Case-medium	186	1	186	0.801	149
Case-low	28	1	28	0.786	22
Control-high	219	0.64	140	0.870	80
Control-medium	987	0.26	257	0.870	80
Control-low	487	0.13	63	0.115	56
	1999		766		614

8.4 Exposure-related Sampling

For the two-stage designs presented in Chapter 3 and in Section 8.2.1 above, the sampling strata were defined by the binary outcome Y and some of the categorical covariates, Z, available for all subjects at the first stage. These components of Z, which we denote by Z_s to indicate that they define the sampling strata, will often be potential confounders, Z_c, but may also include a surrogate measure of exposure. A surrogate exposure (e.g. a crude measure of the true exposure of interest) is an important example of an **auxiliary** variable, i.e. a variable used for defining sampling strata but not of interest in the regression model [179]. If sampling depends on an auxiliary variable Z_a, the logistic model of interest for the weighted analysis is:

$$logit[P(Y = 1|X, Z] = \beta_0 + \beta_x X + \beta_z Z'$$

where Z' excludes Z_a. Where Z_a is a surrogate exposure, it is clear that this variable provides no information about the risk of the outcome once the actual exposure X is available. For example, Z_a could be a simple three-category measure off obesity (normal, overweight, obese) and the exposure to be studied is the actual BMI in kg/m^2. As with stratified case-cohort sampling (Section 8.1.1), sampling of a case-control study within strata defined by a surrogate exposure results in an efficient design. In a comparison of different sampling strategies, a balanced case-control design at the end of follow-up using a surrogate of exposure could be as efficient as a nested case-control design in extracting the information from the cohort [71].

In addition to these modifications of case-cohort and case-control sampling, a number of other exposure-dependent sampling designs have been proposed and these are introduced in the following subsections.

8.4.1 Counter-matching

In the nested case-control study, the small number of controls in the sampled risk set are used to represent all the non-cases in the full risk set at that time point. Where controls are further matched on variables other than time, they represents non-cases with the same matching factors. The amount of statistical 'information' about the exposure-disease relationship contributed by a sampled risk set depends on the variation in the exposure values of the set members: as an extreme example, for an unmatched case-control study, a risk set will not contribute at all to the conditional likelihood if all members have the same exposure. If, in addition to time, the controls are matched on other factors, the risk sets that are concordant for exposure will not contribute to the estimation of the exposure effect but only to the estimation of the coefficients of other variables in the model (provided these variables are not concordant for all members of the risk set!). In a review paper in 1993 describing strategies for sampling from a cohort, Borgan and Samuelsen [16] introduced a design that they called **counter-matched**, where the controls in each risk set are chosen to maximise the variation in exposure. In contrast to matching, where the purpose is to make cases and controls as similar as possible, the purpose of counter-matching is to make them as different as possible.

The counter-matched design, which was described in detail by Langholz and Clayton in 1994 [115], involves stratifying on the exposure or a surrogate of the exposure. This avoids the loss of matched sets from the analysis due to concordant exposure, resulting in better efficiency. In the simple situation where a binary surrogate exposure is available for all members of the study base, but the actual exposure is to be measured on the individuals in a 1:1 nested case-control sample, a counter-matched control will be chosen to have the *opposite* value of the surrogate to that of the case. Where a binary exposure is available for all cohort members, but an expensive confounder or effect modifier is to be obtained for a 1:1 case-control sample, counter-matching on exposure will select a control with the *opposite* value of the exposure to that of the case. This selection of case-control pairs with opposite exposure or surrogate exposure has given rise to the term **counter-**matching, but as will become clear below, counter-matching is not limited to binary exposures (or surrogates) nor to 1:1 case-control studies.

Figure 8.2 (a) illustrates the selection of a 1:1 counter-matched sample, where the two strata are distinguished by the grey and black 'life lines' of their members, and the risk set at any event time is highlighted by the vertical shaded band. The sampled risk set in each year consists of the case and a randomly sampled control from the opposite stratum to the case. Figure 8.2 (b) displays the selection of a 1:3 counter-matched sample from a cohort with four strata, which results in sampled risk sets having one individual from each stratum: once the case is selected and their stratum identified, one individual is chosen at random from each of the other three strata. If a 1:7 case-control study was planned, then to ensure the risk sets of size eight had two individuals in each of the four strata, one control would be selected from the same stratum as the case and two from each of the other three strata.

It is clear that counter-matched sampling will result in a sampled risk set where the distribution of exposure is not representative of that in the background cohort. Indeed the purpose of this sampling design is to deliberately disturb the exposure distribution in an effort to gain efficiency, by selecting an equal number of individuals in each of the sampling strata. But in order to obtain a valid estimate of the exposure effect, the analysis needs to take account of this biased sampling by using appropriate weights.

As for the nested case-control design in Section4.4 of Chapter 4, the estimates from the counter-matched design are obtained from the conditional likelihood of the matched sets. However, Equation 4.21 in Chapter 4 is no longer appropriate as the counter-matched sampled risk set is *not* representative of the full risk set in the background cohort. The likelihood component from a sampled risk set should describe the probability that the event occurred to the case individual, given that there was one case in the set: for 1:1 data, this is the probability that for a given risk set (i.e. case-control pair) the event occurred to the case and not the control individual. Denoting the exposure stratum of the case and control in a sampled pair as X_1 and X_0 respectively, and the

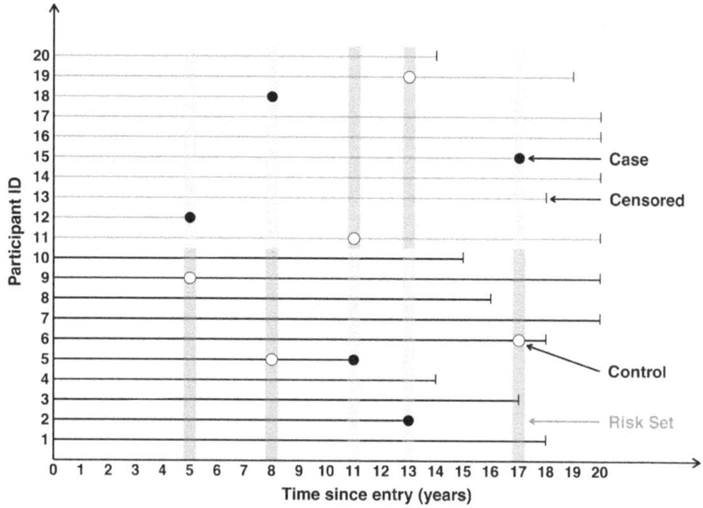

(a) *1:1 counter-match*

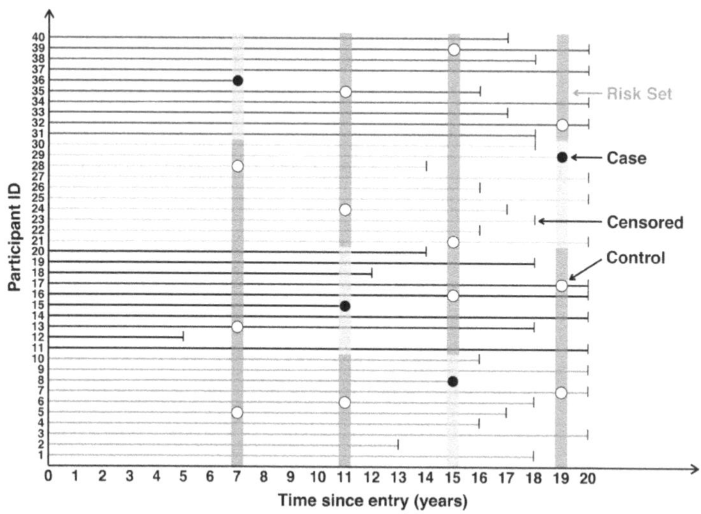

(b) *1:3 counter-match*

FIGURE 8.2: *Illustration of* ***(a)*** *1:1 counter-matched case-control sample from two strata and* ***(b)*** *1:3 counter-matched case-control sample from four strata.*

total numbers in those strata in the full risk set as N_1 and N_0, then the probability of obtaining the sampled risk set is $1/N_0$ as there were N_0 choices for the control. The probability that the event occurred to the case conditional on one event in the pair can be written as:

$$\text{P[case had the event}|\text{one case is observed]} = \frac{e^{\alpha+\beta X_1}.\frac{1}{N_0}}{e^{\alpha+\beta X_1}.\frac{1}{N_0} + e^{\alpha+\beta X_0}.\frac{1}{N_1}}$$

since the probability of obtaining the risk set would have been $1/N_1$ if the event had occurred to the other individual. Multiplying numerator and denominator by $N_1.N_0$, the conditional likelihood component is

$$\frac{e^{\alpha+\beta X_1}.N_1}{e^{\alpha+\beta X_1}.N_1 + e^{\alpha+\beta X_0}.N_0}$$

and the conditional likelihood to be solved involves the product of all such pairs:

$$\textbf{Likelihood for all events} = \prod_{t_i} \frac{e^{\beta X_{1i}}.N_{1i}}{e^{\beta X_{1i}}.N_{1i} + e^{\beta X_{0i}}.N_{0i}} \quad (8.7)$$

where the subscript $1i$ denotes the stratum of the case at time t_i, N_{1i} the number of cohort members in that stratum, and $0i$ denotes the corresponding quantities for the (counter-matched) control. Thus the weight assigned to an individual (whether case or control) depends on their exposure status. For a 1:2 counter-matched case-control study with one individual selected from each of three strata, it can be readily shown that the conditional likelihood is:

$$\prod_{t_i} \frac{e^{\beta X_{1i}}.N_{1i}}{\sum_{k\in R_i^*} e^{\beta X_k}.N_k} \quad (8.8)$$

where the summation in the denominator is taken over the three individuals (case and two controls) in the risk set. In general, a counter-matched study designed to select risk sets containing m_s individuals from stratum s has conditional likelihood:

$$\prod_{t_i} \frac{e^{\beta X_{1i}}.N_{1i}/m_{1i}}{\sum_{k\in R_i^*} e^{\beta X_k}.N_k/m_k} \quad (8.9)$$

where the product is again taken over all risk sets and the sum in the denominator is taken over all the members of the risk set. The conditional likelihood of the counter-matched sample is presented in Table 8.6 where the nested case-control design is included for comparison

TABLE 8.6: *Comparison of risk sets and weights for matched and counter-matched case-control designs.*

Design	Likelihood	Risk Set
Matched	$\prod_{t_i} \frac{e^{\beta X_{1i}+\gamma Z_{1i}}}{\sum_{k\in R^*_{1i}} e^{\beta X_k+\gamma Z_k}}$	$\mathbf{R^*_{1i}}$: All members of the sampled risk set at time t_i who are in the same stratum (i.e. matched set) as the case (denoted by suffix '1i').
Counter-matched	$\prod_{t_i} \frac{e^{\beta X_{1i}+\gamma Z_{1i}}.w_{1i}}{\sum_l^L \sum_{k\in R^*_{li}} w_l e^{\beta X_k+\gamma Z_k}}$	$\mathbf{R^*_{\ell i}}$: All members of the sampled risk set at time t_i who are in stratum ℓ $\mathbf{w}_\ell = \mathbf{N}_\ell/\mathbf{n}_\ell$: the weight assigned to an individual in stratum ℓ, where N_l is the number of cohort members in the stratum and n_l is the number of each sampled risk set to be selected from that stratum.

The implementation of the weighted analysis of counter-matched case-control data is straightforward, as it simply involves assigning a weight to each sampled individual that is the inverse of the sampling fraction of their stratum. As before, a robust variance adjusts for the weights in the regression. A comparison of the matched and counter-matched case-control design is presented in Table 8.7.

Application of counter-matching

In a paper investigating the association of blood group and transfusions with the risk of pregnancy-associated venous thromboembolism [226], the authors reported an increasing risk of postpartum venous thromboembolism (VTE) with the number of red blood cell (RBC) transfusions around delivery. As an illustration, we assume that the details concerning number and type of transfusions had not been available for the full cohort, and that a nested case-control study is to be conducted to estimate the HRs for the different levels of exposure to RBC transfusions. Since transfusion is a rare exposure (approximately 2% of women in this cohort), a nested case-control study is likely to have many uninformative risk sets, where neither the case nor any of their controls have had any transfusion. Assuming that a simple binary indicator for any

TABLE 8.7: *Comparison of matched and counter-matched nested case-control designs.*

	Matched	**Counter-matched**
Purpose	to make cases and controls as *similar* as possible	to make cases and controls as *different* as possible
Matching variables	not of interest, except as adjustment	"matching" done on exposure of interest (or a surrogate)
Analysis	conditional likelihood	weighted conditional likelihood
Information from study base	none	risk set sizes (in sampling strata)
Consequences for estimates	effect of the matching factor is not estimated by conditional analysis	wider range of exposure improves precision

transfusion is available for all members of the cohort, this can be used to select an efficient counter-matched nested case-control sample for which the details about transfusions around delivery are collected.

The first column of results in Table 8.8 presents the estimated HRs from a Cox regression analysis of the cohort of 966,070 deliveries with at least 7 days follow-up postpartum: mothers who had trauma or surgery recorded around delivery were excluded, as well as those with missing smoking information. Transfusion around delivery was associated with postpartum VTE, with evidence of a dose-response effect.

There were 472 cases of VTE during the 6-week follow-up, and in a 1:5 nested case-control sample, 84% of the matched sets were concordant for exposure: the case and all controls had no transfusion around delivery, as might be expected for such a rare exposure. This loss of information is reflected in the wide confidence intervals in the second column of Table 8.8, with the effect of RBC > 5 no longer achieving statistical significance. A more efficient analysis can be conducted by breaking the matching and analysing all cases and controls in a weighted Cox regression with inverse probability weighting (IPW) using the Kaplan-Meier

TABLE 8.8: *Adjusted* hazard ratio estimates (with 95% confidence intervals) for the association of number of RBC transfusions around delivery with postpartum VTE within six weeks of delivery, from full cohort analysis, 1:5 nested case-control study analysed by conditional logistic regression (CLR) and inverse probability weighted (IPW) Cox regression, and 1:5 counter-matched nested case-control study analysed by weighted conditional logistic regression.*

	Cohort	**1:5 NCC CLR**	**1:5 NCC IPW**	**1:5 CM CLR**
RBC units:				
1–2	2.53(1.6,4.1)	2.69(1.5,5.0)	2.58(1.6,4.1)	2.60(1.6,4.2)
3–5	2.79(1.4,5.4)	3.06(1.2,8.0)	2.42(1.2,4.8)	2.84(1.4,5.5)
>5	4.36(1.6,12)	3.65(0.9,15)	4.03(1.5,11)	4.00(1.5,11)
Smoking	1.51(1.1,2.0)	1.42(1.0,2.0)	1.42(1.1,1.9)	1.51(1.1,2.1)
Preeclampsia	2.50(1.8,3.5)	2.15(1.4,3.4)	2.13(1.5,3.1)	1.94(1.3,2.9)
Delivery:				
Instrument	1.08(0.8,1.5)	1.18(0.8,1.8)	1.16(0.8,1.7)	1.26(0.8,1.9)
Elective CS	1.73(1.3,2.4)	1.76(1.2,2.5)	1.74(1.3,2.4)	2.03(1.4,2.9)
Emerg. CS	2.26(1.8,2.9)	2.41(1.8,3.3)	2.37(1.8,3.0)	2.23(1.7,3.0)

**adjusted for maternal age and calendar year, in addition to all other variables displayed in the table*

weights described in Chapter 7. The results of this analysis are presented in the third column of results in Table 8.8, where the confidence intervals are much narrower and the effect of RBC > 5 is again significant. For a 1:5 counter-matched sample, each of the 31 VTE cases who were transfused around delivery was matched to 5 women who had no transfusion and who had not been diagnosed with VTE at the time the cases was identified; each of the 441 cases who had no transfusion was matched to five women who were transfused.The results from the weighted conditional logistic regression of this sample, presented in the final column of Table 8.8, are similar to those from the IPW analysis.

The comparable precision of the estimates from the counter-matched dataset and the IPW analysis of the nested case-control dataset of similar size indicates that the information provided by the surrogate exposure is similar to the cohort information that is provided by the probabilities describing the sampling of the nested controls over time. We might expect that the counter-matched design could be made even more efficient by breaking the matching and analysing with IPW Cox regression. However, unlike the nested case-control design, where the IPW analysis is more efficient than standard conditional logistic regression, it has been found that for counter-matched data, the 'original' method of analysis [114] was more efficient [186]. It may however be of interest to conduct weighted Cox regression of counter-matched data for other potential benefits: overcoming problems with lost/concordant sets since all individuals are used; the time scale can be changed; controls sampled for one study could be reused in another. These are the reasons mentioned before for why IPW weighted Cox regression for nested case-control data may offer advantages in addition to the efficiency gain.

Following the introduction of the counter-matched design, its potential for efficient study of expensive exposures was demonstrated by an application to environmental exposure in 1997 [203], which reported that 3 controls per case in a counter-matched design offered similar efficiency to random sampling with 10 controls per case. The design was also recommended as an efficient means of investigating interactions (effect modification) in case-control studies [40], which is of particular interest for the study of gene-environment interactions [6]. Despite this clear potential for improved efficiency, the straightforward data preparation step, and the ability to get estimates from standard software, the counter-matched design has not been widely adopted by biostatisticians and epidemiologists. While some of this may be due to the difficulty of identifying a surrogate exposure with adequate sensitivity and specificity [114], [6], a commentary in the journal *Epidemiology*, titled 'Counterintuitive Matching' [39], suggested that for practicing epidemiologists the sampling design seemed flawed by its measurement of exposure on individuals who had been selected based on partial knowledge about their exposure! Another factor that may have delayed adoption of the design was that it was discovered at a time when researchers were faced with absorbing numerous new developments in the design and analysis of case-control studies. Although the statistical literature presented these methods in a unified framework, many applied scientists regarded the designs as distinct, each one requiring its own tools for implementation and analysis. However, the common purpose of all designs is to address a research question about the underlying cohort, and the sampling strategy is simply the choice of method for 'representing' the cohort. With this simple insight, the adoption of a new sampling design requires only that it can be analysed by standard software or that user-friendly software tools are developed and provided.

8.4.2 Exposure enriched case-control study

A second-stage sampling design that uses a categorical surrogate of a continuous exposure X, such as the three-level variable (normal, overweight, obese) for BMI, will ensure a good range of the continuous variable in the sample to be analysed and thus a more efficient estimate of the coefficient β_x in a logistic regression model. This is particularly advantageous for a highly skewed continuous exposure, or where interest is focused on the interaction between such an exposure and a categorical factor, especially if that factor is rare in the population. This is exactly the scenario that faces researchers investigating gene-environment interactions: many environmental exposures from air, water, noise and other sources are skewed measures on a continuous scale, and the mutated gene is expected to be rare. The combination of skewed exposure and high cost of (rare) genetic biomarker measurements could lead to very inefficient studies using standard designs. An efficient study should not only over-sample cases (i.e. use a case-control design) but also over-sample controls from the range of exposure levels that have low prevalence. Such was the motivating research problem for the authors who proposed an alternative to the two-stage design, the **exposure enriched case-control design** [90].

In Chapter 3 and Section 8.2.1, valid estimates from such 'two-stage' data required knowledge of the sampling fractions from the underlying cohort. However, the contribution of the magnitude of exposure to the risk of the outcome, and its possible modification by other factors can be validly obtained from the exposure enriched design without the cohort sampling fractions being known. The paper introducing the method [90] used data from an earlier case-control study that had been conducted in 23 villages in Bangladesh to investigate the effect on skin lesions of the arsenic levels in drinking water and genetic polymorphisms [25]. To overcome the skewed distribution of arsenic levels, those investigators had over-sampled controls with low exposure. The following paragraphs will also assume a simple binary surrogate exposure (classified as high or low), but it will be clear that the method extends to any categorical surrogate.

Assume that the risk of a binary outcome is related to an exposure X and an effect modifier E by the logistic model:

$$logit[P(Y = 1|X, E] = \alpha + \beta_X X + \beta_E E + \beta_{int} XE \qquad (8.10)$$

where XE is the interaction term representing the modification of the exposure effect by E. In Section 2.5.5 of Chapter 2, we saw that for case-control sampling, logistic regression provides valid estimates of all the parameters in the model, except for the intercept α. Where a proportion π_1 of cases and π_0 of controls in the population have been selected into the case-control sample, the intercept in the logistic model estimates

$$\alpha_* = \alpha + ln\frac{\pi_1}{\pi_0} \tag{8.11}$$

This equation was derived by using Bayes theorem to express the probability of the outcome *in the sample* (i.e. conditional on being selected into the case-control study), $P(Y = 1|X, S = 1)$ in terms of the probability $P(Y = 1|X)$ in the population, where S is an indicator for membership of the sample. If, as in the arsenic study [25], sampling did not only depend on case-control status, but also on exposure, then for the sampled data, the population model in Equation 8.10 describing the risk of the outcome for an individual with exposure X and effect modifier E becomes:

$$logit[P(Y = 1|X, E, S = 1] = \alpha + \ln\frac{\pi_1(Y, X)}{\pi_0(Y, X)} + \beta_X X + \beta_E E + \beta_{int} XE \tag{8.12}$$

where $\pi_1(Y, X)$ and $\pi_0(Y, X)$ indicate that the sampling probability depends on case-control status and exposure. If the exposure has been dichotomised at a threshold value T, with the sampling fraction of cases and controls depending on whether they are in the 'high' or 'low' category, then following similar steps to those in Equations 2.35 to 2.38 in Chapter 3, the right hand side of Equation 8.12 can be written as follows:

$$\alpha + \ln\frac{\pi_{1H}}{\pi_{0H}} + \beta_X X + \beta_E E + \beta_{int} XE \text{ if X >=T} \tag{8.13}$$

$$\alpha + \ln\frac{\pi_{1L}}{\pi_{0L}} + \beta_X X + \beta_E E + \beta_{int} XE \text{ if X < T} \tag{8.14}$$

where the sampling fractions for cases and controls are π_{H1} and π_{H0} respectively in the high exposure group and π_{L1} and π_{L0} in the low exposure group. Using the low exposure group as reference, this model can be written:

$$\alpha^* + \beta^* I[X \geq T] + \beta_X X + \beta_E E + \beta_{int} XE \tag{8.15}$$

$$\text{where } \alpha^* = \alpha + ln\frac{\pi_{H1}}{\pi_{H0}} \tag{8.16}$$

$$\text{and } \beta^* = ln\frac{\pi_{H1}}{\pi_{H0}} - ln\frac{\pi_{L1}}{\pi_{L0}} \tag{8.17}$$

so that the estimates are obtained from a straightforward logistic regression, by simply including an indicator variable for the dichotomised exposure.

In addition to the asymmetry/skew of the continuous exposure, the gain in power from exposure enriched case-control sampling for investigating effect modification depends on the prevalence of the modifying factor, the ratio of controls to cases and the ratio of high to low exposed individuals selected into the sample. In the investigation of the gene environment interaction in the study of arsenic in drinking water [90], the authors demonstrated dramatic improvements in power compared to simple case-control sampling: for any specific number of cases, the exposure enriched sampling achieved higher power with a much smaller sample size (i.e. lower control to case ratio).

The exposure-enriched design has been extended to propose efficient designs for the study of gene-environment interaction in the risk of a time-varying outcome [211]. A subsample of individuals is selected by retrospective sampling from a longitudinal cohort for genotyping, based on their exposure, covariates and outcome 'trajectory'. The design was demonstrated to have greater efficiency and statistical power than other designs for detecting gene-environment interaction.

8.5 Extreme Case-Control Design

The significant costs of collecting, storing and analysing biological samples has led to the selection of study subjects using some non-standard designs that investigators believe are more informative. These are usually analysed by standard methods, ignoring the interplay between the sampling design and approach to analysis that leads to valid and efficient estimates. For example, a study of biomarkers for lethal prostate cancer [189] proposed that informative biological samples were those from extreme cases and controls: the earliest deaths from prostate cancer and the indolent cancers of long-term survivors. The study compared the prostate cancer deaths within 10 years of diagnosis to controls surviving at least 10 years, using a standard logistic regression analysis.

Readers will recognise that this was simply *exclusive sampling* for a 10-year follow-up and that the OR for the association between biomarkers and prostate cancer death within 10 years was validly estimated by the logistic regression. However, such analysis disregards the time-to-event information which may, as suspected by the investigators, offer some gain in power over a nested design that selected controls at the event times of the cases, rather than the more extreme controls that were chosen. Furthermore, if indeed there is additional information in the more extreme controls, then even further gains in efficiency would be possible by selecting a **more extreme case-control** sample, where the controls all survive a specified minimum time beyond the follow-up time for recruiting cases.

A method has been developed for estimating the underlying HR from extreme case-control designs to estimate the underlying HR [183] from the **extreme case-control (ECC)** design (where the controls are selected by exclusive sampling) and the **more extreme case-control (MECC)** design, where controls must survive at least a specified time interval beyond the follow-up period during which cases are identified. Figure 8.3 provides simple line plots illustrating these two designs.

Assuming a Cox (proportional hazards) model, the data sampled using the ECC or MECC design can be analysed by a weighted likelihood [183], similar to those for other sampling designs, with time-dependent weights (Equation 8.18) assigned to all individuals (cases and controls).

$$\text{Likelihood} = \prod_{t_i} \frac{e^{\beta X_{1i}}.w_{1i}}{\sum_{k \in R_i^*} e^{\beta X_{ki}}.w_{ki}} \tag{8.18}$$

$$\text{where } w_{1i} = \frac{S(t_i|X_{1i})}{S(\tau|X_{1i})} \text{ and } w_{ki} = \frac{S(t_i|X_{ki})}{S(\tau|X_{ki})}$$

Here τ denotes the minimum survival time for controls. For the ECC sample displayed in Figure 8.3(a), $\tau = \tau_0$ is the follow-up time during which events were recorded. The last event time could also be defined

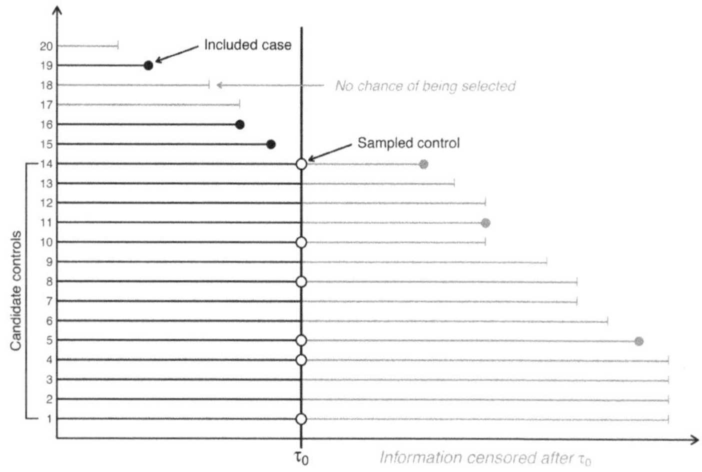

(a) *Extreme case-control (ECC) study of cases by time τ_0, with 2 controls per case who must survive at least to τ_0.*

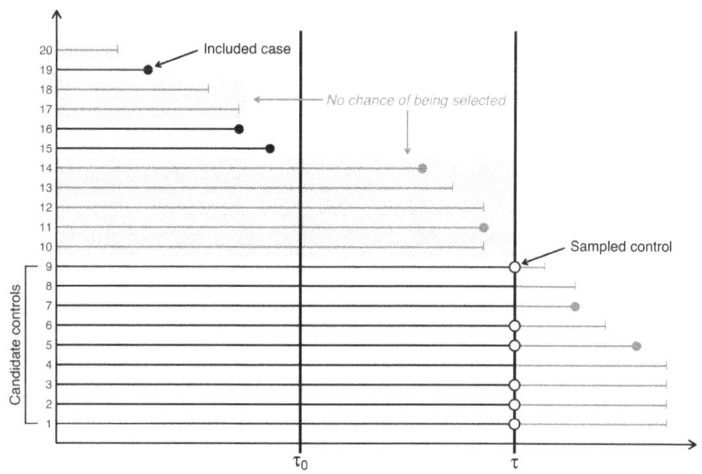

(b) *More extreme case-control (MECC) study of cases by time τ_0, with 2 controls per case who must survive at least to $\tau > \tau_0$.*

FIGURE 8.3: *Illustration of the selection of controls who survive **(a)** at least to the end of follow-up τ_0 for cases (ECC), or (b) at least to a later time $\tau > \tau_0$.*

$$w_{ki} = \frac{S(t_i|X_{ki})}{S(\tau|X_{ki})} \tag{8.19}$$

$$= \frac{S_0(t_i)^{e(\beta X_{ki})}}{S_0(\tau)^{e(\beta X_{ki})}} \tag{8.20}$$

$$= \left[\frac{S_0(t_i)}{S_0(\tau)}\right]^{e(\beta X_{ki})} \tag{8.21}$$

as τ_0, in which case the controls must all survive beyond the last event time. Examining the relative weight of an individual in their risk set, it is simply the ratio of their probabilities of surviving to the event time t_i and to the (later) time τ when they would qualify for selection. A control with a high ratio represents many who were at risk at the time the case occurred but did not survive to be selected. In the special case when controls for risk set R_i^* are selected at the time case i occurs, $w_{1i} = w_{ki} = 1$ and the likelihood is the familiar expression for standard nested case-control sampling. If the ECC/MECC sample is matched on a categorical variable Z, the likelihood is:

$$\prod_{t_i} \frac{e^{\beta X_{1i}+\gamma Z1i}.w_{1i}}{\sum_{k\in R_i^*} e^{\beta X_{ki}+\gamma Z_{1i}} w_{ki}} \tag{8.22}$$

where $Z_{ki} = Z_{1i}$ as a result of the matching. The weight for any individual, which depends on their survival $S(t)$, can be expressed in terms of the baseline survival $S_0(t)$ and covariates as in Equations 8.19–8.21. To compute the weights, S_0 can be estimated by $\hat{S}_0$ using the Kaplan Meier method with all covariates centered.

The conditional likelihood presented in Equation 8.22 is composed of the contributions from matched sets of cases and their extreme controls. If controls are sampled randomly, without matching on a covariate, then assigning them to sampled risk sets as in Equation 8.18 is somewhat artificial as they are all sampled at the same time τ. Without the time-matching to cases, an unconditional likelihood would seem more appropriate than conditional likelihood. Both unconditional and conditional approaches were developed for the ECC designs [183] and the conditional approach was shown to perform well whether applied to matched or unmatched data. The conditional likelihood is also more robust to the censoring mechanism, as it only assumes that censoring is independent

TABLE 8.9: *HR estimates from matched ECC sample of stroke in the Singapore data, using weighted method and conditional logistic regression (CLR).*

		1:2 ECC		Cohort	1:5 NCC
	True	**Weighted**	**CLR**	Cox	CLR
Age 75–84	1.2	-	-	1.17	-
Age 85+	.80	-	-	.65	-
Gender	.80	0.91	0.87	0.80	0.77
Smoking	1.5	1.32	1.43	1.38	1.38
Hypertension	4.5	4.16	4.68	4.65	4.65

of covariates, while the unconditional approach requires censoring to be independent of time or to be very rare before τ. Thus the conditional likelihood is a practical analysis tool for ECC data.

8.5.1 Illustration

The performance of the weighted analysis of ECC data can be illustrated using the 'realistic cohort' introduced in Section 7.2.1, where a stroke outcome was generated using realistic risk factors from a study of older adults in Singapore [214]. For the 34,116 individuals aged 60 or older in the full cohort (50000 individuals), a time to stroke was generated from a Cox proportional hazards model using the hazard ratios shown in the column 'true' in Table 8.9. Hypertension was defined as SBP>=140. The censoring time was generated from an exponential distribution with rate 0.05 and truncated at the end of follow-up (25 years). These settings resulted in 8.78% of individuals aged 60 or more having a stroke. In addition to the true values of the parameters used in the simulation, Table 8.9 presents the estimates from the Cox regression analysis of the full cohort and conditional logistic regression analysis of a 1:5 case-control study matched on age group, to serve as comparison for the ECC estimates. The extreme design included the 1023 cases that occurred in the first 5 years of the 25-year follow-up, each matched to 2 controls who survived at least 5 years (i.e. an ECC design with $\tau_0 = 5$). These data were analysed using the weighted method and by standard conditional logistic regression, and the results are presented in Table 8.9. For the MECC design, the matched controls were chosen from those who survived at least $\tau = K\tau_0, K = 1, 2, 3, 4$ (i.e. 10, 15, 20 and 25 years).

Each design was analysed using the weighted method and conditional logistic regression, and the results presented graphically in Figure 8.4.

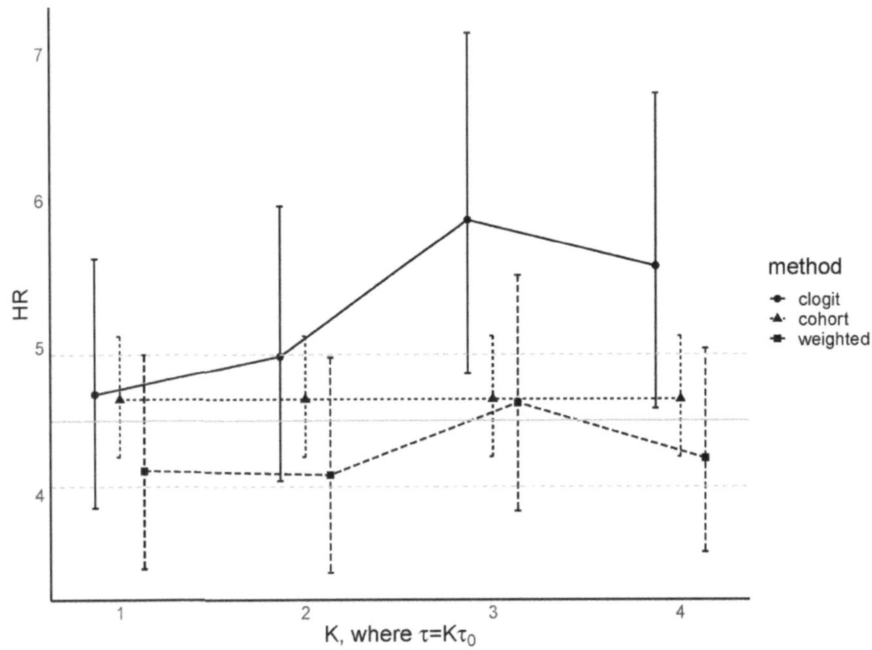

FIGURE 8.4: *Estimated HR for the association between hypertension and stroke in the simulated data (true HR = 4.5), for ECC designs with $\tau = K\tau_0$, $K = 1, 2, 3, 4$.*

The conditional logistic regression analysis of the design with $\tau = \tau_0$ (i.e. exclusive sampling) provides an odds ratio almost identical to the cohort value, as expected. As K increases, the OR from conditional logistic regression becomes more biased, due to ignoring the time gap between the recruitment interval for cases and the sampling time for controls. In contrast, the estimates from the weighted analysis accommodating time information remain close to the cohort value as the designs become more extreme: the dotted lines mark a 10% deviation from the true HR.

8.5.2 Data application

As an illustration of the weighted analysis, ECC and MECC data sampled from the prostate cancer study mentioned earlier [189] were used to estimate the effect of Gleason score and T stage on prostate

TABLE 8.10: *HR estimates from weighted analysis of ECC and MECC samples from prostate cancer patients [189] and from weighted analysis of cases and all eligible controls at year 5 (for ECC) and year 10 (for MECC).*

	Gleason Score		T Stage	
Controls	**ECC**	**MECC**	**ECC**	**MECC**
1:1	1.640	1.637	2.036	2.188
1:2	1.597	1.605	2.046	2.092
All	1.584	1.578	2.022	2.044
Cohort	HR= 1.645		HR= 1.960	
	95 % C.I. (1.46, 1.86)		95% C.I. (1.40,2.74)	

cancer death. For this application, cases of prostate cancer death within 5 years of diagnosis were compared with men who survived at least 5 years (ECC) or at least 10 years (MECC, K=2). Of the 1294 men with biological samples, 108 died from prostate cancer within 5 years of diagnosis. There were 827 candidate controls at $\tau_0 = 5$, after excluding men who were no longer at risk due to death from other causes or censoring. ECC studies with case control ratios of 1:1 and 1:2 were implemented by random sampling from these candidates. For MECC designs with $\tau = 2\tau_0$, 1 control per case and 2 controls per case were sampled from those who survived at least 10 years. In addition to the 1:1 and 1:2 ECC and MECC samples, the weighted method was also applied to an analysis of the cases and *all* candidate controls at 5 or 10 years, as appropriate. The estimates are presented in Table 8.10. The results of the ECC and MECC analyses are in close agreement with the weighted Cox regression using all controls, and with the cohort values. Although not shown here, the larger studies had narrower confidence intervals, as expected.

8.5.3 Power of ECC vs. NCC

The motivation for extreme case-control (ECC) sampling derives from an intuitive belief that there may be more statistical 'information' in controls sampled (much) later in time than the cases. It is indeed reasonable to expect that 'time is information', but the nested case-control (NCC) design has long been known for its efficiency in capturing the information contained in the person-time experience of a cohort. In addition, the NCC design provides estimates of HRs from standard analysis, while the

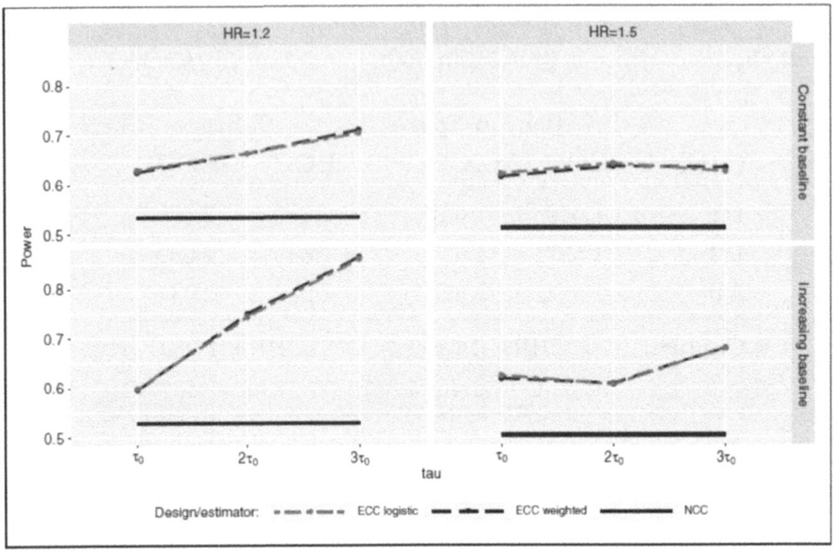

FIGURE 8.5: *Power of ECC design (analysed by weighted likelihood and by simple logistic regression) compared to NCC design, for $\tau = K\tau_0$, $K = 1, 2, 3$ and constant (top row) or increasing (bottom row) baseline hazards ([204], copyright SAGE Publications).*

ECC design requires a non-standard weighted analysis to obtain valid HR estimates. However, an ECC design may be analysed by simple unconditional logistic regression and the OR, rather than HR, used to test for an effect. If the primary objective of an investigator is to maximise power, then two questions arise: (i) does it matter if an ECC design is analysed by simple logistic regression to yield an estimate of OR or by weighted regression to yield a HR? (ii) does the ECC design, using either of these methods of analysis, offer any advantage over the well-known NCC design?

These questions were addressed in a simulation study [204] that investigated how the power depends on the time gap between cases and controls, the magnitude of the HR, the shape of the underlying hazard, and in the case of matching, the strength of the confounder. The ECC design offers a power advantage over the NCC design for smaller HR, which increases with larger time gap, especially when there is an increasing baseline hazard. Examples of the relative power for an ECC design matched on a strong confounder are presented in Figure 8.5. The higher power of the ECC design is a result of a discordant ECC pair having

TABLE 8.11: *Hazard ratio estimates from weighted analysis of ECC and NCC samples from the analysis of the association between the $\varepsilon 4$ allele of APOE and dementia in an elderly cohort [204]. The estimates from a Cox analysis of the full cohort are included for comparison.*

Design	Sample Size	No. of cases	HR (95% C.I.)	SE(ln HR)
NCC 1:1	152	76	2.08 (1.07, 4.03)	0.338
ECC 1:1	152	76	1.68 (1.05, 2.69)	0.240
NCC 1:2	228	76	1.81 (1.01, 3.26)	0.300
ECC 1:2	228	76	2.28 (1.53, 3.40)	0.204
Cohort	466	126	1.96 (1.31, 2.93)	0.206

higher 'information content' than an NCC pair, and the pattern of this relative information over time [204] depends on the exposure prevalence, the magnitude of the hazard ratio, and shape of the underlying hazard. An important practical result for data analysts, is that it was not necessary to use the weighted likelihood method to achieve the power gain, as the simple logistic regression analysis of the ECC data had the same power. Thus for the purposes of hypothesis testing, such as the discovery of new biomarkers, the implementation and analysis of the ECC design are straightforward.

If it is of interest to estimate a HR, for example to contribute to meta-analysis, this can be obtained from the weighted analysis. In an application to an investigation of the association of the APOE gene with dementia, an ECC design with $\tau_0 = 10$ years and $\tau = 15$ years was used to analyse an elderly cohort of 466 individuals who had been followed up for 15–17 years [204]. The ECC design would be expected to have high power for these data, which demonstrated an increasing hazard over time, and indeed the 1:2 ECC design was fully efficient, with the standard error of the ln(HR) being practically identical to the cohort value although based on just half the sample size and half the total cases (Table 8.11).

Despite the advantages of the ECC design, it should be borne in mind that for a specific research question, there are many considerations other than statistical power or efficiency. In particular, for the study of biomarkers using material from a biobank, deterioration in the biological material with storage time or advances in the assay technology might discourage the use of an ECC design in favour of the time-matched NCC study. A detailed discussion of such design considerations is presented as a chapter in a book on methods for biobanking [111].

8.5.4 Variations of extreme sampling

The ECC design presented above assumes that a fixed number of controls per case are to be sampled from a cohort at a fixed time $\tau \geq \tau_0$. However, the ECC approach offers a cost-effective design for an exclusive case-control study that has sufficient resources for any fixed number of controls, perhaps even fewer than the cases [103]. The idea is simple: treating the collection of controls as a single risk set from which individuals are to be matched to cases in 1:m sets. This is achieved by resampling the controls (with replacement) and assigning them randomly to cases to form the risk sets, which are then analysed by the weighted ECC method presented above. As with NCC analysis, the conditional likelihood accommodates controls that appear in more than one risk set.

The perception that observations further out in time provide more information motivated the ECC design and also underlies a sampling strategy called **outcome dependent sampling** [52]. In an application to the study of the effect of environmental contaminants on time-to-pregnancy (subfecundity), the authors first selected a random sample from women in a Norwegian pregnancy cohort who delivered in 2003–2004. This random sample of 550 deliveries was then supplemented by an additional sample of 400 deliveries from women who reported a time-to-pregnancy of at least 12 months, a time range that the authors considered to be informative. The design was more efficient than standard case-cohort sampling, but required a complex likelihood analysis to reap this benefits. In addition to efficiency, the authors pointed out the advantage of estimating a HR instead of an OR that depends on the follow-up, especially for non-rare outcome. However, the ECC design offers both of these advantages: an efficient design and a HR estimate, so that a 1:m ECC sample with $\tau_0 = 12$ and $\tau \geq \tau_0$ could also be used to capture the information in the later time period.

8.6 Exercises

1. In the study of prognostic factors for relapse in ALL patients presented in Section 8.3.1 of Chapter 8, stored DNA was only available for genetic analysis of 251 cases and 363 non-cases. Since the optimal sampling strategy is to sample all cases, then the researchers can only genotype 251 cases, as that is all that are available. However, for non-cases, when patient ID numbers are randomly chosen from each stratum (according to the optimal sampling fractions) for genotyping and some of these found to have no material, the target number could have been achieved by substituting these by other (random) individuals in that stratum who had material. Comment on the validity of this approach.

2. The optimal sampling of a specified number of second-stage observations in a two-stage study (see Chapter 8, Section 8.2) can be computed using the **optfixn** command in Stata or the **optimall** package in R.

   The dataset **pilotcas.dta** contains a pilot sample of 25 observations from each of the four strata in the full CASS data, similar to that described in Table 1 of *Optimal sampling strategies for two-stage studies* by Reilly in Am Jour Epi 1996 (PMID: 8533752). Use these pilot data to suggest an optimal design for a second stage sample of 1000 such as that reported in Table 3 of the paper, where mortality is modelled as a function of age and sex.

3. The dataset **wtpilot.dta** contains a binary outcome (operative mortality) and a number of demographic and clinical covariates (age, sex, weight, surgery, angina, chf, lvedp) for a pilot sample of 118, selected from the full CASS data in Reilly Am Jour Epi 1996. The original plan was to sample 10 observations from each of the twelve strata defined by the outcome, sex, and a 3-category weight variable, but one category had only 8 observations in total (see Table 5 of the paper).

   (i) Use the optimal sampling command with the **wtpilot** data and the population numbers in the 12 strata from Table 5 of the Am Jour Epi paper, to obtain an optimal second-stage sample of 1000 which minimises the variance of left ventricular end diastolic blood pressure (LVEDP) in the following logistic model:

`MORT=c+SEX+WEIGHT+AGE+ANGINA+CHF+LVEDP+SURGERY`

where c is the intercept. You will note some differences from Table 6 in the AJE paper, which used a different pilot sample.

(ii) The full cohort data from which the pilot sample in (i) was drawn is available in `chap8_CASS.dta`. Select another balanced pilot sample of the same size as in (i) and compare the optimal design obtained using this pilot data to the design in (i). (**Note:** some cohort members are missing their LVEDP value, so the optimal sample could also be chosen from individuals who have this variable recorded).

(iii) This and the following parts of the exercise use commands that consider cost, which are available in Stata.

If the study in (i) or (ii) cost an average of \$1 for each first stage and each second stage observation, then the total cost would be approximately \$10,000. Use the **optbud** command in Stata to find the optimal design for this budget if a first-stage observation costs \$5 and a second stage observation costs \$50. What is the total study size, the total and stratum-specific second-stage sample sizes, the total cost of this study and the variance achieved for the coefficient of LVEDP.

(iv) Use the **optprec** command to design a study that would achieve the variance you found in (iii) for minimum cost, assuming the same costs as before for a first and second-stage observation (\$5 and \$50 respectively). What do you notice?

(v) Show that for the same budget as in (iv), if C1=\$5 and C2=\$10 the optimal design is a study approximately 50% larger and would sample at least twice as many controls in each stratum.

(vi) From the logistic regression analysis of the full cohort, calculate the efficiency of each of the designs in (i)-(v) for estimating the coefficient of LVEDP.

4. The dataset **ectopic.dta** is from the study described in Chapter 3, in Section 3.1.1 (*Intentionally missing data*) and Section 3.2.3 (*Computation of sampling fractions*). These data consist of a total of 979 observations from a case-control study of ectopic pregnancy, with the following variables:

   y a binary indicator for case (i.e. ectopic pregnancy) or control

   gonn history of gonnorhea infection

   contr use of contraception

   sexptn multiple sex partners

   chlam positive for chlamydia antibody
   (only available for 327 individuals)

   z stratum variable constructed from **gonn**, **contr** and **sexptn**.

   (i) Repeat the analysis from Exercise 1 of Chapter 3 to estimate the effect of exposure to chlamydia antibody on the risk of ectopic pregnancy, adjusted for the other variables.

   (ii) Verify the numbers and percentages in the final column of Table 8.2 using suitable cross-tabulation commands (or the **coding** command in Stata).

   (iii) Verify that the adjusted OR for chlamydia is approximately the same if the sampling is assumed to depend only on contraceptive use and multiple sex partners. The remaining sections of this exercise will use these two first stage variables (**contr, sexptn**), as in the illustrations in Chapter 8.

   (iv) Treating the available 327 observations as pilot data, verify that for a sample of this size, the minimum achievable variance for the coefficient of chlamydia is .0674. How does this compare to the actual variance achieved in (i)?

   (v) Use the **optprec** command in Stata to verify the design in the second last column of Table 8.3 which minimises the study budget to achieve the same variance as in (iv) if the first and second stage observations cost 5 and 50 units respectively.

   (vi) Use the **optbud** command in Stata to verify that if the costs for first and second stage observations were 5 and

10, respectively, the optimal design for the same cost as the study in (v) would select a larger total sample size and sample all observations in 5 of the strata, as displayed in the last column of Table 8.3.

5. In part (v) of the previous exercise, the optimal sample achieved the same variance as in (iv) if the first and second stage observations cost 5 and 50 respectively. Repeat these computations for the design if the costs were

   (a) 2 and 10
   (b) 5 and 10

   Verify that the sampling fractions that are less than 100% from these two designs are approximately related by a constant. Suggest why this differs from the relative magnitude of $\sqrt{\frac{C_1}{C_2}}$ and $\sqrt{\frac{C_1^*}{C_2^*}}$ that would be expected from Equation 8.5 in Chapter 8.

6. For the likelihood in Equation (2) of *Exposure enriched case-control (EECC) design for the assessment of gene-environment interaction* by Huque et al in Genetic Epidemiol 2016 (doi:10.1002/gepi.21986), verify that:

   (i) if the sampling probability does not depend on case/control status, exposure or genetics (i.e. analysis is based on a simple random sample from the population), then the model in (2) estimates the true population intercept, β_0.

   (ii) if the sampling probability depends only on disease status, the model in (2) can be rewritten with the usual case-control intercept (i.e. Equation 2.42 of Chapter 2).

7. This exercise uses a dataset that was constructed using the Swedish data described in Tables 4.6 and 4.9 in Chapter 4, where the risk factors for postpartum VTE were investigated using various designs. From those data, all identifying information, such as dates and age, have been deleted and only four variables retained: case/control status, a 3-level BMI category, and indicator variables for smoking and preeclampsia. The time in weeks from delivery to VTE (within one year) was replaced by a random day from a 4-week or 8-week window, which although fictitious, preserved sufficient relationship

with the categorical exposures to generate an interesting exercise. The data are available in `chap8_pe&vte.dta`. (NOTE: depending on your software, the selection of the nested case-control sample below may take some time because of the large cohort! In this case, you could proceed with this exercise using a 25% or 50% sample of the cohort.)

(i) Estimate the hazard ratios for PE, smoking and BMI category from the constructed cohort in `chap8_pe&vte.dta`.

(ii) Select a 1:2 and 1:5 nested case-control study from the cohort and estimate the HRs from each design using conditional logistic regression.

(iii) Select three 1:1 extreme case-control designs where the earliest cases (within 10 weeks) are each matched to extreme controls who survive longer than (a) 10 weeks, (b) 20 weeks and (c) 30 weeks. For each design, estimate the ORs from unconditional logistic regression and compare to the HRs from conditional logistic regression of the matched pairs.

(iv) Repeat the sampling and analysis in (iii) for a 1:2 and 1:5 case-control ratio, comparing the unconditional analysis to the conditional analysis of the matched sets.

(v) **Note:** In this and the following task, the correct robust standard error is available in the R package `https://github.com/nyilin/SamplingDesignTools`

Prepare a table with the estimates and standard errors from (iv) and compare to Figure 8.4 of Chapter 8.

(vi) Prepare a table with estimates and standard errors from the full cohort, the nested case-control samples and a selection of the extreme case-control samples. Comment on the efficiency.

9

More Complex Data Structures

9.1 Clustered Data

The designs presented in Chapters 3–8 all concern the selection and analysis of a study sample from an underlying population or cohort of independent individuals. However, there are many applications in health research where the population under study consists of clusters of individuals who are related by some important shared characteristics. Clusters can be small, such as members of the same family who are correlated due to their shared genetic and lifestyle factors, or can be of large and varying size, such as patients attending the same health facility or members of a community subjected to a health intervention. In the following subsections, we will see that in clustered data settings, the concepts of case-control and two-stage designs presented in previous chapters can facilitate efficient study design and analysis.

9.1.1 Two-stage design using aggregate cluster data

The two-stage designs introduced in Chapter 3 dealt with samples selected from a cohort of independent individuals where the first-stage information was available for each of the individuals and the second stage information was collected on the subsample. The first-stage information was a binary outcome and some basic information such as sex, age group and perhaps other categorical confounders. However there are settings where the information available at the design stage is in the form of aggregate data describing the clusters from which the study individuals are to be selected. For example, health facilities such as clinics or hospitals may routinely record summaries of patient numbers, percentage male and female, average age and numbers and/or proportion with various outcomes of interest. Where these data are only available in aggregate form, they can still be used to define strata from which to draw an efficient second-stage sample of individuals for analysis.

TABLE 9.1: *Numbers of the total 82,887 individuals in Malawian ART treatment program [75] who are adherent to treatment (controls) and lost to care (cases), stratified by clinic type (numbers underlined) and calendar year.*

	Cases N=16,141	Controls N=66,746
Private	*302*	*2095*
2005	22	247
2006	167	1006
2005	113	842
Public	*15,839*	*64,651*
2005	3492	11,991
2006	6014*	22,887
2005	6333	29,773

* *typed as 6104 in Table 2 of [75].*

Such a design was described for the evaluation of the Malawian national antiretroviral treatment (ART) program, involving more than 80,000 patients in 650 clinics [75]. Interest was focused on the loss of an individual from care at six months post registration (a binary outcome) and its association with patient characteristics, region, type of clinic (public/private) and year of registration. Since patient-level data were not available in electronic form, the Malawian Ministry of Health conducted a one-time cross-sectional survey of a sample of patients for whom data were retrieved from their paper records. However, this survey did not make use of the information that was available at all clinics describing their cohort of patients every 3 months in terms of the numbers retained and lost, and summaries of variables of interest: patient age, sex, WHO disease stage and year of registration. This summary information could have been used to define strata from which to draw a second stage sample of individuals for whom details would be obtained from their medical records. For example, the binary outcome and clinic type (public/private) define 4 strata from which to sample; the outcome together with year of registration (2005–2007) and clinic type (public/private) define 12 strata ranging in size from 22 to 29,773 (see Table 9.1).

The authors investigated the performance of balanced two stage designs with different choices of stratification, illustrating the gain in efficiency compared to a simple case-control sample or random sample of the same size. To achieve a power of 80% for detecting the interaction between type of clinic and calendar year, the case-control design would need to sample 40,000 individuals (approximately half the cohort), while similar power could be achieved from a balanced design of 5000 individuals from the four strata defined by case/control status and public/private clinic. On further stratifying by calendar year, a balanced sample of only 500 has 80% power and a sample of 2000 individuals captures almost all the information in the full cohort of 82,887 individuals.

In this example, the balanced sampling across clinic type and calendar year provides a huge gain in efficiency for estimating the interaction between these two factors, but the authors illustrate that this can come at a cost of reduced precision in the estimates of coefficients for variables not involved in the stratification (e.g. age, WHO disease stage) compared to a simple case-control design. For a given application, the choice of design, and of stratification scheme, will depend on the magnitude of this trade-off and the relative importance of the different coefficients in the model.

9.1.2 Efficient adjustment for cluster interventions

Health services research will often be concerned with interventions that are implemented at the level of a health facility such as a clinic or hospital, a community served by the same public-health team, or a geographic area managed by a regional health authority. For example, the delivery of antiretroviral therapy (ART) for persons living with HIV will usually be clinic-based, while counselling services for this population might be community-based. Although all individuals in a cluster share the same exposure, interest will be focused on the health outcomes of the individuals and how this relates to various demographic and clinical characteristics. Clustered data will also arise where a treatment or intervention is randomly assigned to groups, rather than to individuals, i.e. a cluster-randomised trial.

Whether an intervention is assessed from an observational study or randomised trial, the association between the treatment and the outcome of interest needs to be adjusted for individual characteristics that are potential confounders. In an observational study, some basic information may be available from administrative databases (e.g. patient lists) and in a randomised trial, the enrolment of participants routinely involves the collection of information on characteristics that are deemed essential. In either an observational study or randomised trial of an intervention that has been allocated to clusters, investigators may recognise some additional characteristics that should be considered as potential confounders or that provide opportunity for further meaningful analysis. In this situation, the collection of the additional data on all individuals in all clusters, which could be very costly, may be unnecessary, and investigators may conduct a substudy on a sample of individuals chosen randomly from the full cohort or stratified by cluster.

Such a two-stage approach was taken in the Familia Salama study in Tanzania in 2012–2014 [200], which evaluated the effect of health worker education on antenatal care. The clusters to which the intervention or standard care were randomly assigned were 60 wards, which between them had more than 200,000 pregnancies registered during the study period. As the information available for these pregnancies from the ward registers was limited, an in-depth survey was conducted for a random sample of 2042 (approximately 2%) of the pregnancies, and information gathered on important confounders, including maternal health and reproductive history. While a valid analysis could be conducted using this random survey sample, statistical power can be much improved by using the available basic information for all pregnancies as first-stage data and conducting a two-stage analysis.

By using the mother's ID and ward, the authors were able to link 1239 of the survey participants to a total study base of almost 75,000 pregnancies. For all these pregnancies, data were available on the outcome and intervention, as well as two potential confounders (district and gestational age). The numbers of pregnancies in the strata defined by these first-stage variables and the corresponding numbers in the second-stage survey sample enable the weights to be obtained for a two-stage analysis of the 1239 pregnancies. This analysis accommodates the potential confounding effects of the variables that are only available in the survey sample, which include maternal health, reproductive history and other factors. The results from the two-stage analysis are compared to those from analysis of only the 1239 individuals on Table 9.2, which illustrates that a two-stage analysis of only about 2% of the study cohort enabled adjustment for many potential confounders with no loss of statistical power.

TABLE 9.2: *Estimates for the association between health worker education and compliance with WHO recommendations for antenatal care, using a random sample of individual pregnancies from a cluster-randomised trial and a two-stage analysis that incorporates first-stage information available from antenatal registers [200].*

	Survey Sample only **n=1239**		Survey Sample and first-stage data **n=74,824**	
	OR (95% C.I.)	p	OR (95% C.I.)	p
Crude	1.66 (1.03,2.67)	.04	2.51 (1.72,3.68)	$\leq$ .001
*Adjusted**	1.97 (1.13,3.42)	.02	2.88 (1.75,4.75)	$\leq$ .001

* *adjusted for: district, mother's education, gestational age, maternal and child health knowledge, history of hypertension and HIV indicators.*

9.1.3 Case-control sampling within clusters

In the examples in the previous two subsections, the second-stage individuals were selected without regard to the specific cluster to which they belonged. Section 9.1.1 involved balanced case-control sampling within strata defined by calendar year and clinic type (public or private), and Section 9.1.2 involved a simple random sample of approximately 2% of the study individuals who were linked to the wards (clusters) in which they received antenatal care. Although the clusters (wards or clinics) would be known for the sampled individuals, neither of these analyses accommodated a cluster effect in the model. The estimates from these models will be valid provided there are no unmeasured cluster-level confounders. For example, if the clusters were primary care clinics serving different patient populations, then the age distribution of patients may be an important cluster-level confounder. Where there is potential correlation between members of a cluster that is not captured by the available data, a naive analysis of a random sample (overall or stratified by cluster) or a simple/overall case-control sample has little or no bias and valid confidence intervals [76]. However, a two-stage sampling design that depends on case-control status *and* cluster needs to have cluster effects accommodated in the analysis [76].

For the study of a rare outcome, we have seen many examples of the statistical efficiency of the case-control design. However, in a clustered data setting, such as the communities served by different clinics, it is logistically inefficient to first identify the individuals to be included in the second-stage sample and then extract the detailed records for each of these from the records in their clinic. In contrast, a case-control design stratified by cluster would determine the numbers of individuals to be selected from each clinic and then each clinic would contribute a random sample of the required number of cases and non-cases from their records for the study. A two-stage analysis of the combined data could then be implemented using the inverse of the sampling fractions as weights. This design would not only be more efficient in a practical sense, but can also have good statistical efficiency.

For effects that have large between-cluster variation compared to within-cluster variation, the case-control sampling design has the potential to offer high statistical efficiency compared to other sampling designs. For example, the 'clinic type' variable in the evaluation of the Malawi ART program, which is constant (zero variation) within cluster, would have a standard error less than 50% of that obtained from a study of the same size using a simple/overall case-control design or random sampling within cluster [76]. However, the gain in efficiency for such effects comes at the cost of a loss of efficiency for estimating the effects of factors whose variation within cluster is large compared to variation between cluster: in the Malawi ART example, the efficiency for estimating the effect of participant's age was greatest for a simple case-control design, and even a random second-stage sample was more efficient than the case-control sample within clusters.

Before choosing the sampling design for a second-stage sample from clustered data, investigators need to consider if the variables of primary interest have larger variation between cluster or within cluster. Since a cluster-randomised intervention has high between-cluster variation (zero within-cluster variation) and the intervention effect is of primary interest, a second-stage case-control sample within clusters offers the most efficient estimate of the intervention effect from such a trial. For observational studies, if the within-cluster variation is higher than the between-cluster variation for the parameter of interest, or if this cannot be determined, sampling within cluster may not be useful, and a simple random sample (or for rare outcome, a simple case-control design) would avoid the trade-off in power between the variables.

9.2 Two-stage Augmentation Sampling

In all the examples of two-stage studies so far, the second-stage sample on whom the additional variables were measured was a subsample of the total/first-stage study sample. Thus the second-stage sample was nested within the first-stage sample, or in the case of stratified two-stage sampling, nested within first-stage strata. This is the standard two-stage (also called two-phase) design that is implemented in epidemiological studies. While such sampling designs provide a way of enriching available data, there are situations where the additional information required to optimise the use of data from an existing study, whether cohort, cross-sectional or case-control, is not the collection of additional variables on some participants but the collection of additional participants **(augmentation sampling)** to enable a new research question to be addressed with sufficient power or the same research question to be addressed in a wider population. For example, the original study may have highlighted a small subgroup of interest, for whom a larger sample size would be required to obtain precise estimates, or there may be aspects of the original research question that the investigators wish to examine in an **expanded population**, i.e. a wider target population than that from which the original study sample was chosen.

As a simple example, suppose an investigation of risk factors for cardiovascular disease was conducted in the population over 50 years of age and it was subsequently of interest to conduct a more in-depth investigation for women, then any women selected for the original study can contribute information. However, these may not only offer limited statistical power due to sample size, but investigators may be interested in all adult women, not only those over 50. By augmenting the available data with additional observations sampled from all adult women, the question can be addressed in the larger target population and interactions with age explored.

In some applications of augmentation sampling, it is meaningful to select the additional participants from the same target population as the original study. More generally, the augmentation sampling design selects additional participants from both the original target population and an expanded target population. As with the simpler two-stage designs already encountered in this book, valid estimates can be obtained provided

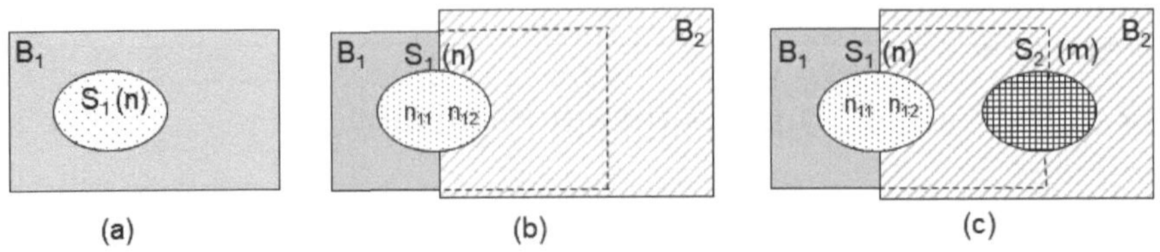

FIGURE 9.1: *Illustration of overlapping study bases B_1 and B_2, with a sample of size n selected at Stage 1 from B_1, augmented at Stage 2 with a sample of size m. The ij suffixes indicate membership of underlying study bases B_1 and B_2.*

TABLE 9.3: *Number of individuals in the population who fulfil the inclusion criteria for Study 1 (N) and Study 2 (N'), with observations in the augmentation sample from B_2 underlined.*

	B_1 **only**	**Overlap**	B_2 **only**	Total
Study Base B_1	N_{10}	N_{11}		N
Sample 1	n_{10}	$\underline{n_{11}}$		n
Study Base B_2		$N'_{11} = N_{11}$	N'_{01}	N'
Augmented		$N_{11} - n_{11}$	N'_{01}	$N'_{01} + N_{11} - n_{11}$
Sample 2		m_{11}	m_{01}	$\underline{\text{m}}$

the differential sampling is accommodated by appropriate weights, which are explained in the following paragraphs.

Assume that a study has been conducted where a sample of n participants was selected from individuals in the population with a specific characteristic, which we will refer to as study base B_1 (Figure 9.1(a)). If it is of interest to subsequently address a research question concerning individuals with another characteristic (i.e. from study base B_2), then some observations in the available sample from the first study, S_1, can only represent the overlapping study bases $B_1 \cap B_2$ (see Figure 9.1(b)). The idea of augmentation sampling is to use the overlapping individuals from the first study sample and to augment them by further sampling from all *other* members of the B_2 study base (see Figure 9.1(c) and Table 9.3).

The augmented sample for Study 2 includes the n_{11} observations sampled from the population for Study 1 that are relevant for Study 2 and the additional m observations sampled at step 2 from study base B_2 with these n_{11} removed. Thus, individuals in the overlap of the two study bases, who have not already been selected for Study 1, have an opportunity to be sampled at the second step. Simple random sampling of a proportion p_1 of individuals at Stage 1 and a proportion p_2 of individuals at Stage 2 yields the final sample of size $n_{11} + m$ from study base B_2 for a weighted analysis, where the weights are:

$$w = 1 \text{ if sampled at Stage 1} \tag{9.1}$$

$$w = \frac{1}{p_2} \text{ if at sampled Stage 2} \tag{9.2}$$

The reader will notice the similarity to the weighting of data from a case-cohort design, where the overlapping study base $B_1 \cap B_2$ can be regarded as a subcohort of B_2, and all individuals in the first stage sample who belong to this subcohort are retained (with weight=1) in the final analysis dataset. Thus being selected at the first stage is the 'event' that guarantees inclusion in the analysis dataset.

If the final analysis is relevant to the population $B_1 \cup B_2$, and not only to B_2, then the n observations from Stage 1 and m observations from Stage 2 need to be reweighted to represent the combined study base. Study base B_1 can be reconstructed by weighting the observations of Sample 1 by $\frac{1}{p_1}$ and Study base B_2 can be reconstructed from Sample 2 using Equations 9.1 and 9.2. However, if these weights are used to reconstruct $B_1 \cup B_2$, the individuals in the overlapping study base $B_1 \cap B_2$ are counted twice. To overcome this double counting, these individuals can each be assigned half their weight [128]:

$$B_1 \text{ only: } w = \frac{1}{p_1} \tag{9.3}$$

$$B_2 \text{ only } : w = \frac{1}{p_2} \tag{9.4}$$

$$B_1 \cap B_2 : w = \frac{1}{2}(\frac{1}{p_1} + 1) \text{ if sampled at Stage 1} \tag{9.5}$$

$$= \frac{1}{2}(\frac{1}{p_2}) \text{ if sampled at Stage 2} \tag{9.6}$$

More generally, augmentation designs can use stratified random sampling, perhaps with different stratification factors for the stratified sampling of individuals at the first and second step. In applications where it is meaningful to select the additional participants from the same target population as the original study, but to use different sampling strata for the augmentation sampling than for the original study, this is known as the **restratification design** in the ecology literature. Here, we will consider the most general design where the augmentation sampling is from an expanded population, and the use of different stratification factors is indicated in Table 9.4 by the strata h=1,2, ... H for the sampling at Stage 1, and strata k=1,2, ... K for the sampling at Stage 2. The weights in the final column of the table would reconstruct the populations from which the Stage 1 and Stage 2 samples were selected, i.e. the N individuals in study base B_1 and the M individuals in study base B_2 who have not already been sampled at Stage 1.

The stratified random sampling of n individuals from study base B_1

TABLE 9.4: *Number of individuals in the sampling strata for Study 1 and Study 2, with corresponding samples sizes and the weights to represent the N and M individuals from whom the samples were selected.*

	Stage 1		
Stratum	Study Base (N)	**Sample 1** (n)	Weights
1	N_1	n_1	N_1/n_1
2	N_2	n_2	N_2/n_2
...		...	...
H	N_H	n_H	N_H/n_H

	Stage 2		
Stratum	Study Base $\notin$ Sample 1 (M)	**Sample 2** (m)	Weights
1	M_1	m_1	M_1/m_1
2	M_2	m_2	M_2/m_2
...	...	...	
K	M_K	m_K	M_K/m_K

at Stage 1 and m individuals from study base B_2 at Stage 2 yields the final sample of size $n_{11} + m$ from study base B_2 for a weighted analysis, with weights:

$$w = 1 \text{ if sampled at Stage 1} \tag{9.7}$$

$$w = \frac{M_k}{m_k} \text{ if sampled at Stage 2} \tag{9.8}$$

As before, the observations sampled at Stage 1 enter the analysis with weight=1, but each stage 2 observation now has a weight that depends on the stratum k to which it belongs.

For analysis relevant to the population $B_1 \cup B_2$, re-weighting the combined sample of $n + m$ observations results in the individuals in the overlapping study base being counted twice. As before, this is corrected by taking half the weight, which will depend on whether the observation was sampled at Stage 1 or Stage 2.

$$B_1 \text{ only: } w = \frac{N_h}{n_h} \tag{9.9}$$

$$B_2 \text{ only } : w = \frac{M_k}{m_k} \tag{9.10}$$

$$B_1 \cap B_2 : w = \frac{1}{2}(\frac{N_h}{n_h} + 1) \text{ if sampled at Stage 1} \tag{9.11}$$

$$= \frac{1}{2}(\frac{M_k}{m_k}) \quad \text{ if sampled at Stage 2} \tag{9.12}$$

In the paper proposing the weights in Equations 9.9 to 9.12 [128], the application involved the investigation of risk factors for incident HPV infection during follow-up of a cohort of unvaccinated participants in a HPV vaccine trial. Interest was focused on HPV16 and HPV18, which account for 50% and 20% respectively of cervical cancer cases, and the risk factors included age, number of sexual partners and baseline levels of antibodies to HPV16 or HPV18, which indicate previous exposure to those infections. Study base B_1, consisting of women who were free of HPV16 infection at baseline, was expanded to include women who were free of HPV18 (Study Base B_2). A stratified sample of women was selected from B_1 using baseline levels of HPV16 antibodies to define three strata (H=3 in Table 9.4). This sample of women free of HPV16 infection was augmented at Stage 2 by stratified sampling from an expanded population (women free of HPV18), this time using baseline levels of

HPV18 antibodies to define three sampling strata ($K = 3$ in Table 9.4). The joint study base ($B_1 \cup B_2$) from which this two-stage sample was drawn, consisting of women who were free of one or both of the infections (HPV16 and HPV18) at baseline, was reconstructed using the weights in Equations 9.9 to 9.12. The weight assigned to women who were free of both infections at baseline ($B_1 \cap B_2$) depends on their HPV16 antibody if sampled at Stage 1 and their HPV18 antibody if sampled at Stage 2. Analysis of the augmented samples is straightforward, using weighted logistic regression.

9.3 Time-dependent Exposure

The Cox proportional hazards regression model introduced in Chapter 4 assumed that the exposure of interest, X, was known at baseline for all cohort members and remained the same throughout follow-up. For the various cohorts presented in subsequent chapters, such a time-independent exposure was also assumed. In Chapter 4, the proportional hazards model was represented by the simple partial likelihood in Equation 4.15 or the more general equation in the first row of Table 4.10, which is the following product over all event times

$$\prod_{t_i} \frac{e^{\beta X_i + \gamma Z_i}}{\sum_{k \in R_i} e^{\beta X_k + \gamma Z_k}} \tag{9.13}$$

where t_i denotes the event times, X is the exposure and Z the other covariates in the model. At each event time, the partial likelihood component consists of the ratio of the hazard of the case, which depends on X and Z, and the total hazard of all members of the cohort who are still at risk. Any individual in the denominator will be characterised by their same covariate profile at all times where they contribute as a member of the risk set. However, there are many applications where an exposure of interest occurs for some individuals during follow-up, so that these persons contribute unexposed time before becoming exposed. Such a **time-dependent exposure** is illustrated in Figure 9.2, where a small cohort of 15 individuals is followed for 20 years.

Only three of the individuals (numbered 2, 8 and 12) are exposed at baseline, a further four (numbered 5, 7, 10 and 15) become exposed

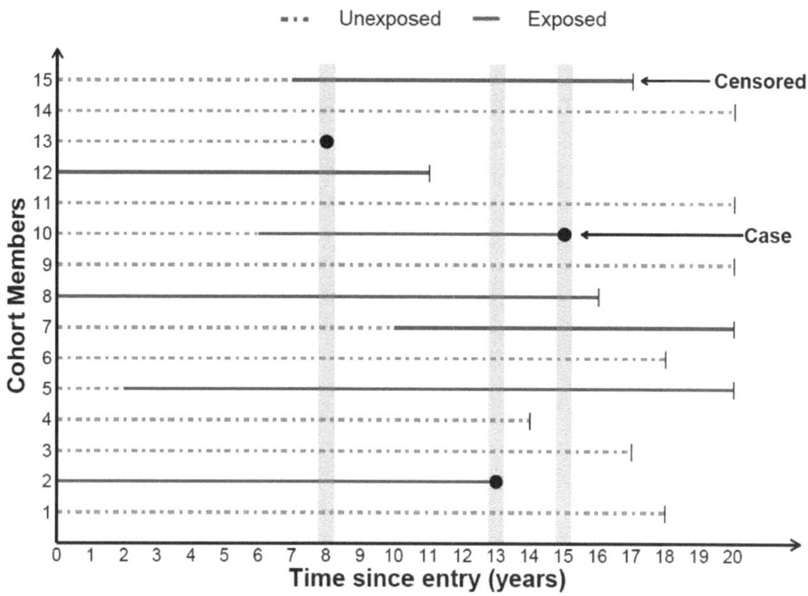

FIGURE 9.2: *Illustration of a cohort with time-dependent exposure.*

at various times during the follow-up, and the remaining eight are unexposed throughout follow-up. Individual 7 is unexposed at the time of the first event in year 8, but exposed at the time of the second event in year 13, so their contribution to the partial likelihood will be different on these two occasions. The correct exposure status at each event time can be readily obtained from the comparison of the exposure time to the event times.

The simplest way to analyse such data with statistical software is to split the records of any individual who changed exposure status during follow-up, so that they contribute unexposed person time and exposed person time (see Table 9.5). The unexposed record is censored and the exposed record is defined as an event or censoring depending on the final outcome status of the individual: the first (unexposed) record for individual 15 in Figure 9.2 is censored at year 7 and the second (exposed) record begins at year 7 and is censored at year 17; in contrast, the first (unexposed) record for individual 10 is censored at 6 years and the second (exposed) record starts from year 6 and is defined as an event at year 15. Once the dataset has been rearranged, it can be analysed by standard Cox regression.

TABLE 9.5: *Rearrangement of data from the cohort in Figure 9.2 with outcome Y, where records from individuals who changed exposure status X are split into unexposed and exposed person-time.*

ID	Enter	Exit	Z	X	Y
15	0	7	Z_{15}	0	0
15	7	17	Z_{15}	1	0
14	0	20	Z_{14}	0	0
13	0	8	Z_{13}	0	1
12	0	11	Z_{12}	1	0
11	0	20	Z_{11}	0	0
10	0	6	Z_{10}	0	0
10	6	15	Z_{10}	1	1
...	...	...	...	...	...

X: *time-dependent exposure*
Z: *time-independent covariates*

9.3.1 Exposure density sampling

Matched cohort data was introduced in Section 6.1 of Chapter 6 as a design for the study of the association between an exposure available at baseline and a binary outcome. Where exposed and unexposed subjects are frequency matched, analysis is conducted using an unconditional logistic regression model that includes the matching variable(s) together with the exposure and other variables of interest. Where the data have been individually-matched, a conditional logistic regression model is used. To estimate the HR for a time-to-event outcome in a matched cohort, stratified Cox regression fits different baseline hazards in the matched strata, thus providing an adjusted estimate under the assumption of a common HR across the strata.

When an exposure is time-dependent, one approach has been to analyse the HR of exposed individuals from the time they become exposed, by comparing them to a (possibly matched) sample of those who do not become exposed. While this is conceptually simple, involving only the setting of the 'time zero', it is biased due to 'borrowing from the future' if the unexposed persons are chosen from those who do not become exposed during the observation period. Despite this weakness, this design has often been used in hospital epidemiology to study the effect of exposures acquired during hospitalisation [233], such as hospital-acquired infection. If Figure 9.2 represents a cohort of 15 hospitalised patients, where the event is in-hospital death (and discharged patients are censored), then patients 2, 8 and 12 enter the analysis as exposed on day 0 (representing their acquisition of the exposure on the day of admission), while patients 5, 10, 15 and 7 enter the analysis from day 2, 6, 7 and 10 respectively. If a matched cohort study such as just described was implemented, then any of the remaining eight unexposed individuals could be selected to be compared to any of the exposed except number 7: for exposed individual 7, number 13 is not among the unexposed who could be selected, as they have been censored earlier.

Readers will recognise that a more appropriate comparison group for a person who acquires the exposure at a specific time t is a set of controls chosen from the individuals who are unexposed *at time* t, i.e. for individual 5 in Figure 9.2, anyone except numbers 2,8 and 12 can be selected; for individual 10, number 5 is now also excluded, etc. The dataset assembled in this way will contain a matched cohort of exposed and unexposed individuals, matched on their time in the study, where some of the unexposed may later become exposed. This is the exact equivalent of the incidence density sampling of controls (who can later become cases) in a nested case-control study, hence **exposure density sampling**. If some of the selected unexposed individuals later become exposed, then the data needs to be analysed using the methods for time-dependent exposure presented in Section 9.3. If additional matching was used in the selection of the unexposed individuals, these factors must also be included in the model.

9.3.2 Nested case-control sampling

The partial likelihood in Equation 9.13 compared the case at each event time to the full risk set at that time. As seen in Chapter 4, the risk set could instead be represented by the case and a small number of individuals sampled from the non-cases at the event time. The partial likelihood then becomes:

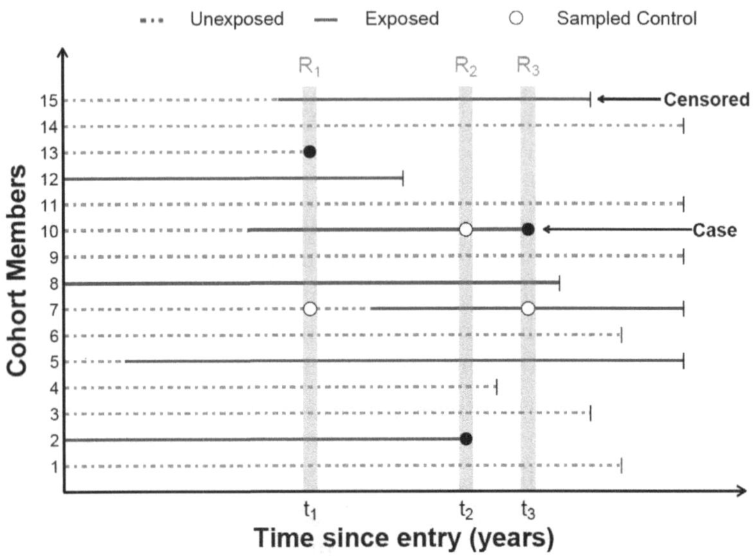

FIGURE 9.3: *Illustration of the cohort from Figure 9.2 with with a 1:1 nested case-control sample: cases marked as solid circles and time-matched controls as open circles.*

$$\prod_{t_i} \frac{e^{\beta X_i + \gamma Z_i}}{\sum_{k \in R_i^*} e^{\beta X_k + \gamma Z_k}} \tag{9.14}$$

where R_i^* is the *sampled* risk set, consisting of the case and their matched controls. Figure 9.3 presents the same cohort as in Figure 9.2, with the times of the first three events marked as t_1, t_2, t_3 and a single control selected at each of these event times. The partial likelihood contributions will involve the three pairs of individuals, (13,7), (2,10) and (10,7), and their exposure status at the event time. The exposure status of controls in the analysis is determined by comparing their exposure time to their sampling time. Alternatively, if the cohort is first split as presented in the previous paragraph, nested case-control sampling from the *records* in the split data will result in randomly selected controls with the correct exposure status for their selection time. The equivalence of these two sampling approaches can be readily seen from Figure 9.3.

Illustration: Prostate Cancer Screening

The data for this illustration is from a study of the risk of cancer in siblings of Swedish patients diagnosed between 1958 and 2009 [120]. For the analysis of prostate cancer risk among the brothers of a man who has been diagnosed with the disease, the first man diagnosed in the family is referred to as the "index" case and the cohort consists of the brothers of these 14,446 index cases. The 20,953 brothers were followed up from the index date to December 2009, during which time a total of 1589 (7.6%) had a diagnosis of prostate cancer. In contrast, the rate of prostate cancer diagnosis was only 2.2% in a cohort of brothers of 'index' controls who were cancer-free at the time of diagnosis of the cases. This corresponds to case brothers having more than three times the risk (IRR=3.69, 95% CI: 3.46–3.93) when adjusted for calendar time, age and number of brothers [120]). The findings were similar when using age as the time scale.

To investigate whether the introduction of prostate specific antigen (PSA) testing in Sweden in the mid-1990s resulted in a 'screening effect', the authors presented a graphical comparison of the incidence in siblings of index cases and controls diagnosed/sampled pre- and post-1997. In both of these periods, case siblings had a significantly higher incidence of prostate cancer than control siblings, but the difference was larger in the post-1997 period. Here we repeat the analysis of the case siblings, treating the availability of PSA screening as a time-dependent exposure: any follow-up time prior to 1998 is defined as unexposed time and follow-up during or after 1998 as exposed time. The changing risk of prostate cancer with age can be accommodated by adjustment or by using age as the time scale. Depending on the choice of time scale, either the calendar year (or the age of a man) prior to 1998 will be defined as unexposed and calendar years (or ages) from 1998 as exposed.

Discarding follow-up time prior to 40 years of age, when there are very few prostate cancer diagnoses, the cohort consisted of 19,491 siblings, among whom there were 1498 diagnosed with prostate cancer during follow up, with the youngest age at diagnosis being 42 years. The separate Kaplan-Meier plots of the cancer-free survival in the periods before and after PSA screening are presented in Figure 9.4. From this plot it can be seen that there is limited information available for the period prior to screening (1998), due to the start-up date of the Swedish registers used for the data linkage. Although the Swedish Cancer Register records all cancer diagnoses since 1958, the identification of family members relies on the MultiGeneration Register, which records the

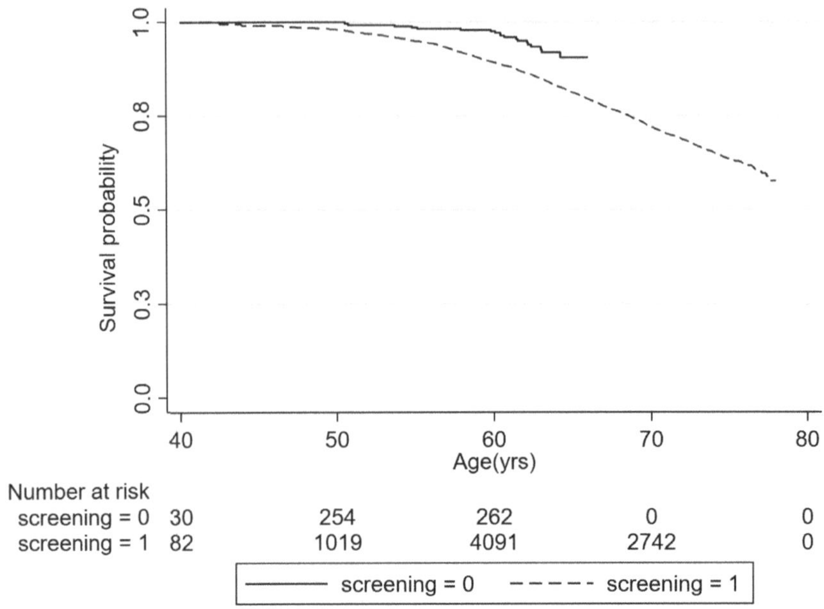

FIGURE 9.4: *Kaplan-Meier plot of prostate cancer in brothers of cases diagnosed in Sweden before and after the widespread availability of PSA screening.*

parents of all people born in Sweden since 1932. Thus the brothers in the prostate cancer analysis are at most 66 years old in 1998.

Among the 19,491 men, there were 17,557 whose follow-up began in 1998 or later and 1934 whose follow-up started before 1998 and finished after 1998, generating two records (one exposed and one unexposed). On splitting the data as explained above, there was a total of 21,425 records available for analysis of the introduction of screening as a time-dependent exposure. A Cox regression analysis, adjusting for the number of siblings, yielded a hazard ratio of 2.29 on the age scale and 2.59 on the time scale (see Table 9.6). A nested case-control sample can be selected either from the cohort of individuals or from the split records as explained above. The results of conditional logistic regression of a 1:3 nested case-control sample gave similar estimates to the full cohort with wider confidence intervals as expected (second row of Table 9.6). Due to the imbalance in exposure, the nested case-control sample has many concordant sets. In such situations, statistical power may be improved by breaking the matching and conducting a weighted Cox regression of the individuals with the time-dependent exposure pre/post 1998. The

TABLE 9.6: *Hazard ratios (and 95% confidence intervals) for prostate cancer in brothers of index cases diagnosed in 1998 or later compared to earlier years.*

	Age Scale		Time Scale	
	HR	**95% C.I.**	**HR***	**95% C.I.**
Cohort	2.29	(1.45, 3.63)	2.59	(1.64, 4.10)
1:3 Nested case-control				
CLR	2.28	(1.38, 3.75)	2.53	(1.57, 4.09)
IPW	2.32	(1.44, 3.71)	2.62	(1.64, 4.17)

* *adjusted for age and number of brothers.*

results of such analysis of the nested case-control sample are presented on the third row of Table 9.6, where for the analysis on the age scale, the estimated HR has improved precision compared to the conditional logistic regression. For the time scale analysis, the potential improvement is offset by the need to adjust for the age at entry.

9.3.3 Detailed history of exposure in case-control studies

In a nested case-control study, details of exposure are gathered at the time of event (for the case) or selection (for the matched control). Where the study subjects are sampled within a well-defined study base, there may also be aspects of exposure available at baseline. In contrast to the baseline (time-independent) exposure measures, measures of exposure that occur during follow-up are time-dependent. Taking cigarette smoking as an example, cohort members may be classified at baseline as never-smokers, ex-smokers or current smokers, but at the time of event/sampling the smoking status may have changed and other details may be of interest to the investigators. In a nested case-control study, cases and controls may be asked for details regarding the duration of smoking (if currently smoking), the time since quitting (if an ex-smoker) and the accumulated exposure over their lifetime or in specific age-bands. If the case-control data is analysed by conditional logistic regression, then the likelihood contribution of each risk set consists of a comparison of the exposure history of the cases to that of their time-matched controls (Table 4.10 in Chapter 4). In contrast, Cox regression of the full cohort will treat the exposure as a time-dependent covariate as discussed above. Thus, at each event time, the selected controls in the nested case-control study are used to represent the full risk set that would contribute to a Cox regression with time-dependent covariates.The Cox regression analysis has greater efficiency than conditional logistic regression, not only from the larger sample size, but also from the fact that all non-cases contribute to the risk set at each event time, while matched case and control individuals enter the conditional logistic regression only at their own event/selection time, and in addition, a set is dropped from analysis if the individuals are concordant for exposure. We have seen in Chapter 6 how this greater efficiency of Cox regression can be exploited by using an appropriately weighted regression to analyse nested case-control data.

An important feature of the weighted analysis is that the controls must be followed up past their selection time in order for the reweighted case and control records to reconstruct the cohort experience over the follow-up time. In the earlier examples of such analyses in Chapter 6, the additional information required for the controls was the time of any 'future cases', i.e., the event times for any controls who became a case at any time from their selection time until the end of the study period. Where the exposure of interest is time-dependent, a weighted Cox regression will also require the 'future' exposure information for controls from their selection time to the end of the study.

In the prostate cancer example above, the weighted Cox regression gave a small improvement in precision compared the conditional logistic regression. In that example, the time-dependent exposure was a simple indicator for pre- or post-1998, when PSA screening for prostate cancer became widely available in Sweden. Since this information can be readily determined simply from knowing entry, exit and event dates, a nested case-control sample from the cohort of brothers can be analysed by weighted Cox regression provided the times of future events among the selected controls are known. However, for a time-dependent exposure that requires effort and expense to ascertain for cases and their matched controls, such as the (changing) exposure to cigarette smoking, the weighted Cox regression methods presented so far are unlikely to be of interest. The question then arises if one can use exposure data from the individuals in a nested case-control study, not just at the event/selection time but also *prior* information, to obtain valid estimates from a Cox regression with an alternative weighting system. In the absence of any weighting, simply treating the available case and control records as a cohort is likely to result in a downward bias of the HR compared to the estimate based on comparing each case to the large number of controls in the underlying population. It should also be clear that a conditional logistic regression of the matched sets that excludes any future cases will likely result in an upward bias from this comparison of cases to these 'pure controls', while inclusion of all future cases in all risk sets will generate a downward bias. The bias from such naive analyses was explored for a simple binary exposure in a simulated cohort of 100,000 individuals, of whom 20% were exposed at baseline and a further 25% were assigned a random exposure time during 10 years of follow-up. With a constant baseline hazard for the outcome, and a HR of 2 for its association with exposure, the event rate in the cohort was approximately 15%. Table 9.7 presents the HR estimate from the full cohort in the first row, valid analyses of a 1:1 nested case-control sample in the second and third row, and naive analyses in the fifth and sixth rows. The results in the last row were obtained from the approach discussed in detail in the following paragraphs.

An intuitively appealing method that avoids the extremes of complete inclusion or exclusion of future cases argues that all cases and controls in the nested case-control sample can be used to represent the underlying cohort *at all times prior to their selection* provided the "imbalance" in the case/control ratio is overcome by appropriate weighting

TABLE 9.7: *Hazard ratios (and 95% confidence intervals) for a time-dependent exposure in a simulated cohort with HR = 2 and a 1:1 nested case-control sample from the cohort.*

	Analysis	**HR**	**95% C.I.**
Cohort	Cox regression	2.01	(1.94, 2.08)
1:1 Nested case-control			
	Conditional logistic regression (CLR)	2.04	(1.91, 2.18)
	Weighted cox regression (IPW)	1.94	(1.84, 2.05)
	Naive Cox regression[1]	1.57	(1.50, 1.64)
	Naive CLR[2]	2.20	(2.06, 2.36)
	Weighted Cox (Leffondre)[3]	1.87	(1.76, 1.99)

[1] *sampled individuals treated as 'cohort' up to selection time*
[2] *future cases excluded from risk sets*
[3] *stratified weights proposed by [122]*

[122]. In the simple illustration in Figure 9.3, this means that the records of individuals 2, 7, 10 and 13 would contribute their follow-up from entry to event or selection to the weighted Cox regression. In fact, there would be 6 records available for weighting, since the proposed method [122] assigns distinct identification numbers to 'multiple' subjects such as individuals 7 and 10: number 7 would contribute two censored records, one at t_1 and one at t_3 (i.e. t=8 an t=15 from Figure 9.2), and number 10 would contribute one censored at t_2 (t=13) and a record with event at t_3 (t=15). Note that this approach is recommended for a rare disease, whereas there are 3 cases in the cohort of 15 individuals in the simple graphical example.

The proposed weights [122] can be obtained from external resources such as population survival estimates, and are motivated as follows. At any event time, the individuals selected for the nested case-control study consist of a ratio of (current and future) cases to non-cases that is determined by the study design, for example a ratio of 1:2 for a study with 2 controls per case. However, this ratio in the full cohort would be $\frac{N(t)\pi(t)}{N(t)*(1-\pi(t))}$ where $N(t)$ is the number at risk at the event time t, and $\pi(t)$ is the probability of having the event at or after time t. Assuming all cases in the cohort are sampled into the nested case-control study, the weights to restore the balance are then:

$$w(t) = 1 \text{ for cases}$$
$$w(t) = \frac{(1-\pi(t))}{\pi(t)} . \frac{n_1(t)}{n_0(t)} \text{ for controls} \tag{9.15}$$

where $n_1(t)$ and $n_0(t)$ are the numbers of cases and controls at time t, e.g. $\frac{n_1(t)}{n_0(t)} = 1/2$ for a case-control ratio 1:2. If age is the time scale, $\pi(t)$ can be estimated from population survival tables. Where such information is not available, a simplified version of the weights using just the overall probability π in place of $\pi(t)$ provides reasonable estimates of the HR in settings where $\pi(t)$ does not change much over the study period. These simple weights also have the advantage that they can be implemented in Cox regression analysis in any statistical package, while the weights in Equation 9.15 require a package that accommodates time-dependent weights, such as R. The results from the Cox regression using the simple weights are included in the last row of Table 9.7. This estimate is somewhat biased, but unlike the naive Cox regression and naive conditional logistic regression, the confidence interval almost includes the true value of 2.

9.4 Time-varying Associations

All the Cox models presented so far assume that the underlying hazard is increased by a constant factor at all times during follow-up by an exposure X, the so-called 'proportional hazards' assumption. However, it may be more reasonable to assume a changing effect over time for some exposures, such as the protection offered by a vaccine in the time period following vaccination. Where age is used as the time scale, an increasing or decreasing risk/benefit of an exposure with advancing age are examples of **non-proportional hazards**. A simple approach to relaxing the proportional hazards assumption is to split the records of each individual into 'epochs' and fit a different coefficient in each epoch (see Chapter 7 of [171]). In this way, the age is effectively being handled as a 'time-dependent' exposure with a number of categories. For example, if we wish to estimate the HR in four age categories (<50, 50–60, 60–70, >70), then the records for an individual will be split into their contributions to these strata. The top panel of Table 9.8 displays the records of four individuals in the original data, followed from their age at the start of follow-up (start age) to their age at the event or censoring (end age). To fit a different HR in each of the age categories, these individuals will have their records split into the contributions shown in the bottom panel of Table 9.8. A stratified Cox regression with the four indicators **m1–m4** will estimate the hazard ratio for males in each age category. An application of the method to the Framingham data is presented in Example 9.1, where the estimates indicate a decline in the differential risk of CHD in men and women with advancing age. The HR estimated from a simple Cox regression of the same data was 2.10 (95% C.I. 1.81–2.23).

The non-proportional hazards in this simple introduction is the most general, in that it makes no assumption of the functional relationship between the HR and time. However, it requires the data analyst to choose an appropriate categorisation to capture the underlying change in the HR, without using too crude or too fine a resolution. One can also model the ln(HR) as a linear function of time by using an interaction

TABLE 9.8: ***Top:*** *A sample of individual records from two males and two females;* ***Bottom:*** *the corresponding split records over four age categories.*

ID	male	start age	end age	event
101	1	43	68	1
102	1	55	75	0
103	0	52	65	1
104	0	61	71	0

ID	stratum	enter	exit	status	m1	m2	m3	m4
101	1 (<50)	43	50	0	1	0	0	0
101	2 (50–60)	50	60	0	0	1	0	0
101	3 (60–70)	60	68	1	0	0	1	0
102	2 (50–60)	55	60	0	0	1	0	0
102	3 (60–70)	60	70	0	0	0	1	0
102	4 (>70)	70	75	0	0	0	0	1
103	2 (50–60)	52	60	0	0	0	0	0
103	3 (60–70)	60	65	1	0	0	0	0
104	3 (60–70)	61	70	0	0	0	0	0
104	4 (>70)	70	71	0	0	0	0	0

columns m1, m1, m3 and m4 are indicator variables for whether an individual is a male in age stratum 1, 2, 3 or 4

term created from the product of exposure and time in a standard Cox model. Where more complex relationships are to be modelled, parametric functions or cubic splines [84] are alternatives to the piece-wise step functions[176] used in the simple example above.

9.4.1 Time-varying associations and case-control designs

Consider a cohort of individuals who are classified as exposed/unexposed at baseline, and from which the cases occurring during a specified time period are identified. If these cases are compared to a sample of non-cases selected randomly during the same time period, then the OR of

Example 9.1. *Application of the approach illustrated in Table 9.8 to the Framingham teaching data to estimate the age-specific HR of CHD in men compared to women.*

Age Group	Indicator	HR	95 % C.I
<50	male1	4.23	(2.73, 6.56)
50–60	male2	2.48	(2.01, 3.06)
60–70	male3	1.76	(1.50, 2.07)
70–80	male4	1.89	(1.51, 2.35)
>80	male5	1.05	(0.65, 1.70)

the exposure in different time intervals can be estimated using logistic regression, by first splitting the control records into the chosen time intervals. To avoid enriching the controls in any time interval with 'future cases', the cases contribute only one record, which could still result in some residual bias due to the under-representation of such individuals if the outcome is not rare. If the time scale is age, then the arrangement of the control records will follow the same procedure as Table 9.8, with the case record being assigned to the age stratum in which they were diagnosed. By modelling the interaction between stratum and exposure in a similar way to Example 9.1, the ORs for the different periods are estimated. If the prevalence is not assumed to be the same across the time intervals, then a stratum effect (i.e. different α values) should be included in the model. For this logistic regression analysis, a robust variance estimate is appropriate, since the same control can contribute to different time-periods.

While the method presented above enables the estimation of an OR in different time intervals, it does not allow the assessment of whether the effect of exposure over time follows a smooth trend: for example, the Framingham analysis in Example 9.1 suggests a steady decline in the association with age, that might be of interest to test formally. Another disadvantage of the data-splitting approach is the choice of appropriate time-intervals and the assumption of a common OR during the interval with change at the boundary. This problem could be mitigated by choosing many narrow intervals, but would then require a large sample size, which is contrary to the spirit of why a case-control study was done in the first place!

A simple and elegant approach for assessing the form of a time-varying association is to regard the controls as a subcohort, and conduct a case-cohort analysis [101]. The controls in this setting are not an exact subcohort, as they do not include controls who later became cases (see Chapter 4, Section 4.5). However, if the disease is rare, these 'pure' controls will be a close representation of the underlying cohort. In the standard case-cohort design, the sample for analysis consists of the subcohort together with any cases outside the subcohort, and members of the subcohort serve as the reference group at each event time when they are still at risk. The Prentice likelihood introduced in Chapter 4 (see Example 4.13) is the product of the partial likelihood components at each event time t_i

$$\prod_{t_i} \frac{e^{\beta X_i + \gamma Z_i}}{\sum_{j \epsilon S_i} e^{\beta X_j + \gamma Z_j} + I[i \notin S_i] e^{\beta X_i + \gamma Z_i}} \tag{9.16}$$

where S_i denotes the subcohort members at risk at event time t_i, X denotes the exposure and Z the other predictor variables in the model. Thus, the likelihood to be solved is similar to a Cox partial likelihood, except that a case occurring outside the subcohort enters the risk set in the denominator only at their own event time. This can be easily implemented in statistical software by assigning such cases an entry time just before their event time and then conducting a standard Cox regression analysis. In the case of the imperfect subcohort in the setting being discussed here, all of the cases are outside the subcohort.

The case-cohort likelihood offers great flexibility for the modelling of time-varying effects, since β can be any function of time. For example, a simple linear trend in the HR with time would result in the likelihood:

$$\prod_{t_i} \frac{e^{(\beta_0 + \beta t_i) X_i + \gamma Z_i}}{\sum_{j \epsilon S_i^*} e^{(\beta_0 + \beta t_i) X_j + \gamma Z_j}} \tag{9.17}$$

where the denominator in Equation 9.16 has been replaced by the notation from Chapter 4, with S_i^* denoting the members of the subcohort (and the case, if outside the subcohort) at risk at time t_i.

For a time-dependent exposure, the case-cohort model allows the HR to depend on the duration of exposure, by modelling β as a function of this time rather than the time scale used for analysis. For a simple linear function, the likelihood in Equation 9.17 can be written as Equation 9.18,

$$\prod_{t_i} \frac{e^{(\beta_0+\beta u_{ii})X_i+\gamma Z_i}}{\sum_{j\epsilon S_i^*} e^{(\beta_0+\beta u_{ji})X_j+\gamma Z_j}} \tag{9.18}$$

where u_{ji} is the duration of exposure for individual j at risk at event/analysis time t_i, and the double subscript 'ii' distinguishes the case at that time from the other members of the risk set. As before, X_i denotes the exposure status of the case at time t_i and X_j the exposure status for non-cases in the risk set. For example, where age is the time scale and individuals are exposed from different ages, the preparation of the data for analysis involves arranging each control in multiple records that accommodate their change in exposure status during follow-up (if such change occurred) as well as duration of exposure at the event times.

A nested case-control sample can also provide valid estimates of a time-dependent exposure and time-varying associations, by using conditional logistic regression models with interaction terms. This approach is presented in detail for an application to varicella vaccine effectiveness in children [163], where the impact of time since vaccination and age at vaccination are considered. In addition to simplicity, conditional logistic regression has the advantage that it applies to non-rare outcomes. However, in contrast to the exclusive sampling followed by case-cohort analysis above, it does not make use of the exposure history at event times prior to the control's own selection time. This potential loss in efficiency was the motivation for the weighted Cox regression of nested case-control data introduced earlier (Equations 9.15) in the context of a time-dependent binary exposure [122]. Provided the necessary population data is available, the same approach can be used for more complex models. In the example included in the publication introducing the method [122], the authors investigate multiple aspects of smoking history for their association with lung cancer: ever-smoker, time since cessation and cigarette years in all individuals; smoking intensity and duration in current smokers. Like the case-cohort approach in the previous paragraph, this method also requires an assumption of rare outcome.

9.5 Combining Matched and Unmatched Case-control Data

In the designs presented in previous chapters, it was assumed that all the data for analysis arose from conducting a single study, that was either matched or unmatched. However, it is also possible that both matched and unmatched case-control data are available from two or more studies of the same (or a related) research question. Such data arose from the study of risk factors for cervical cancer and cervical intraepithelial neoplasia (CIN III) in Spain and Columbia: the study of cervical cancer [17] included 436 cases and 387 controls randomly selected from the population; the CIN study [156] compared 525 cases to 512 controls that had been individually matched on age ± 5 years, place of recruitment and the date ± 1 day of specimen collection. Below we present a joint likelihood for the analysis of such data using two different approaches that are easy to implement in practice. These methods are not only useful for the pooling of two or more studies, but also have potential for handling missing exposure data in matched studies, instead of the "all or nothing" approach of either conducting a conditional regression of the complete sets or breaking all the matching and using an unconditional (weighted) analysis. The joint analysis of matched and unmatched data allows for the alternative of only breaking the matching of the 'problem' sets and combining these observations with the matched observations in the 'intact' sets. The incomplete sets that would be excluded from a conditional analysis can be due to missing exposure for the case, missing exposure for the matched control (or for all matched controls in a 1:m case-control study) or the inability to identify controls with the required matching factors for some cases.

9.5.1 Joint likelihood of matched and unmatched data

In the logistic regression model for a binary outcome Y, the likelihood components for a case ($Y = 1$) and non-case/control ($Y = 0$) with exposure X are:

$$P(Y = 1|X) = \frac{e^{\alpha+\beta X}}{1 + e^{\alpha+\beta X}} \tag{9.19}$$

$$P(Y = 0|X) = \frac{1}{1 + e^{\alpha+\beta X}} \tag{9.20}$$

so that the likelihood for n_1 cases and n_0 controls is the product:

$$\prod_{i=1}^{n_1} \frac{e^{\alpha+\beta X_i}}{1+e^{\alpha+\beta X_i}} \prod_{i=n_1+1}^{n_1+n_0} \frac{1}{1+e^{\alpha+\beta X_i}} \tag{9.21}$$

$$= \prod_{i=1}^{n} \left[\frac{e^{\alpha+\beta X_i}}{1+e^{\alpha+\beta X_i}}\right]^{Y_i} \left[\frac{1}{1+e^{\alpha+\beta X_i}}\right]^{1-Y_i} \tag{9.22}$$

For a matched pair (one case and one control), denoting the exposure values of the case and control as X_1 and X_0 respectively, the logistic regression model results in Equation 2.53 in Chapter 2 for the probability that the event happens to the individual with exposure X_1, conditional on one event in the pair

$$\frac{P(Y=1|X_1)}{P(Y=1|X_1)+P(Y=1|X_0)} = \frac{e^{\beta X_1}}{e^{\beta X_1}+e^{\beta X_0}} \tag{9.23}$$

$$= \frac{e^{\beta(X_1-X_0)}}{1+e^{\beta(X_1-X_0)}} \tag{9.24}$$

This expression is similar to Equation 9.19 above for an 'observation' with exposure equal to the difference in the case and control exposure values. If there are m pairs, the likelihood is the product:

$$= \prod_{i=1}^{m} \frac{e^{\beta(X_{i1}-Xi0)}}{1+e^{\beta(X_{i1}-X_{i0})}} \tag{9.25}$$

where X_{i1} and X_{i0} indicate the exposure status of the case and control in the ith pair. Thus with appropriate data preparation, we can analyse the unmatched and matched data together [153] by combining the likelihood contributions from 9.22 and 9.25. The steps to prepare the data for analysis are presented in the box on the next page. In the paper proposing this method [153], the authors conducted a joint analysis of the unmatched study and matched study of risk factors for cervical cancer [17, 156] introduced above, to estimate the risk associated with multiple sexual partners (three levels). The ORs from the separate unconditional and conditional analysis are presented in Table 9.9, where they are compared with the estimates from the model without interaction. The unmatched and matched studies both provide strong evidence of a trend in risk with more sexual partners, with little evidence of confounding by education level. The likelihood ratio test of homogeneity

- prepare the matched data as one record per set with outcome=1, and covariates = difference in case and control values
- append these records to the unmatched records
- use an indicator for whether record is from the matched or unmatched study, to allow different intercept
- use more indicators if more than two studies are combined
- conduct standard logistic regression
- assumption of a common OR for the studies can be tested using interaction between exposure and study group

of the studies was not significant, so it is reasonable to report the results from the pooled analysis without interaction. Readers will note that the interaction model reproduces the exact ORs for the reference group in the crude analysis but not in the adjusted analysis. This is a result of the contribution of education level in the two studies, and exact agreement can be produced by including an interaction between study and education level. The pooled OR lies between those from the unmatched and matched analysis and is a reasonable estimate of the (common) underlying OR when the interaction is not significant.

TABLE 9.9: *Crude and adjusted (for education level) ORs for association of cervical cancer with multiple sexual partners, from separate and pooled analysis of one unmatched and one matched case-control study [153].*

	Crude		**Adjusted**		**p (trend)**
No. partners (Ref <=1)	2–5	6+	2–5	6+	
Unmatched (n=823)	1.94	6.62	2.17	7.73	< .001
Matched (n=1037)	1.61	4.73	1.64	4.69	< .001
Pooled	1.78	5.52	1.89	5.86	< .001
Interaction[1]					
CIN (Ref)	1.61	4.73	1.67	4.76	< .001
ICC vs. CIN	1.21	1.40	1.27	1.56	(.42, .27)[2]

[1] *Likelihood ratio test (vs. pooled model, no interaction) p=0.47*
[2] *p-values = 0.42 (crude) and 0.27 (adjusted)*

9.5.2 Missing indicator method

Another approach to the analysis of matched and unmatched pairs in a case-control study involves using a missing indicator variable and redefining exposure in a way that allows the required relationships to be modelled [88]. Using M_1 and M_0 to denote missing exposure for the case and control, respectively, and setting the value of the missing exposure to zero (i.e. $X_1 = 0$ if $M_1 = 1$ and $X_0 = 0$ for $M_0 = 1$), the conditional probability of the event occurring to the case in a pair can be written:

$$= \frac{e^{\beta X_1 + \gamma M_1}}{e^{\beta X_1 + \gamma M_1} + e^{\beta X_0 + \gamma M_0}} \tag{9.26}$$

and the full likelihood, i.e. the product over all pairs

$$= \prod_i \frac{e^{\beta X_{i1} + \gamma M_{i1}}}{e^{\beta X_{i1} + \gamma M_{i1}} + e^{\beta X_{i0} + \gamma X_{i0}}} \tag{9.27}$$

The paired observations are of three kinds, since the exposure data is either complete, missing for the case or missing for the control: pairs with missing exposure for the case and control do not contribute any information about the association between exposure and outcome. The likelihood components from Equation 9.27 for these three types of pairs are presented in Table 9.10, from which it can be seen that fitting the conditional logistic regression model in 9.27 (after setting the missing exposures to zero) is equivalent to fitting the conditional likelihood to the intact pairs and the unconditional likelihood to the incomplete pairs. The contribution to the likelihood of pairs with missing exposure for both case and control will be a constant that does not depend on β.

For the estimate of β from the logistic regression model 9.27 to be valid, the complete pairs (conditional) analysis must be valid and the incomplete pairs (unconditional) analysis must be adequately adjusted for confounding. To formally test whether it is reasonable to assume a common OR is being estimated from the conditional and unconditional components, an interaction term can be used as in Section 9.5.1, using an indicator for whether an observation is from a complete or incomplete pair. A statistically significant interaction would indicate that the complete and incomplete pairs do not represent the same association between outcome and exposure, so that a pooled estimate is not meaningful. An example of how this might occur is where the matching has eliminated

TABLE 9.10: *The likelihood components from Equation 9.27 for each kind of case-control pair, using the missing indicator M and setting missing exposures to zero.*

Complete Pair	**Case missing X**	**Control missing X**
$M_{i1} = 0,\ M_{i0} = 0$	$M_{i1} = 1, X_{i1} = 0,\ M_{i0} = 0$	$M_{i1} = 0,\ M_{i0} = 1, X_{i0} = 0$
$\frac{e^{\beta X_{i1}}}{e^{\beta X_{i1}}+e^{\beta X_{i0}}}$	$\frac{e^{\gamma}}{e^{\gamma}+e^{\beta X_{i0}}}$	$\frac{e^{\beta X_{i1}}}{e^{\beta X_{i1}}+e^{\gamma}}$
	$= \frac{1}{1+e^{-\gamma+\beta X_{i0}}}$	$= \frac{e^{-\gamma+\beta X_{i1}}}{1+e^{-\gamma+\beta X_{i1}}}$
Conditional Probability (usual)	Unconditional Probability for control	Unconditional Probability for case

some source of confounding that cannot be completely adjusted in the unconditional model.

The estimate of β from the missing indicator method is the weighted average of the estimates from the separate conditional and unconditional analyses, with the sample sizes as weights [88]. It can be easily verified that the ln(OR) from the pooled analysis in Table 9.9 is also approximately equal to the weighted average of the separate estimates. This is unsurprising, as the likelihood that is solved for this missing indicator method differs from the joint likelihood in Section 9.5.1 only in the appearance of the parameter γ, which represents the ln(odds) associated with missingness and is not of intrinsic interest. Another method derived for estimating the OR from complete and incomplete pairs [149] uses a weighted average of the estimates from the separate conditional and unconditional analyses, with the inverse of the separate variance estimates as weights. Since variance is inversely proportional to sample size, it is unsurprising that simulation studies found the performance of this estimator for a crude OR to be similar to the missing indicator method [149]. For the adjusted ORs that are most often of interest in epidemiological studies, the missing indicator method is more convenient.

For simplicity, the presentation above has assumed a single exposure measure X, but the method can also be used for matched pairs where more than one exposure and/or confounder variable is to be modelled. In this situation, the X above represents all the predictor variables in the logistic model of interest, and if any of these components are missing, the observation is assigned a missing indicator $M = 1$ and *all* the predictor variables are set to zero. While this ignores the information available in the partially incomplete observations, it nonetheless uses more information than a conditional analysis of complete pairs which would drop both members of the pair.

9.5.3 Cases with matched and unmatched controls

In the previous subsections, the matched and unmatched data were from different individuals, so that the joint estimate could be expressed as a simple weighted average. In contrast, if some or all of the study cases have both a matched and an unmatched control, the estimates from the conditional and unconditional analyses are correlated due to the inclusion of the same cases in both. Examples of such data are studies that include both a sibling and non-sibling control for cases, or studies that compare cases to their partner and to an age-matched control from the general population. In this situation, the estimates from the matched and unmatched analysis can again be combined in a weighted average, but the weights now depend on the correlation as well as the variance of the individual estimates [116]. Obtaining a valid estimate of the standard error of the combined estimate is non-trivial as the covariance matrix must first be estimated using sandwich estimators or bootstrap methods.

9.6 Exercises

1. The cluster-based case-control sample stratified by clinic discussed in Section 9.1.1 of Chapter 9 could be viewed as a matched case control sample (matched on clinic). Thus, a standard conditional logistic regression could be used for analysis.

   (i) Explain which effects considered in the paper *Strategies for monitoring and evaluation of resource-limited national antiretroviral therapy programs: the two-phase design* by Haneuse et al in BMC Med Res Meth 2015, could and could not be estimated in this way.

   (ii) In particular, how might you address their question about the change in the effect of public/private clinic over calendar time, using only such a conditional logistic regression analysis.

2. Simulate clustered data using the same setup described in the appendix of *On the Analysis of Case-Control Studies in Cluster-correlated Data Settings* by Haneuse and Rivera-Rodriguez in Epidemiology 2018. Select cluster-based case-control samples as in the paper, and conduct a weighted logistic regression analysis and a weighted GEE analysis (that accommodates the cluster). Repeat the sampling a large number of times and summarise the performance of the two analyses in terms of bias, standard error and coverage.

3. The numbers necessary to complete Table 9.3 of Chapter 9 for the study of HPV16-negative and HPV18-negative women can be found in one or both of the following papers:

   Logistic analysis of epidemiologic studies with augmentation sampling involving re-stratification and population expansion by Li et al, in Biostatistics 2015

   Glutathione S-transferase L1 multiplex serology as a measure of cumulative infection with human papillomavirus by Robbins et al in BMC Infectious Disease 2014.

   Verify that there are 3058 women in the population who are negative for HPV16 or HPV18 or both.

4. For the augmentation sampling in Section 9.2 of Chapter 9, Equations 9.7 and 9.8 are the weights used for analysis to address a research question in Study Base 2:

   (i) What are the appropriate observations and weights for analysis of data to address a research question in Study Base 1?

   (ii) Compare the augmentation weights to the weights for a case-cohort design.

5. In the paper *Association of Autism Spectrum Disorder With Prenatal Exposure to Medication Affecting Neurotransmitter Systems* by Janecka et al in JAMA Psychiatry 2018, the Methods section describes the selection of the population-based case-control sample (in the **Sample** subsection), and the weighted analysis (in the **Statistical Analysis** subsection). The authors specifically state that they used inverse probability weighting to account for the probability of an individual from the birth cohort being included in the study. Justify the weights in the supplementary figure (**eFigure 5**).

6. This exercise uses the same Framingham data as in Chapter 7 of the text book *Statistical Modeling for Biomedical Researchers* by William Dupont. The dataset (named `2.20.Framingham.dta` as it was first used in section 2.20 of the 2002 edition of the book) is from a cohort of men and women followed-up for cardiovascular disease. Here we will examine how CHD is related to sex and age.

   (i) Plot the Kaplan-Meier curves for men and women.

   (ii) Run a simple Cox model with sex as predictor and verify that men have approximately twice the risk of CHD as women.

   (iii) Calculate age at exit from the age at entry and follow-up time, and split the data so that each individual has a record for follow-up in each of the following 5 age categories: <50, [50-60), [60-70), [70-80), >=80 (i.e. decades of age except the youngest and oldest groups). Generate 5 indicator variables for men in these categories. Fit a simple Cox regression with these 5 variables and verify that the hazard ratio for men (compared to women) decreases with age.

(iv) Test the proportional hazards assumption by testing if all 5 coefficients are the same

7. The dataset **addicts.dta** contains data from a study comparing two clinics for the time that heroin addicts continue to attend for their treatment (i.e. the 'survival' time is the time to drop out). The variables are:

   id Patient ID

   survt time to drop out or censoring (in days)

   status 1=drop-out, 0=censored

   clinic coded 1 or 2

   prison indicator of whether the patient had been in prison

   dose maximum methadone dose (mg/day)

   (i) Compare the retention of the two clinics on a Kaplan-Meier plot and test whether the difference is significant using the log rank test.

   (ii) Fit a Cox proportional hazards model with clinic, dose, and prison as covariates.

   (iii) Assess the proportional hazards (PH) assumption for the effect of clinic graphically (one way of doing this is by plotting the adjusted survival curves, stratified by clinic, and comparing to the Kaplan-Meier).

   (iv) Test the PH assumption for the three covariates using an appropriate statistical test.

   (v) Fit a Cox model where the effect of clinic is time-varying, with the HR assumed to increase or decrease monotonically over time.

8. **Note:** to save computational time, this exercise could be conducted using a random 10% of the cohort.

   The dataset `sim_tve_cens.dta` is a simulated cohort of 100,000 individuals followed up for 20 years with a random uniform censoring time assigned with probability 0.5. At the start of follow-up, 20% of the individuals are already exposed and 25% of the remaining 80% acquire the exposure at a random time in the first 10 years of follow-up. The data has been simulated with a HR of 2.0 for the association between the time-dependent exposure and outcome.

(i) run an appropriate Cox model to verify the HR of 2.0

(ii) Select a 1:1 nested case-control study, note the number of controls replicated as cases in the dataset, and estimate the HR from (a) conditional logistic regression and (b) weighted Cox regression. Compare the results.

9. Using the simulated data in the previous exercise, select a sample by exposure density sampling and estimate the HR. Compare the results to the estimate from the full cohort and from a nested case-control study of similar size.

10. In Exercise 6 above, the HR for men compared to women in the Framingham dataset was found to decrease steadily across the age groups (i.e. a 'dose-response' with age). An alternative method of assessing the proportional hazards assumption (i.e., investigating if the risk factor is time-dependent) is to test for an interaction between the risk factor and time.

    (i) Select a case-control sample from the Framingham dataset from Exercise 6, fit a Cox model on the age scale, and test formally for a linear trend in the HR for male sex by including an interaction with time. Compare your results and conclusions to Exercise 6 above.

    (ii) Select a case-control sample by exclusive sampling and assess the proportional hazards assumption (on the age scale) for male sex using the case-cohort approach in *Estimating time-varying exposure-outcome associations using case-control data: logistic and case-cohort analyses* by Keogh et al in BMC Med Res Meth 2016.

11. Outline how you would design and analyse a case-control study to investigate if there was a waning of the effectiveness of a Covid-19 mRNA booster vaccine in people who had previously had two shots of the Astra-Zeneca vaccine. Pay particular attention to:

    (a) the definition of the cohort from which the sample is taken

(b) the time scale for analysis

(c) the use of a case-cohort approach to the analysis

(d) the model(s) used

(e) whether frequency matching by age would be useful

(f) potential bias from changes in population prevalence or behaviour

12. The dataset `prostate_sibs` contains a simplified extract from the data on brothers of prostate cancer patients from the paper *Patterns of changing cancer risks with time since diagnosis of a sibling* by Lee et al in International Journal of Cancer 2015. All variables are provided in integer years rather than specific dates, and a small random time increment has been added to the exit age to break the ties between the diagnosis year of an index case and the exit year of a sibling.

    (i) Treating the age in 1998 as a time-dependent exposure, fit a Cox model on the age scale to estimate the hazard ratio adjusted for number of siblings.

    (ii) Repeat the analysis in (i) with elapsed years as the time scale and adjusting for age at entry as a continuous variable.

    (iii) Select a 1:1 nested case-control sample from the cohort and estimate the hazard ratio associated with the time-dependent exposure using conditional logistic regression.

    (iv) Use the full cohort information to obtain the Kaplan-Meier weights and conduct a weighted Cox regression of the nested case-control sample from (iii) (**Note:** if any controls are censored at an event time, these ties need to be broken with small random increments to compute the correct weights).

13. Follow-up of a clinical cohort of AIDS patients on first-line ART (anti-retroviral treatment) is conducted at approximately yearly visits. During follow-up, some patients switch to a different treatment, INSTI (integrase strand transfer inhibitor). This new treatment is a time-dependent exposure of interest, to be investigated for its association with a diagnosis of insulin resistance during follow-up. However, this treatment is

also thought to be a risk factor for increase in BMI, which in turn is associated with risk of insulin resistance (i.e. acts as a mediator).

To investigate the association between insulin resistance and switching to INSTI (with INSTI-naïve as the reference group), the investigators wish to consider alternatives to the analysis of the whole cohort, and so they are considering:

(a) a case-control sample: what is the appropriate time axis for the sampling?

(b) a matched cohort of INSTI 'switchers' vs. INSTI-naive: suggest some appropriate matching factors?

10

Other Controlled Epidemiological Studies

10.1 Self-controlled designs

10.1.1 Case-crossover design

The paper that introduced the case-crossover design in 1991 for the study of transient exposures [135] compared the exposure of a case just before the event to their exposure status at a previous comparable time interval: thus, in the words of the author, the design provides a scientific way to answer the question 'why now?' rather than the question 'why me?' addressed by the more familiar epidemiological designs. The reprint of this 'historical' article by the same journal (American Journal of Epidemiology) in 2017 [136], with an invited commentary in the same issue [228], is a testament to the contribution that the design has made to health research. The actual 'historical' background to the design has been described in a review article [137], where the authors explain how the original design arose from their difficulties with identifying a suitable control group.

Ideally, controls should represent the study base in which the cases occurred, i.e. if they had the outcome of interest, they would have been identified as cases. Controls that meet this criterion for selection are straightforward to identify for a study conducted in a well-defined study base. However, there are many situations where investigators have difficulty in identifying an appropriate control group and such a situation arose in a 1988 study of MI that led to the case-crossover design. The purpose of the study was to investigate why the risk of MI was higher in the morning, and after considering (and discarding) several conventional control groups, the investigators concluded that the best comparison group was the patients themselves on the previous day [137]. Thus was born the case-crossover design, where a patient's exposure on their 'case day' was compared with their exposure on one or more 'control days' [135]. The design is ideally suited to the study of acute onset of an outcome for which a transient exposure is to be investigated as a 'trigger': short-term effects of environmental conditions such as extreme weather conditions [70] and air pollution [97]; adverse events associated with pharmaceuticals or vaccines [230]; cardiovascular events following stressful life events [154, 61].

A clear advantage of the case-crossover design is the removal of confounding by fixed covariates, not only genetic (which would also be removed by comparing identical twins) but also other characteristics of the case that can be particularly challenging in conventional case-control (or even cohort) designs, such as indication for exposure to a medication or treatment [207]. But there are still many sources of confounding to consider in a case-crossover study in order to protect against selection bias, information bias and confounding bias [152]. As a simple example, the usual concern about recall bias is still present in a case-crossover design, due to the 'case period' exposure being more recent and perhaps also a patient's effort to understand why they have been diagnosed 'now' rather than 'then'.

Although intuitively simple, the case-crossover design can be very challenging with respect to the choice of time periods to be compared. Much has been written about the importance of the choice of the 'referent' or control time period, as described in detail for some studies of air pollution [97, 151]. Choosing times that maximise the contrast [135], or investigating of various choices [207] would likely suffer from 'winner's curse' bias [228] and compromise the validity of the results, but where subject-matter knowledge enables a reasonable choice of time period, time-stratified analysis offers a useful sensitivity analysis [97]. Other aspects of time that are critical, and that may also have an impact on the choice of referent period, are the timing and duration of exposure and the timing of the outcome. Even if the timing and duration of exposure are precisely known, there may be insufficient biological knowledge to accurately define the lag from (accumulated) exposure to its physiological action (active period) and ultimate effect, or to propose a reasonable duration of such effect. The difficulty of choosing the active period and effect period is highlighted in a study of clarithromycin and cardiovascular outcomes [234], where the prior studies that were summarised in the introduction used many different choices of time periods, ranging from days to weeks or years.

The case-crossover design is a paired design, where the 'control' is the case individual him/herself at an earlier reference time. Thus, using the same notation as in Chapter 2, the exposure and outcome information

TABLE 10.1: *2-by-2 table of case-crossover data.*

	Exposed in reference period: Yes	Exposed in reference period: No
Exposed in index period	n_{11}	n_{10}
Unexposed in case period	n_{01}	n_{00}

can be presented on a 2-by-2 table (Table 10.1),
and as in Chapter 2 (Equation 2.47), the crude OR is simply the ratio of the cross-diagonal discordant terms:

$$OR_{paired} = \frac{n_{10}}{n_{01}} \tag{10.1}$$

As explained in Section 2.6 of Chapter 2, this OR can also be obtained from a conditional logistic regression, which maximises the likelihood:

$$\prod_{i=1}^{N} \frac{e^{\beta X_{i1}}}{e^{\beta X_{i1}} + e^{\beta X_{i0}}} \tag{10.2}$$

where X_1 and X_0 now denote the exposure of the same individual in the index (case) period and reference (control) period, whereas in Chapter 2, these denoted the exposure of the case and control individual in the matched pair.

10.1.2 Extensions to the case-crossover design

The validity of the OR estimate from a case-crossover study depends on the choice of appropriate reference time. Where it is reasonable to assume the exposure is stationary or exchangeable, then greater efficiency can be obtained by comparing exposure in the index period to the previous 'usual frequency' rather than to just a single control day or other short period [137]. If information is obtained from electronic records rather than from the study subject, this not only eliminates the potential for recall bias, but enables seasonal or circadian fluctuations to be accommodated. However, there are many situations where the contribution of time cannot be ignored, and following the introduction of the case-crossover design, a number of extensions have been developed to accommodate time effects.

Case-time-control design

The first design to adjust for time trends was the case-time control design [207], where the sample of cases in the case-crossover study is augmented with a sample of controls. These controls have their exposure ascertained for the same two time periods as the cases, which we will refer to as the index time and the reference time. The availability of a control group enables the contribution of time and the adjusted (for time) effect of exposure to be estimated from a joint analysis of the case and control data, using conditional logistic regression as explained in the following. Table 10.2 represents the time at which cases were observed (T_1) and their earlier reference time (T_0), and the exposure status of the individual at these two times, X_1 and X_0, respectively. The controls, who are observed at these same index and reference times, have outcome $Y = 0$ on both occasions, while the cases have $Y = 1$ at the index time and $Y = 0$ at the reference time.

Assuming a logistic regression model, the conditional likelihood for the cases is given by Equation 10.2 or Equation 10.3.

$$\prod_{i=1}^{N} \frac{e^{\beta(X_{i1}-X_{i0})}}{1+e^{\beta(X_{i1}-X_{i0})}} \tag{10.3}$$

Using the period ($T = 1$ or $T = 0$) instead of Y as the outcome, results

TABLE 10.2: *Representation of data gathered at an index time T_1 and a previous reference time T_0 from cases and time-matched controls.*

→ time →

Time	T_0	T_1
Exposure	X_0	X_1
Outcome:		
Case	0	1
Control	0	0

in the same likelihood component. More importantly, by using the time period as outcome, the conditional likelihood components for the controls capture the association between time and exposure. Thus the combined data records from cases and controls allow the fitting of the underlying model:

$$logit(T = 1) = \alpha + \beta X \quad \text{for controls} \tag{10.4}$$
$$= \alpha + (\beta + \gamma)X \quad \text{for cases} \tag{10.5}$$

This is fit by conditional logistic regression, with time period as outcome with an interaction term between the exposure X and an indicator variable for the type of pair ($C = 1$ for a case pair, $C = 0$ for a control pair). The interaction term is of primary interest, since e^{γ} is the OR associated with exposure, adjusted for the time effect e^{β}. Thus the model enables the overall OR from the case-crossover analysis to be partitioned into the product of the OR for exposure and OR for time.

The model just described was applied to data from a case-crossover study of the association between inhaled beta-agonist use and life-threatening asthma episodes among persons whose asthma required ongoing treatment [207]. The investigators identified 129 cases in the cohort of treated persons and compared their exposure to beta-agonists in the year prior to the event and in the preceding year. Among the 129 cases, there were 29 who were exposed in the index year but not in the reference year, and 9 cases who were exposed in the reference year but not in the index year, giving a crude OR=3.2. Augmenting the 129 cases with 655 time-matched controls, and implementing the conditional logistic regression analysis described above, resulted in the estimates presented in Table 10.3.

This example illustrates how the case-crossover estimate fails to separate the effect of the exposure to the drug from other factors. Even when matching for important risk factors and adjusting for a number of proxy measures of disease severity, a conventional logistic regression model provided similar results [207]. However, as Table 10.3 shows, the case-time-control design provided a much reduced estimate of the association of the drug with the outcome and a significant contribution from other factors to the change over time.

Case-case-time control design

For the case-time-control estimates to be valid, it is assumed that the controls and cases have the same underlying exposure prevalence and

TABLE 10.3: *Odds ratio estimates from conditional logistic regression of paired observations from asthma cases and conditional logistic regression model with interaction effect from analysis of the same cases supplemented with paired observations from time-matched controls (from [207]).*

	OR (95% C.I.) controls	**OR (95% C.I.) cases**
Dichotomous		
Case-crossover		3.2 (1.5 - 6.8)
Case-time-control	2.6 (1.6 - 4.1)	1.2 (0.5 - 3.0)
Continuous		
Case-crossover		2.8 (1.6 - 4.5)
Case-time-control	1.6 (1.2 - 2.2)	1.7 (0.9 - 3.0)

pattern. In other words, the controls should reflect the exposure pattern over time of the cases if there was no association between exposure and outcome. While this would usually be true in an environmental epidemiology study, there may be several issues with such an assumption in pharmacoepidemiology, such as a change in an individual's behaviour with the onset of a health event, or treatment of early symptoms of an impending, but not yet confirmed, diagnosis. In such situations, a separate sample of randomly chosen external controls will provide a biased representation of the exposure profile of cases. A method for overcoming the potential bias extends the ideas of the case-time-control design, by comparing the case's exposure, not to an external sample of controls, but to the 'control time' of **future cases** The method assumes that these future cases have the same trend in exposure over calendar time as the current cases.

The analysis of case-case-time control data proceeds in the same way as for the case-time-control design, with the interaction term in the conditional logistic regression model again providing the estimate of primary interest. The only difference between the two designs is that the controls for the case-time-control design are selected from individuals who may or may not develop the outcome, while for the case-case-time control design, controls are selected from those who *are known* to develop the outcome later.

In the paper proposing the case-case-time control design [227], the authors applied the method to a study of the association between vitamin use and stroke, where the data indicated an increased exposure to vitamins in the year prior to the stroke. The exposure of cases to vitamins for at least three days in the thirty days prior to admission for stroke (the index date) was compared to the exposure in matched controls chosen from those admitted 90 days later (i.e. future cases), resulting in no evidence of an association, whereas a standard case-time-control analysis estimated a 50% increase in stroke risk after brief exposure to vitamins. Since a case-time-control design adjusts for a temporal trend that is common to cases and non-cases, it does not make the necessary adjustment for the trend that is specific to cases in this example, resulting in a biased, and biologically unreasonable, estimate.

As with all case-crossover type designs, the selection of the appropriate time intervals is crucial in case-case-time control studies. In this design, the investigator must not only consider the time window for the case and referent exposure, but also select how close/far a future case's event should be in order for their current time to be an appropriate match for current cases. Selection of an appropriate time gap requires knowledge of the biological mechanisms underlying how the transient exposure might have an impact on the risk of the outcome. The length of the time gap has consequences for the power of the study, as a larger gap will result in fewer (or perhaps no) controls available for cases that occur later in follow-up, which will be further exasperated in the case of matching.

10.1.3 Self-controlled case series

The self-controlled case series method, like the case-crossover design, uses only data from cases. However, unlike the simple case-crossover design, individuals in the case series can have more than one event during the observation time and the method provides an estimate of the IRR or HR following a transient exposure. An important aspect of the design is that the exposure does not need to be assumed stationary or exchangeable as in the case-crossover design, as age or time are handled in much the same way as in a cohort study. The method was developed to investigate whether meningitis was associated with MMR vaccination in young children [230]. The cases of meningitis, identified from hospital and laboratory records, could be easily linked to their vaccination records, but the selection of control children had several difficulties, including a lack of clarity regarding the appropriate underlying population from which to sample. Using only the cases and their vaccination records, the case series method highlighted an increased risk of meningitis approximately 2–3 weeks after vaccination with a specific MMR vaccine, resulting in a change in the MMR vaccines used in the UK. The method has since been used to investigate the safety of numerous other vaccines, including many studies of adverse reactions following vaccination against SARS-Cov2.

The earliest work on case series data [172] analysed the 'cohort' of cases using simple Cox regression, ignoring the fact that only cases were selected for analysis. The more correct method for analysing the case series is conditional likelihood, where the likelihood of the outcome for each individual is conditional on the event(s) having been observed during the individual's observation time. The approach to data analysis is very similar to the methods encountered in Chapter 9 for handling a time-dependent exposure (see Table 9.5 in Chapter 9): the observation time of each individual is split into intervals, one of which is the risk period (i.e. the exposed period), and perhaps also split by age categories, so that each individual has multiple records in the expanded data.

The underlying incidence rate during the unexposed period is assumed to be constant (within each age group), and the estimate of interest is the increased incidence (IRR) in the exposed time interval. The incidence for individual i in stratum j and exposure level k is assumed to be a log-linear function:

$$\lambda_{ijk} = e^{\gamma_i + \alpha_j + \beta_k} \tag{10.6}$$

where γ_i is the individual effect, α_j is the effect of stratum j and β_k is the effect of exposure level k. For simplicity, we will consider a dichotomous exposure, i.e. k= 1 or 0, so that for an individual in the reference stratum, the incidence is e^{γ_i} during the unexposed time and $e^{\gamma_i+\beta}$ while exposed, so that the $IRR = e^{\beta}$. Thus the exposure effect is automatically adjusted for characteristics of the individual, such as sex, health, frailty or genetic factors, although these may be considered as effect modifiers by including interaction terms in the model. The number of events, n_{ijk}, experienced by individual i in stratum j at exposure level k will depend on how much of their follow-up time is spent in that state. Denoting this time as e_{ijk}, then the expected number of events in the interval is $\lambda_{ijk}e_{ijk}$ and the observed number n_{ijk} can be modelled as a simple Poisson regression (Equations 10.7–10.9) once the time intervals have been calculated for the records of all individuals.

$$n_{ijk} = Poisson(\lambda_{ijk} e_{ijk}) \quad (10.7)$$
$$ln(\lambda_{ijk}) = \gamma_i + \alpha_j + \beta_k \quad (10.8)$$
$$\text{offset} = e_{ijk} \quad (10.9)$$

The data preparation and model fitting are presented in a step-by-step tutorial [230] for the MMR example mentioned above, for which the data and code are available on an Open University web site dedicated to the case series method (http://stats-www.open.ac.uk/sccs/index.htm). A text book from the same group [62] provides a detailed modelling guide, with extensive practical applications, together with R code and datasets.

10.1.4 Exposure-crossover design

The previous section introduced a number of case-only designs (case-crossover, case-time-control, self-controlled case series) for studying the transient increase in risk associated with an acute exposure. However, many acute exposures may be associated with a *sustained* change in risk, such as health outcomes following social upheaval or economic crisis, psychological trauma, medical interventions or initiation of long-term treatment. In addition, the case-only designs investigate a single case-defining event whereas the risk associated with an exposure may often manifest as recurring events, such as infections in immunocompromised patients or flares in arthritis patients. The **exposure-crossover design** overcomes both of these limitations of case-only designs by comparing the risk in the same individuals, both cases and non-cases, in the periods before and after the exposure[178].

In comparing the baseline health events of an individual (i.e. before exposure) to events subsequent to an exposure, it is common in defining the baseline time to exclude some time immediately prior to the exposure (the 'induction time') in order to reduce any confounding by indication or other reverse causation. This potential confounding may be visible on a time-series type plot of events versus appropriate time intervals, such as days or weeks. Such plots also help direct the subsequent analysis, which will be simpler where the event rates are reasonably constant in the pre- and post- exposure intervals (excluding the induction time), as a simple mean will suffice to represent the outcome in the two intervals. Where there are time trends within one or both of the intervals, this will need to be accommodated by using methods of analysis appropriate for 'repeated measures' [66].

For a very rare event, no meaningful patterns can be observed and a simple analysis can be conducted using a paired 2-by-2 table, where now the rows and columns represent the 'before' and 'after' time intervals and the counts are the numbers of individuals who had the event (any occurrence) in one, both, or neither of those intervals. The association can be assessed with a McNemar test and quantified with a paired OR as in Chapter 2.

10.2 Test-negative Design

To assess a health intervention against a disease of low incidence, a randomised clinical trial is not practical. If the case definition for the disease includes laboratory confirmation, then electronic medical records offer a convenient study base in which to conduct an observational study. Such was the approach taken by a 1980 investigation of the efficacy of a pneumococcal vaccine in immunocompromised individuals [27] using only cases of pneumococcal infection. The study included all individuals with a pneumococcal pathogen identified by the CDC between 1978 and 1980, who were classified as to whether or not they were vaccinated and whether their pneumococcal isolate was of a type included in the vaccine. Of the 35 vaccinated individuals, a surprising 63% (n = 22) had an isolate that was covered by the vaccine, compared to 263 (67%) of the 392 unvaccinated individuals (OR = 0.83, 95% C.I. 0.39, 1.86). This suggests little or no benefit of vaccination in this special subgroup (immunocompromised individuals) who would usually not be represented in clinical trials. Since the introduction of this approach, known now as the 'indirect cohort' method, it has been used to evaluate pneumococcal vaccines in several countries.

The 'test-negative design' [51] adopts a somewhat similar approach, but compares individuals testing positive and negative for the pathogen of interest and is thus a special case of a case-control design using 'other patient controls'. Using other patients as the reference group in a case-control study can mitigate various biases that can result from using a random sample of controls from the population that gave rise to the cases: selection bias (by investigators or study subjects), measurement bias (such as recall bias) and confounding bias (for example from disease severity or indication in pharmacoepidemiology). In the test-negative design, the other patients who serve as controls are usually chosen from those presenting with similar symptoms, often at the same health facility, but who test negative for the disease under investigation. Further insights regarding the potential of a vaccine against a virus circulating in the population can be gained by comparing the cases to different control groups: for example, influenza-positive cases could be compared to influenza-negative individuals who are positive for other specific respiratory viruses, or who are negative for all tested viruses [219] [193].

The test-negative design was introduced as an efficient method for assessing the effectiveness of influenza vaccination using surveillance records [196] for individuals who presented to a physician with flu-like illness. For such vaccine effectiveness studies, the test-negative design has advantages over a standard cohort approach where outpatient (flu) visits and/or positive tests are compared in vaccinated and unvaccinated individuals, or a standard case-control approach where vaccination rates are compared in patients seeking care for flu to persons not seeking such care. Both of these standard designs are susceptible to selection bias when vaccination is optional, as it is reasonable to hypothesise that more health-conscious persons may be more likely to seek vaccination and also to seek health care. By sampling only from those seeking care, the test-negative design overcomes this source of bias and estimates the OR of vaccination among those who *would seek care.* Despite being conducted in this restricted study base, the test negative design provides a valid estimate of the OR in the wider population under the same reasonable assumptions as for the validity of 'other patient' case-control studies [95], i.e.

- the distribution of the causes of the symptoms of non-cases does not depend on vaccination status
- the vaccine effectiveness does not depend on health-seeking behaviour

Where there are seasonal trends for the illness of interest and/or the vaccination coverage (as for influenza), it is also important that the control group is selected during the same calendar time as the cases and that the estimates of efficacy are adjusted for calendar time. For a seasonal illness, this adjustment can be achieved by using incidence density sampling (i.e. a nested case-control study) with calendar time as a matching factor [67] Where vaccine coverage is stable over time, inclusion of out-of-season controls may improve power, although adjustment for seasonality in the illness can result in such controls contributing very little information. Where there are no temporal trends of concern, the assumptions above for the validity of the test-negative estimate can be formally tested if data are available from prior randomised clinical trials of the vaccine.

10.2.1 Bias in test-negative designs

The test-negative design is expected to reduce the selection and measurement bias of standard cohort or case-control studies. However, these biases are not necessarily eliminated, and as already mentioned, a careful choice of the control group is essential to avoid other biases [222]. Much of the discussion of bias in vaccine effectiveness estimates from test-negative designs concerns confounding due to various health-seeking behaviour scenarios [2]. Where community controls are available, the magnitude of this bias can be assessed by comparing the results using test-negative and community controls [69].

Although the bias from health-seeking behaviour may not be eliminated by the test-negative design [210], the design has been demonstrated to be robust in a wide range of practical settings [64]. Since the controls represent those who would have sought care for the outcome of interest, the estimate obtained is valid for clinically-presented disease, provided vaccination does not alter the probability of attending care for the disease under study [2]. If a measure of disease severity is available, adjustment for this variable can reduce the bias in the estimate without the need to assume a fixed level of health-seeking behaviour for the subjects in the test-negative study [32]. Test-negative studies may also be subject to bias from various trends in calendar time [46], but the bias due to temporal trends in vaccine coverage is of small magnitude for rare diseases.

The test-negative design has been particularly useful in the era of Covid-19 to study risk and preventative factors for the disease and the effectiveness of vaccines. In the earlier days of the epidemic when testing was mostly of symptomatic patients, efforts to identify risk or preventative factors for infection with SARS-Cov-2 [191] could benefit from the inclusion of an additional population-based control group [220], in order to discriminate between risk factors for infection and for symptomatic disease. As testing was rolled out to be available to asymptomatic persons, there was no need for an additional control group. For the assessment of the efficacy of vaccines against Covid-19, the test-negative design offered an efficient method of assessing the newly-developed vaccines in the period after their approval for widespread use, when randomised clinical trials would have been ethically questionable due to the risk of serious illness and the imposition of societal restrictions. Randomised clinical trials would also have been impractical for estimating efficacy in the narrow subgroups that were prioritised in the roll-out of vaccination in many countries. The validity of the design for clinically-presenting disease made it especially suitable for evaluating the impact of the vaccines and vaccine programs, as the primary concern of health authorities was the burden on the health-care system and the management of hospitalised Covid-19 patients.

The validity of the efficacy estimates from test-negative designs is subject to the same caveats concerning selection, measurement bias and confounding bias as presented in the previous section. The public-health and individual response to Covid-19 testing and vaccination also highlighted many other factors that need to be considered [126], including the sensitivity and specificity of the laboratory tests used and temporal confounding due to the roll-out of the vaccination and the shift to lower risk groups over time [96]. Since breakthrough infections are not uncommon after Covid-19 vaccination, a test-negative study needs to meet the criteria for incidence density sampling in order to avoid bias due to the 'leaky vaccine' effect [45]. While these criteria are straightforward to describe, they raise practical challenges in a setting where sub-clinical infections are common and result in person-time that is naturally immune and should be censored [127].

The test-negative design also offers an efficient method of comparing the effectiveness of a different number of doses/boosters of vaccine and/or the protection offered by a specific vaccine against different variants, such as the Delta and Omicron variants of SARS-Cov-2 [1]. Although these questions are of high relevance for public health authorities around the world, there were relatively few studies investigating the cross-protection offered by the available vaccines as new variants emerged, perhaps due to the speed with which these became dominant.

10.2.2 Cluster-randomised test-negative design

Many Covid-19 vaccination protocols were targeted to well-defined groups, such as essential workers, college students and care-home residents. Despite this group focus, vaccination was mostly provided to individuals, often prioritised by age. A cluster-randomised trial using these and other natural clusters in the population, would not only reduce transmission within clusters, but also offer a cost-efficient test-negative design that could overcome many of the biases [4] discussed in the previous section. The data contributing to the estimate of effectiveness are the test results (positive and negative) of individuals in the randomised clusters, where the association of test-negativity with the intervention (such as vaccination) is represented by a RR or OR. Assuming that the test-negative design samples all cases and m controls per case from each cluster, valid estimates of the OR can be very simply obtained from the average proportion of positives in the intervention clusters compared to the control clusters. If an equal number of clusters is assigned to intervention and control, the expected proportions of test-positives are

$$\text{Intervention:} \quad \frac{RR}{RR + \frac{m}{2}(RR+1)} \tag{10.10}$$

$$\text{Control:} \quad \frac{1}{1 + \frac{m}{2}(RR+1)} \tag{10.11}$$

The difference between these two quantities is a quadratic equation in RR, which can be solved to provide the RR estimate. The confidence interval can then be obtained by an appropriate transformation of the confidence interval for the difference in the average proportions of positives in the two arms.

Disregarding the clustering, analysis of the individual-level data provides a valid OR, but to assess significance or construct valid confidence intervals requires permutation methods [4]. Alternatively, if there is a reasonable number of clusters, the correlation between members of a cluster can be accommodated by generalised estimating equations [4], which involves a straightforward logistic regression that specifies the cluster identifier and the correlation structure (e.g. exchangeable) and provides robust standard errors [98].

10.3 Negative Controls

In experimental studies such as clinical trials, randomisation is used to balance the potential confounders that might lead to spurious associations between the outcome and the exposure of interest. In observational studies, this 'adjustment' is achieved by restricted, stratified or matched designs and/or adjustment in statistical models. Despite careful design and analysis, there often remains a potential for residual confounding, due to factors that were not possible to include in the design or analysis, or the nature of the data source. Laboratory experiments often use 'negative controls', for which the scientist does not expect any response, to demonstrate conditions when the outcome should not, and *does not*, occur according to the hypothesis being tested. For example, it is routine practice in Elispot assays to include negative control wells that do not contain the active substance being tested (saline is often used) and any response from these wells can be used as a correction for background due to aspects of the experiment not related to the exposure of interest: for example, the laboratory environment, technical variation in the equipment, or spontaneous activity in the cells.

10.3.1 Confounding bias

Taking inspiration from the common practice of using negative controls in laboratory experiments, a similar approach was proposed for assessing bias due to confounding in epidemiological studies [129], and the same principles hold for other sources of bias such as selection bias and measurement bias. In laboratory science, the choice of negative control can usually be classified as one of the following:

- leaving out an essential ingredient
- checking for a response that would be unexpected or impossible under the hypothesised mechanism

The first of these approaches represents a **negative exposure** and the second a **negative outcome**. Both approaches were used to address the controversy surrounding influenza vaccination in 2006 [94], which reported that after careful adjustment for confounders, vaccination was found to have a protective effect against influenza before the flu season, during the season, and after the season had passed, with the magnitude of the effect *decreasing* across these three time periods, contrary to what would be expected. This is an example of a negative exposure, where the 'essential ingredient' that is left out of the analysis in the earlier period(s) is influenza! In additional analyses, the authors investigated the association between vaccination and outcomes unrelated to influenza, such as hospitalisation for injury or trauma, and found a protective effect of vaccination, an impossible causal pathway, providing clear evidence of unadjusted confounding.

The use of negative controls is well-recognised in some areas of epidemiological research, such as family studies and perinatal epidemiology. The risk of cancer (or other disease) in the family members of a patient is often the first step in identifying genetic risk factors. The estimate of risk to relatives will usually be adjusted for age, sex (of the proband and the relative) and the degree of relationship, all of which are easily ascertained. However, the increased risk in family members can also be due in part to shared non-genetic factors such as habits and lifestyle, which are difficult to quantify or even observe. In such studies, spouses of patients can be used as negative controls [177], where the 'essential ingredient' (shared genetic factors) is excluded. In perinatal epidemiology, studies of maternal exposures will often include paternal exposure as a negative control: for example, paternal smoking, alcohol consumption or stress represent impossible causal pathways for the effect of maternal exposure. The control exposure may also be measured on the mother herself, in the pre-pregnancy or post-delivery period or during a subsequent unexposed pregnancy [187].

The purpose of a negative control is to represent as far as possible the common causes of the exposure and outcome being investigated, especially the unobserved causes that cannot be accommodated by adjustment. Thus a negative control exposure should share these common causes with the outcome and a negative control outcome should share these common causes with the exposure. Choosing an appropriate negative control requires a thorough understanding of the epidemiology of the area of investigation and of potential biological mechanisms. An unexpected association with a negative control outcome might reveal some overlooked common causes with the exposure that are not shared by the outcome under investigation.

10.3.2 Selection bias

In addition to confounding bias, negative control exposures and outcomes can be used to assess selection bias and measurement bias in epidemiological studies. Bias can result where selection into the study depends on exposure (or a cause of exposure) and outcome (or a cause of the outcome), as in a case-control study where the probability of an exposed subject being included is different for cases and controls. In a case-control study that includes all cases and the identification of cases is independent of exposure, the study will provide a biased estimate of the odds ratio in the population if the controls are not representative of the distribution of exposure. Such bias led to some controversy about coffee consumption and pancreatic cancer in the 1980s [63] following a case-control study where controls were selected from individuals attending the same clinical practice as the cases, but with different complaints. Among the many potential sources of bias identified, it was suggested that the various digestive disorders of the controls may have resulted in them consuming lower amounts of coffee than healthy persons in the population. A sensitivity analysis of such bias can be conducted [197] where a range of estimates are available that describe the exposure (coffee drinking) in the selected controls with and without digestive disorders, and the risk of digestive disorders in the selected controls compared to those not selected. An online calculator (`http://selection-bias.louisahsmith.com`) facilitates such sensitivity analysis by calculating (i) bounds for the bias under assumed/estimated relationships between exposure and an unmeasured factor, and (ii) E-values for the selection bias, describing the minimum extent of the relationships that would suffice to explain the bias.

Selection bias can also be assessed by using negative controls that are chosen so that they represent the same selection process and so will depend on a thorough understanding of the area of investigation, in terms of clinical knowledge and epidemiology. The appropriate choice of negative controls may be very specific to the outcome, exposure and research study question. For example, case-control studies of vaccines against diarrhoeal diseases such as rotavirus or cholera that compare cases who present at health facilities to community controls, may be subject to selection bias due to vaccinated individuals or those with the infection of interest being more likely to seek care [92]. In such settings, diarrhoea that is negative for the organism can be used as a potential negative control outcome and vaccination against some other infectious disease is a potential negative control exposure. Although selection bias is a particular concern in case-control studies, especially where cases are identified among patients who are hospitalised or attending outpatient care, this bias can also arise in cohort studies where there is differential participation among the exposed and unexposed members of the cohort. For example, in a cohort study of the association between statin use and diabetes, the diabetes patients were identified from a large computerised database of medical records [44]. Selection could thus depend on one or more conditions leading to a diagnosis of the outcome (diabetes) and the result would be prone to bias if selection also depended on exposure (e.g. if statin users were better monitored). To assess this potential bias, the authors used peptic ulcers as a negative exposure, as there is no known association between peptic ulcers and diabetes. A comparison of cases to these negative controls did not detect any evidence of such bias.

The potential biases and the choice of negative controls in these examples and many more can be understood by using DAGs to represent the causes and 'descendants' (i.e. consequences) of the exposure and outcome under investigation [8].

10.3.3 Measurement error bias

Many exposures and outcomes are subject to measurement error, due to practical limitations of data collection. For example, outcomes will sometimes be recorded from the report of a patient or caregiver rather than confirmed by medical imaging or laboratory analysis. Exposures are even more difficult to measure precisely, even those that are simple to define, such as smoking and environmental pollution. Since it is the measured outcome that is analysed but the underlying 'true' outcome that is of interest, then an exposure that influences the measured outcome can result in bias. The purpose of blinding in randomised clinical trials is to protect against such bias in the analysis of health outcomes recorded by a clinical investigator: if the treatment/exposure of the patient is known to the clinician, this may prompt more or less diligence in assessing symptoms. As a result of blinding, any measurement errors in the outcome will be non-differential.

Where the measurement error of concern is in the exposure, then bias can result from an outcome that influences the measured exposure. A well-known example of such differential measurement error is the recall bias in case-control studies that rely on 'remembered' exposures as a reasonable measure of the true exposure. However, the case-control study is not the only design that may have bias due to differential measurement error in an exposure [8].

Whether the differential measurement error occurs in the exposure or outcome, the potential bias can be investigated by using either an appropriate negative control exposure or negative control outcome. For example, to investigate bias due to outcome measurement error in reported diarrhoea by swimmers who are exposed to water with enterococcus bacteria, one could use the levels of enterococcus assigned to non-swimmers as a negative control exposure [99], or a condition unrelated to bacterial infection as a negative control outcome. The negative control should follow the same principle as above: to capture the same 'nuisance' correlations while 'breaking' the causal chain by removing an essential ingredient or representing an impossible pathway under the proposed hypothesis.

10.3.4 Negative self-control

A study subject can serve as their own control where a suitable negative control exposure or outcome is identified. A self-controlled negative outcome was proposed recently for the analysis of naturally acquired immunity [164] from prior rotavirus infection, where the outcome (rotavirus-positive diarrhoea), but not the negative-control outcome (non-rotavirus diarrhoea) would be expected to have lower risk in those previously infected with rotavirus. This design differs from the case-time-control design in the purpose and choice of the negative control. The negative control outcome is not simply the absence of the outcome being studied, but an alternative outcome that would not be possible under the proposed mechanism.

Negative control exposures may also be measured on the study subject themselves, as in studies of intrauterine exposures that use pre-pregnancy or post-delivery exposures as negative controls. A recent nested case-control study of the association between autism and air pollution in the pre-pregnancy, pregnancy and postnatal periods, used as a negative (self-control) exposure the pollution levels measured post-outcome (28–36 months)[138]. In contrast to the exposure-crossover design which compares individuals for their outcome(s) during exposed and unexposed periods, the negative self-controlled exposure is used to conduct additional analyses on study subjects sampled in a standard design (here a nested case-control study) to assess the estimates for residual confounding.

10.4 Active Comparators

The active comparator design can be thought of as the selection of a 'positive control' exposure that would be expected to give a positive, or perhaps similar, result if the underlying causal hypothesis is true. In contrast to the negative control designs where a null effect is expected, the focus of the active comparator design is on observing the effect of the exposure in another setting that is consistent with the causal hypothesis.

Active comparators are of particular importance in pharmacoepidemiology, where the evidence from real-life use of a new drug (i.e. observational data) is an important complement to the results from the clinical trials conducted in more idealised and restricted conditions, that led to the adoption of the drug. Pharmacoepidemiology uses a number of active comparator designs, that differ in the selection criteria for the individuals using the study drug or the comparator drug [232]. The simplest of these is the **active comparator new user design**, which compares initiators of the study drug to initiators of the comparison drug. This defines a rather restrictive population and more practical scenarios can be represented by various relaxations of the inclusion/exclusion criteria. The **prevalent new user** design includes all study drug initiators, whether or not they previously used the comparator, reflecting a common situation in the treatment of chronic diseases as new drugs become available. This design allows for numerous contrasts of interest, as it represents individuals who are prescribed the new/study drug as an alternative or additional treatment, those for whom it is the first and only treatment, and those initiating or continuing only the comparator drug. For example, a comparison of prevalent users of the comparator who do and do not switch to the study drug, will provide key evidence for prescribing protocols. The sampling of comparators can be stratified on prior use (e.g. duration and volume) of the comparator and propensity score matching used to reduce confounding by indication.

10.4.1 Self-controlled active comparator

While the original purpose of the case-time-control design was to adjust for confounding by indication [207], this measure is assumed to cancel out in the paired data. However, there are many examples in pharmacoepidemiology where confounding by indication will often not be removed by a case-time-control or self-controlled case series analysis, due to the indication (and hence also the exposure to treatment) being time-dependent. The extent of such bias can be estimated from the self-controlled design by using an active comparator that would be prescribed for the same indication but whose action is unrelated to the hypothesis being tested. For example, the association between penicillin and venous thromboembolism (VTE) would be prone to confounding by respiratory infection, an indication for antibiotics and a know risk factor for VTE. If an association of similar magnitude is observed for an alternative antibiotic prescribed for the same indication (e.g. patients

TABLE 10.4: *Odds ratio estimates from three self-controlled designs for a (Drug1) and an active comparator (Drug2).*

Design	**Drug1**	**Drug2**	**Ratio**[1]	**Interaction**[2]
Case-crossover	3.35	3.56	0.94(0.87,1.03)	1.03(0.95,1.13)
Case-time-control	2.98	3.14	0.95(0.84,1.07)	1.06(0.94,1.15)
Self-controlled case series	2.93	3.37	0.87(0.82,0.92)	0.95(0.89,1.01)

[1] *ratio (95% C.I.) of estimates from analyses of the two groups exposed to only one drug;* [2] *from joint models; associations all significant*

with allergy to penicillin), this would provide evidence of confounding by indication. An illustrative analysis using Danish national databases analysed this question using the case-crossover, case-time-control and self-controlled case series designs [74]. Each design estimated a strong association of VTE with penicillin and with an alternative antibiotic (see Table 10.4), similar to the results from interaction analyses. These findings suggest confounding by indication, with some weak evidence from the self-controlled case series of reduced risk in the group receiving the study drug.

10.5 Summary

From the early work of survey sampling and case-control studies up to the present, there is a continued interest in extending the designs for selecting an informative sample from a cohort and the methods for its analysis, in pursuit of the valuable 'bargain' of an efficient design. The designs vary widely in their mathematical and computational complexity and many are inaccessible to practitioners. However, there are others that fit neatly into familiar structures and that can be understood intuitively and statistically by anyone familiar with the classic epidemiology designs. This chapter has focused on such designs, in keeping with the purpose of the book: to encourage epidemiologists and biostatisticians to analyse observational data using better controlled observational designs that can be implemented by exploiting or repurposing standard statistical methods and software.

Bibliography

[1] EK Accorsi, A Britton, KE Fleming-Dutra, and ZR Smith et al. Association between 3 doses of mrna covid-19 vaccine and symptomatic infection caused by the sars-cov-2 omicron and delta variants. *JAMA*, 327:639–651, 2022.

[2] KEC Ainslie, M Shi, M Haber, and WA Orenstein. A dynamic model for evaluation of the bias of influenza vaccine effectiveness estimates from observational studies. *Am J Epidemiol.*, 188:451–460, 2019.

[3] K Akre, AM Ekström, LB Signorello, LE Hansson, and O Nyrén. Aspirin and risk for gastric cancer: a population-based case-control study in sweden. *Br Jour Cancer*, 84:965–968, 2001.

[4] KL Anders, Z Cutcher, I Kleinschmidt, and CA Donnelly et al. Cluster-randomized test-negative design trials: a novel and efficient method to assess the efficacy of community-level dengue interventions. *Am J Epidemiol*, 187:2021–2028, 2018.

[5] EB Andersen. *Conditional Inference and Models for Measuring*, page 69. Mental Hygieisk Forlag., Copenhagen, 1973.

[6] N Andrieu, AM Goldstein, DC Thomas, and B Langholz. Counter-matching in studies of gene-environment interaction: efficiency and feasibility. *Am J Epidemiol*, 153:265–274, 2001.

[7] P Armitage. The use of the cross-ratio in aetiological surveys. In J Gani, editor, *Perspectives in Probability and Statistics*, pages 349–355. Academic Press, London, 1975.

[8] BF Arnold, A Ercumen, J Benjamin-Chung, and JM Colford (Jr). Brief report: negative controls to detect selection bias and measurement bias in epidemiologic studies. *Epidemiology*, 27:637–641, 2016.

[9] WE Barlow, L Ichikawa, D Rosner, and S Izumi. Analysis of case-cohort designs. *J Clin Epidemiol*, 52:1165–72, 1999.

[10] R Bender and M Blettner. Calculating the 'number needed to be exposed' with adjustment for confounding variables in epidemiological studies. *J Clin Epidemiol*, 55:525–530, 2002.

[11] R Bender, O Kuss, M Hildebrandt, and U Gehrmann. Estimating adjusted nnt measures in logistic regression analysis. *Statistics in Medicine*, 26:5586–5595, 2007.

[12] J Berkson. Limitations of the application of fourfold table analysis to hospital data. *Biometrics Bulletin*, 2:47–53, 1946.

[13] SN Bhupathiraju, F Grodstein, MJ Stampfer, and WC Willett et al. Exogenous hormone use: oral contraceptives, postmenopausal hormone therapy, and health outcomes in the nurses' health study. *Am J Public Health*, 106:1631–1637, 2016.

[14] DA Binder. Fitting Cox's proportional hazards models from survey data. *Biometrika*, 79:139–147, 1992.

[15] O Borgan, B Langholz, SO Samuelsen, and L Goldstein et al. Exposure stratified case-cohort designs. *Lifetime Data Anal*, 6:39–58, 2000.

[16] O Borgan and SO Samuelsen. A review of cohort sampling designs for cox's regression model: Potentials in epidemiology. *Norsk Epidemiologi*, 13:239–248, 2003.

[17] FX Bosch, N Munoz, S de Sanjose, and I Izarzugaza et al. Risk factors for cervical cancer in colombia and spain. *Int J Cancer*, 52:750–758, 1992.

[18] A Bradford-Hill. The environment and disease: association or causation? *P Roy Soc Med*, 58:295–300, 1965.

[19] F Bray, J Ferlay, I Soerjomataram, and RL Siegel et al. Global cancer statistics 2018: Globocan estimates of incidence and mortality worldwide for 36 cancers in 185 countries. *CA-Cancer J Clin*, 68:394–424, 2018.

[20] NE Breslow. Design and analysis of case-control studies. *Ann Rev Public Health*, 3:29–54, 1982.

[21] NE Breslow. Statistics in epidemiology: The case-control study. *J Am Stat Assoc*, 91:14–28, 1996.

[22] NE Breslow and KC Cain. Logistic regression for two-stage case-control data. *Biometrika*, 75:11–20, 1988.

[23] NE Breslow and N Chatterjee. Design and analysis of two-phase studies with binary outcome applied to wilm's tumour prognosis. *Applied Statistics*, 48:457–468, 1999.

[24] NE Breslow and NE Day. *Statistical Methods in Cancer Research: Volume 1 - The analysis of case-control studies.* IARC Scientific Publications No. 32, 1980.

[25] CV Breton, W Zhou, ML Kile, and EA Houseman et al. Susceptibility to arsenic-induced skin lesions from polymorphisms in base excision repair genes. *Carcinogenesis*, 28:1520–1525, 2007.

[26] M Brisson, JJ Kim, K Canfell, and M Drolet et al. Impact of hpv vaccination and cervical screening on cervical cancer elimination: a comparative modelling analysis in 78 low-income and lower-middle-income countries. *Lancet*, 395:575–590, 2020.

[27] CV Broome, RR Facklam, and DW Fraser. Pneumococcal disease after pneumococcal vaccination: an alternative method to estimate the efficacy of pneumococcal vaccine. *N Engl J Med*, 303:549–552, 1980.

[28] KC Cain and NE Breslow. Logistic regression analysis and efficient design for two-stage studies. *Am J Epidemiol*, 128:1198–1206, 1988.

[29] MS Chase and MR Klauber. A graph of sample size for retrospective studies. *Am J Publ Health*, 55:1993–1996, 1965.

[30] K Chen. Generalized case–cohort sampling. *J R Stat Soc B*, 63:791–809, 2001.

[31] KH Chu, NJ Brown, A Pelecanos, and AFT Brown. Simpson's paradox: a statistician's case study. *Emerg Med Australas*, 30:431–33, 2018.

[32] I Ciocanea-Teodorescu, M Nason, A Sjölander, and EE Gabriel. Adjustment for disease severity in the test-negative study design. *Am J Epidemiol.*, 90:1882–1889, 2021.

[33] S Cnattingius, CM Hultman, M Dahl, and P Sparén. Very preterm birth, birth trauma, and the risk of anorexia nervosa among girls. *Arch Gen Psychiat*, 56:634–8, 1999.

[34] WG Cochran. *Sampling Techniques.* Wiley, New York, 2nd edition, 1963.

[35] D Coggon, G Rose, and DJP Barker. *Epidemiology for the Uninitiated.* BMJ, 4th edition, 1997.

[36] CR Cohen, J Gichui, R Rukaria, and SS Sinei et al. Immunogenetic correlates for chlamydia trachomatis–associated tubal infertility. *Obstet Gynecol*, 101:438–444, 2003.

[37] CR Cohen, SS Sinei, EA Bukusi, and JJ Bwayo et al. Human leukocyte antigen class ii dq alleles associated with chlamydia trachomatis tubal infertility. *Obstet Gynecol*, 95:72–77, 2000.

[38] GA Colditz, SE Philpott, and SE Hankinson. The impact of the nurses' health study on population health: prevention, translation, and control. *Am J Public Health*, 106:1540–1545, 2016.

[39] J Cologne. Counterintuitive matching. *Epidemiology*, 8:227–229, 1997.

[40] J Cologne and B Langholz. Selecting controls for assessing interaction in nested case-control studies. *J Epidemiol*, 13:193–202, 2003.

[41] S Cruchet, MC Obregon, G Salazar, E Diaz, and M Gotteland. Effect of the ingestion of a dietary product containing lactobacillus johnsonii la1 on helicobacter pylori colonization in children. *Nutrition*, 19:716–721, 2003.

[42] P Cummings, B McKnight, and S Greenland. Matched cohort methods for injury research. *Epidemiol Rev*, 25:43–50, 2003.

[43] E Dahlqwist, J Zetterqvist, Y Pawitan, and A Sjölander. Model-based estimation of the attributable fraction for cross-sectional, case–control and cohort studies using the r package af. *Eur J Epidemiol*, 31:575–582, 2016.

[44] G Danaei, LA García Rodríguez, OF Cantero, and MA Hernán. Statins and risk of diabetes: an analysis of electronic medical

records to evaluate possible bias due to differential survival. *Diabetes Care*, 36:1236–1240, 2013.

[45] NE Dean. Re: Measurement of vaccine direct effects under the test-negative design. *Am J Epidemiol*, 188:806–810, 2019.

[46] NE Dean, ME Halloran, and IM Longini Jr. Temporal confounding in the test-negative design. *Am J Epidemiol*, 189:1402–1407, 2020.

[47] B Delcoigne, E Colzani, M Prochazka, and G Gagliardi et al. Breaking the matching in nested case-control data offered several advantages for risk estimation. *J Clin Epidemiol*, 82:79–86, 2017.

[48] B Delcoigne, N Hagenbuch, MEC Schelin, and A Salim et al. Feasibility of reusing time-matched controls in an overlapping cohort. *Stat Methods Med Res*, 27:1818–1829, 2016.

[49] B Delcoigne, NC Stoer, and M Reilly. Valid and efficient subgroup analyses using nested case-control data. *Int J Epidemiol*, 47:841–849, 2018.

[50] AP Dempster, NM Laird, and DB Rubin. Maximum likelihood from incomplete data via the em algorithm. *J R Stat Soc B*, 39:1–38, 1977.

[51] G DeSerres, DM Skowronski, XW Wu, and CS Ambrose. The test-negative design: validity, accuracy and precision of vaccine efficacy estimates compared to the gold standard of randomised placebo-controlled clinical trials. *Euro Surveill*, 18:20585, 2013.

[52] J Ding, H Zhou, Y Liu, J Cai, and MP Longnecker. Estimating effect of environmental contaminants on women's subfecundity for the moba study data with an outcome-dependent sampling scheme. *Biostatistics*, 15:636–650, 2014.

[53] R Doll and A Bradford Hill. Lung cancer and other causes of death in relation to smoking: a second report on the mortality of british doctors. *Brit Med J*, 2:1071–1081, 1956.

[54] T Dwyer and AL Ponsonby. Sudden infant death syndrome and prone sleeping position. *Ann Epidemiol*, 19:245–249, 2009.

[55] K Einarsdottir, K Humphreys, C Bonnard, and J Palmgren et al. Linkage disequilibrium mapping of chek2: common variation and breast cancer risk. *PLoS Med*, 3:e168, 2006.

[56] A Ekbom. The swedish multi-generation register. *Methods Mol Biol*, 675:215–220, 2011.

[57] AM Ekström, M Eriksson, LE Hansson, and A Lindgren et al. Occupational exposures and risk of gastric cancer in a population-based case-control study. *Cancer Res*, 59:5932–5937, 1999.

[58] AM Ekström, M Held, LE Hansson, L Engstrand, and O Nyrén. Helicobacter pylori in gastric cancer established by caga immunoblot as a marker of past infection. *Gastroenterology*, 121:784–791, 2001.

[59] ENCEPP. Guide on methodological standards in pharmacoepidemiology (revision 9). ema/95098/2010. 2021. `https://www.encepp.eu/standards_and_guidances/documents/1.ENCePPMethodsGuideRev.9.pdf`, 2021. Accessed: 2019-10-24.

[60] M Endler, S Cnattingius, M Granfors, and AK Wikström. The inherited risk of retained placenta: a population based cohort study. *Brit J Obstet Gynaec*, 125:737–744, 2018.

[61] F Fang, K Fall, MA Mittleman, and P Sparen et al. Suicide and cardiovascular death after a cancer diagnosis. *N Engl J Med*, 366:1310–1318, 2012.

[62] P Farrington, Heather Whitaker, and YG Weldeselassie. *Self-Controlled Case Series Studies A Modelling Guide with R*. Chapman and Hall/CRC, 2018.

[63] AR Feinstein, RI Horwitz, WO Spitzer, and RN Battista. Coffee and pancreatic cancer. the problems of etiologic science and epidemiologic case-control research. *J Am Med Assoc*, 246:957–61, 1981.

[64] JM Ferdinands, IM Foppa, AM Fry, and BL Flannery et al. Re: Invited commentary: beware the test-negative design. *Am J Epidemiol.*, 185:613, 2017.

[65] J Ferguson, A Alvarez-Iglesias, J Newell, J Hinde, and M O'Donnell. Estimating average attributable fractions with confidence intervals for cohort and case-control studies. *Stat Methods Med Res*, 27:1141–1152, 2016.

[66] GM Fitzmaurice, NM Laird, and JH Ware. *Applied Longitudinal Analysis, 2nd Edition.* Wiley Series in Probability and Statistics, 2011.

[67] IM Foppa, M Haber, JM Ferdinands, and DK Shay. The case test-negative design for studies of the effectiveness of influenza vaccine. *Vaccine*, 31:3104–3109, 2013.

[68] R Franca, P Rebora, G Basso, and A Biondi et al. Glutathione s-transferase homozygous deletions and relapse in childhood acute lymphoblastic leukemia: a novel study design in a large italian aieop cohort. *Pharmacogenomics*, 13:1905–1916, 2012.

[69] MF Franke, JG Jerome, WR Matias, and R Ternier et al. Comparison of two control groups for estimation of oral cholera vaccine effectiveness using a case-control study design. *Vaccine*, 35:5819–5827, 2017.

[70] WQ Gan, SB Henderson, G Mckee, and W Yuchi et al. Snowfall, temperature, and the risk of death from myocardial infarction: a case-crossover study. *Am J Epidemiol*, 189:832–840, 2020.

[71] F Graziano, MG Valsecchi, and P Rebora. Sampling strategies to evaluate the prognostic value of a new biomarker on a time-to-event end-point. *BMC Med Res Methodol*, 21:93, 2021.

[72] G Gustafsson, P Kogner, and M Heyman. Childhood cancer incidence and survival in sweden 1984-2010. Report 2013, Karolinska Institutet, 2013.

[73] WA Guy. Contributions to a knowledge of the influence of employments upon health. *Journal of the Statistical Society of London*, 6:197–211, 1843.

[74] J Hallas, H Whitaker, JA Delaney, and SM Cadarette et al. The use of active comparators in self-controlled designs. *Am J Epidemiol*, 190:2181–2187, 2021.

[75] S Haneuse, B Hedt-Gauthier, F Chimbwandira, and S Makombe et al. Strategies for monitoring and evaluation of resource-limited national antiretroviral therapy programs: the two-phase design. *BMC Med Res Methodol*, 15:31, 2015.

[76] S Haneuse and C Rivera-Rodriguez. On the analysis of case-control studies in cluster-correlated data settings. *Epidemiology*, 29:50–57, 2018.

[77] JH Hankin, DO Stram, K Arakawa, and S Park et al. Singapore chinese health study: Development, validation, and calibration of the quantitative food frequency questionnaire. *Nutrition and Cancer*, 39:187–195, 2001.

[78] JA Hanley and B Foster. Avoiding blunders involving 'immortal time'. *Int J Epidemiol*, 43:949–961, 2014.

[79] JA Hanley, E Turner, C Bellera, and D Teltsch. How long did their hearts go on? a titanic study. *Brit Med J*, 327:1457–1458, 2003.

[80] LE Hansson, AM Ekström, R Bergström, and O Nyrén. Carcinoma of the gastric cardia: surgical practices and short-term operative results in a defined swedish population. *World J Surg*, 24:473–478, 2000.

[81] RF Heller, AJ Dobson, J Attia, and J Page. Impact numbers: measures of risk factor impact on the whole population from case-control and cohort studies. *J Epidemiol Commun H*, 56:606–610, 2002.

[82] B Herity, M Moriarty, LE Daly, J Dunn, and GJ Bourke. The role of tobacco and alcohol in the aetiology of lung and larynx cancer. *Brit J Cancer*, 46:961–964, 1982.

[83] MA Hernán, D Clayton, and N Keiding. The simpson's paradox unraveled. *Int J Epidemiol*, 40:780–785, 2011.

[84] KR Hess. Assessing time-by-covariate interactions in proportional hazards regression models using cubic spline functions. *Stat Med*, 13:1045–1062, 1994.

[85] M Hildebrandt, R Bender, U Gehrmann, and M Blettner. Calculating confidence intervals for impact numbers. *BMC Med Res Methodol*, 6:32, 2006.

[86] MJ Holmberg and LW Andersen. Collider bias. *J Am Med Assoc*, 327:1282–1283, 2022.

[87] N Houssami and K Hunter. The epidemiology, radiology and biological characteristics of interval breast cancers in population mammography screening. *NPJ Breast Cancer*, 3:12, 2017.

[88] M Huberman and B Langholz. Application of the missing-indicator method in matched case-control studies with incomplete data. *Am J Epidemiol*, 150:1340–1345, 1999.

[89] M Hultman, P Sparén, N Takei, RM Murray, and S Cnattingius. Prenatal and perinatal risk factors for schizophrenia, affective psychosis, and reactive psychosis of early onset: case-control study. *Brit Med J*, 318:421–426, 1999.

[90] MH Huque, RJ Carroll, N Diao, DC Christiani, and LM Ryan. Exposure enriched case-control (eecc) design for the assessment of gene-environment interaction. *Genet Epidemiol.*, 40:570–578, 2016.

[91] JA Hutcheon, A Chiolero, and JA Hanley. Random measurement error and regression dilution bias. *Brit Med J*, 340:c2289, 2010.

[92] LC Ivers, IJ Hilaire, and JE Teng CP Almazor et al. Effectiveness of reactive oral cholera vaccination in rural haiti: a case-control study and bias-indicator analysis. *Lancet Glob Health*, 3:e162–e168, 2015.

[93] J Ferguson and M O' Connell. Estimating and displaying population attributable fractions. `https://cran.r-project.org/web/packages/graphPAF/vignettes/graphPAF_vignette.pdf`, 2022. Accessed: 2022-10-21.

[94] LA Jackson, ML Jackson, KM Neuzil, and NS Weiss. Evidence of bias in estimates of influenza vaccine effectiveness in seniors. *Int J Epidemiol*, 35:337–344, 2006.

[95] ML Jackson and JC Nelson. The test-negative design for estimating influenza vaccine effectiveness. *Vaccine*, 31:2165–2168, 2013.

[96] ML Jackson and KJ Rothman. Effects of imperfect test sensitivity and specificity on observational studies of influenza vaccine effectiveness. *Vaccine*, 33:1313–1316, 2015.

[97] H Janes, L Sheppard, and T Lumley. Case-crossover analyses of air pollution exposure data: referent selection strategies and their implications for bias. *Epidemiology*, 16:717–726, 2005.

[98] NP Jewell, S Dufault, Z Cutcher, CP Simmons, and KL Anders. Analysis of cluster-randomized test-negative designs: cluster-level methods. *Biostatistics*, 20:332–346, 2019.

[99] JM Colford (Jr), KC Schiff, JF Griffith, and V Yao et al. Using rapid indicators for enterococcus to assess the risk of illness after exposure to urban runoff contaminated marine water. *Water Res*, 46:2176–2186, 2012.

[100] H Keogh and IR White. A toolkit for measurement error correction, with a focus on nutritional epidemiology. *Stat Med*, 33:2137–2155, 2014.

[101] RH Keogh, P Mangtani, L Rodrigues, and DP Nguipdop. Estimating time-varying exposure-outcome associations using case-control data: logistic and case-cohort analyses. *BMC Med Res Methodol.*, 16, 2016.

[102] RS Kim. A new comparison of nested case-control and case-cohort designs and methods. *Eur J Epidemiol.*, 30:197–207, 2015.

[103] YM Kim and J Im. Cost-effective extreme case-control design using a resampling method. *Evol Bioinform*, 15:1–9, 2019.

[104] BR Kirkwood and JAC Sterne. *Essential Medical Statistics, 2nd Edition.* Wiley-Blackwell, 2003.

[105] M Kivi, AL Johansson, M Reilly, and Y Tindberg. Helicobacter pylori status in family members as risk factors for infection in children. *Epidemiol Infect.*, 133:645–652, 2005.

[106] M Kivi, AL Johansson, A Salim, Y Tindberg, and M Reilly. Accommodation of additional non-randomly sampled cases in a study of helicobacter pylori infection in families. *Stat Med*, 24:4045–4054, 2005.

[107] M Kivi, Y Tindberg, M Sörberg, and TH Casswall et al. Concordance of helicobacter pylori strains within families. *J Clin Microbiol*, 41:5604–8, 2003.

[108] MJ Knol, M Egger, P Scott, MI Geerlings, and JP Vandenbroucke. When one depends on the other:reporting of interaction in case-control and cohort studies. *Epidemiology*, 20:161–166, 2009.

[109] MJ Knol, S Le Cessie, A Algra, JP Vandenbroucke, and RHH Groenwold. Overestimation of risk ratios by odds ratios in trials and cohort studies: alternatives to logistic regression. *Can Med Assoc J*, 184:895–899, 2012.

[110] L Kupper. Matching. In *Encyclopedia of Biostatistics*. John Wiley & Sons Ltd., 2005.

[111] E Laara. Study designs for biobank-based epidemiologic research on chronic diseases. In *Methods in Biobanking*. Humana Press, Totowa, NJ, 2011.

[112] JE Lane-Claypon. A further report on cancer of the breast with special reference to its associated antecedent conditions. *Reports on Public Health and Medical Subjects*, 32, 1926.

[113] Langholz and O Borgan. Estimation of absolute risk from nested case-control data. *Biometrics*, 53:767–774, 1997.

[114] B Langholz and O Borgan. Counter-matching: a stratified nested case-control sampling method. *Biometrika*, 82:69–79, 1995.

[115] B Langholz and D Clayton. Sampling strategies in nested case-control studies. *Environ Health Persp*, 102:47–50, 1994.

[116] S leCessie, N Nagelkerke, FR Rosendaal, and KJ van Stralen et al. Combining matched and unmatched control groups in case-control studies. *Am J Epidemiol*, 168:1204–1210, 2008.

[117] AJ Lee, L McMurchy, and AJ Scott. Re-using data from case-control studies. *Stat Med*, 16:1377–1389, 1997.

[118] BK Lee, I Le Ray, JY Sun, and A Wikman et al. Haemolytic and nonhaemolytic neonatal jaundice have different risk factor profiles. *Acta Paediatrica*, 105:1444–1450, 2016.

[119] J Lee, CS Tan, and KS Chia. A practical guide for multivariate analysis of dichotomous outcomes. *Ann Acad Med Singapore*, 38:714–719, 2009.

[120] M Lee, K Czene, P Rebora, and M Reilly. Patterns of changing cancer risks with time since diagnosis of a sibling. *Int J Cancer.*, 136:1948–1956, 2015.

[121] PH Lee. Is a cutoff of 10% appropriate for the change-in-estimate criterion of confounder identification? *J Epidemiol*, 24:161–167, 2014.

[122] K Leffondre, W Wynant, Z Cao, and M Abrahamowicz et al. A weighted cox model for modelling time-dependent exposures in the analysis of case-control studies. *Stat Med*, 29:839–850, 2010.

[123] M Leu, K Czene, and M Reilly. Bias correction of estimates of familial risk from population-based cohort studies. *Int J Epidemiol*, 39:80–88, 2010.

[124] M Leu, M Reilly, and K Czene. Evaluation of bias in familial risk estimates: a study of common cancers using swedish population-based registers. *J Natl Cancer Inst*, 100:1318–1325, 2008.

[125] D Levy. *50 Years of Discovery: Medical Milestones from the National Heart, Lung, and Blood Institute's Framingham Heart Study.* Dumont, N.J. Center for Bio-Medical Communication, Inc., 1999.

[126] JA Lewnard, MM Patel, NP Jewell, and JR Verani et al. Theoretical framework for retrospective studies of the effectiveness of sars-cov-2 vaccines. *Epidemiology*, 32:508–517, 2021.

[127] JA Lewnard, C Tedijanto, BJ Cowling, and M Lipsitch. The authors reply. *Am J Epidemiol*, 188:807–808, 2019.

[128] Y Li, M Safaeian, HA Robbins, and BI Graubard. Logistic analysis of epidemiologic studies with augmentation sampling involving re-stratification and population expansion. *Biostatistics*, 16:169–178, 2015.

[129] M Lipsitch, E Tchetgen Tchetgen, and T Cohen. Negative controls: a tool for detecting confounding and bias in observational studies [published correction appears in epidemiology. *Epidemiology*, 21:383–388, 2010.

[130] S Lisonkova and KS Joseph. Left truncation bias as a potential explanation for the protective effect of smoking on preeclampsia. *Epidemiology*, 26:436–440, 2015.

[131] I-M Liu. Breslow-day test. In Peter Armitage and Theodore Colton, editors, *Encyclopedia of Biostatistics*, volume 1, page 560. John Wiley & Sons Ltd., 2nd edition, 2005.

[132] L Löfgren, S Eloranta, K Krawiec, and A Asterkvist et al. on behalf of the steering group of the National Register for Breast Cancer. Validation of data quality in the swedish national register for breast cancer. *BMC Public Health*, 19:495, 2019.

[133] JF Ludvigsson, C Almqvist, AK Edstedt Bonamy, and R Ljung et al. Registers of the swedish total population and their use in medical research. *Eur J Epidemiol.*, 31:125–136, 2016.

[134] J Luo, H-O Adami, M Reilly, and A Ekbom et al. Interpreting trends of pancreatic cancer incidence and mortality: a nation-wide study in sweden (1960-2003). *Cancer Cause Control*, 19:89–96, 2008.

[135] M Maclure. The case-crossover design: a method for studying transient effects on the risk of acute events. *Am J Epidemiol*, 133:144–153, 1991.

[136] M Maclure. The case-crossover design: a method for studying transient effects on the risk of acute events. *Am J Epidemiol*, 185:1174–1183, 2017.

[137] M Maclure and MA Mittleman. Should we use a case-crossover design? *Annu Rev Public Health*, 21:193–221, 2000.

[138] H Magen-Molho, MG Weisskopf, D Nevo, and A Shtein et al. Air pollution and autism spectrum disorder in israel: a negative control analysis. *Epidemiology.*, 32:773–780, 2021.

[139] SS Mahmood, D Levy, RS Vasan, and TJ Wang. The framingham heart study and the epidemiology of cardiovascular disease: a historical perspective. *The Lancet*, 383:999–1008, 2014.

[140] G Maldonado and S Greenland. Simulation study of confounder-selection strategies. *Am J Epidemiol*, 138:923–936, 1993.

[141] MA Mansournia, NP Jewell, and S Greenland. Case-control matching: effects, misconceptions, and recommendations. *Eur J Epidemiol*, 33:5–14, 2018.

[142] MG Marmot, DG Altman, DA Cameron, and JA Dewar et al. The benefits and harms of breast cancer screening: an independent review. *Br J Cancer*, 108:2205–2240, 2013.

[143] MA McIsaac and RJ Cook. Adaptive sampling in two-phase designs: a biomarker study for progression in arthritis. *Stat Med*, 34:2899–2912, 2015.

[144] B McKnight, LS Cook, and NS Weiss. Logistic regression analysis for more than one characteristic of exposure. *Am J Epidemiol*, 149:984–992, 1999.

[145] L Meng, S Oberg, A Sandstrom, C Wang, and M Reilly. Identification of risk factors for incident cervical insufficiency in nulliparous and parous women: a population-based case-control study. *BMC Medicine*, 20:348, 2022.

[146] O Miettinen. Stratification by a multivariate confounder score. *Am J Epidemiol*, 104:609–620, 1976.

[147] O Miettinen. Design options in epidemiologic research: an update. *Scand J Work Environ Health*, 8:7–14, 1982.

[148] O Miettinen. The 'case-control' study: valid selection of subjects. *J Chron Dis*, 38:543–548, 1985.

[149] KM Miller and SW Looney. A simple method for estimating the odds ratio in matched case-control studies with incomplete paired data. *Stat Med*, 31:3299–3312, 2012.

[150] EA Mitchell, R Scragg, AW Stewart, and DMO Becroft et al. Results from the first year of the new zealand cot death study. *New Zeal Med J*, 104:71–76, 1991.

[151] MA Mittleman. Optimal referent selection strategies in case-crossover studies: a settled issue. *Epidemiology*, 16:715–716, 2005.

[152] MA Mittleman and E Mostofsky. Exchangeability in the case-crossover design. *Int J Epidemiol*, 43:1645–1655, 2014.

[153] V Moreno, ML Martín, FX Bosch, and S de Sanjose et al. Combined analysis of matched and unmatched case-control studies: comparison of risk estimates from different studies. *Am J Epidemiol*, 143:293–300, 1996.

[154] E Mostofsky, M Maclure, JB Sherwood, and GH Tofler et al. Risk of acute myocardial infarction after the death of a significant person in one's life: the determinants of myocardial infarction onset study. *Circulation*, 125:491–496, 2012.

[155] DC Muller, TL Larose, A Hodge, and F Guida a et al. Circulating high sensitivity c reactive protein concentrations and risk of lung cancer: nested case-control study within lung cancer cohort consortium. *Brit Med J*, 364:k4981, 2019.

[156] N Munoz, FX Bosch, S de Sanjose, and A Vergara et al. Risk factors for cin iii in spain and colombia. *Cancer Epidem Biomar*, 2:423–431, 1993.

[157] MH Murad, N Asi, M Alsawas, and F Alahdab. New evidence pyramid. *Evid Based Med*, 21:125–127, 2016.

[158] NJD Nagelkerke, S Moses, FA Plummer, and RC Brunham. Logistic regression in case–control studies: the effect of using independent as dependent variables. *Stat Med*, 14:769–775, 1995.

[159] J Nam. Optimum sample sizes for the comparison of the control and treatment. *Biometrics*, 29:101–108, 1973.

[160] J-M Nam and TR Fears. Optimum allocation of samples in strata-matching case-control studies when cost per sample differs from stratum to stratum. *Stat Med*, 9:1475–1483, 1990.

[161] H Needleman. Low level lead exposure: history and discovery. *Ann Epidemiol*, 19:235–238, 2009.

[162] R Ness. Introduction. *Ann Epidemiol*, 19:225, 2009.

[163] LM Niccolai, LG Ogden, CE Muehlenbein, and JD Dziura et al. Methodological issues in design and analysis of a matched case-control study of a vaccine's effectiveness. *J Clin Epidemiol.*, 60:1127–1131, 2007.

[164] GR Northrup, L Qian, K Bruxvoort, and FM Marx et al. Inference of naturally acquired immunity using a self-matched negative-control design. *Epidemiology*, 32:168–178, 2021.

[165] D Oakes. Survival times: spects of partial likelihood (with discussion). *Int Stat Rev*, 49:235–264, 1981.

[166] G Oakley. The scientific basis for eliminating folic acid-preventable spina bifida: a modern miracle from epidemiology. *Ann Epidemiol*, 19:226–230, 2009.

[167] J Palmgren. Regression models for bivariate binary responses. Technical Report No. 101, Department of Biostatistics, School of Public Health and Community Medicine, University of Washington, Seattle., 1989.

[168] N Pearce. Classification of epidemiological study designs. *Int J Epidemiol*, 41:393–397, 2012.

[169] C Persson, L Engstrand, O Nyrén, and LE Hansson et al. Interleukin 1-beta gene polymorphisms and risk of gastric cancer in sweden. *Scand J Gastroenterol*, 44:339–345, 2009.

[170] Physicians' Health Study Research Group. Preliminary report: findings from the aspirin component of the ongoing physicians' health study. *New Engl J Med*, 318:262–264, 1988.

[171] WD Du Pont. *Statistical Modeling for Biomedical Researchers: A Simple Introduction to the Analysis of Complex Data, Second edition.* Cambridge University Press, 2009.

[172] RL Prentice. A case-cohort design for epidemiologic cohort studies and disease prevention trials. *Biometrika*, 73:1–11, 1986.

[173] RL Prentice and R Pyke. Logistic disease incidence models and case-control studies. *Biometrika*, 66:403–411, 1979.

[174] M Prochazka, P Hall, G Gagliardi, and F Granath et al. Ionizing radiation and tobacco use increases the risk of a subsequent lung carcinoma in women with breast cancer: case-only design. *J Clin Oncol*, 23:7467–7474, 2005.

[175] A Qaseem, JS Lin, RA Mustafa, and CA Horwitch et al.: Clinical Guidelines Committee of the American College of Physicians. Screening for breast cancer in average-risk women: A guidance statement from the american college of physicians. *Ann Intern Med*, 170:547–560, 2019.

[176] C Quantin, M Abrahamowicz, T Moreau, and G Bartlett et al. Variation over time of the effects of prognostic factors in a

population-based study of colon cancer: comparison of statistical models. *Am J Epidemiol*, 150:1188–200, 1999.

[177] P Rebora, M Lee, K Czene, MG Valsecchi, and M Reilly. High risks of familial chronic lymphatic leukemia for specific relatives: signposts for genetic discovery? *Leukemia*, 26:2419–21, 2012.

[178] D Redelmeier. The exposure-crossover design is a new method for studying sustained changes in recurrent events. *J Clin Epidemiol*, 66:955–963, 2013.

[179] M Reilly and M Sullivan Pepe. A mean score method for missing and auxiliary covariate data in regression models. *Biometrika*, 82:299–314, 1995.

[180] KL Sainani. Understanding odds ratios. *PM R*, 3:263–267, 2011.

[181] A Salim, B Delcoigne, K Villaflores, and W-P Koh et al. Comparisons of risk prediction methods using nested case-control data. *Stat Med*, 36:455–465, 2017.

[182] A Salim, C Hultman, P Sparen, and M Reilly. Combining data from 2 nested case–control studies of overlapping cohorts to improve efficiency. *Biostatistics*, 10:70–79, 2009.

[183] A Salim, X Ma, K Fall, O Andrén, and M Reilly. Analysis of incidence and prognosis from extreme' case-control designs. *Stat Med*, 33:5388–5398, 2014.

[184] A Salim, Q Yang, and M Reilly. The value of reusing prior nested case–control data in new studies with different outcome. *Stat Med*, 31:1291–1302, 2012.

[185] SO Samuelsen. A pseudolikelihood approach to analysis of nested case-control studies. *Biometrika*, 84:379–394, 1997.

[186] SO Samuelsen, H Anestad, and A Skrondal. Stratified case-cohort analysis of general cohort sampling designs. *Scand J Statistics*, 34:103–119, 2007.

[187] E Sanderson, C Macdonald-Wallis, and G Davey Smith. Negative control exposure studies in the presence of measurement error: implications for attempted effect estimate calibration. *Int J Epidemiol.*, 47:587–596, 2018.

[188] S Sandin, P Lichtenstein, R Kuja-Halkola, and H Larsson et al. The familial risk of autism. *J Am Med Assoc*, 311:1770–1777, 2014.

[189] A Sboner, F Demichelis, S Calza, and Y Pawitan et al. Molecular sampling of prostate cancer: a dilemma for predicting disease progression. *BMC Medical Genomics*, 3:8, 2010.

[190] JJ Schlesselman. *Case Control Studies: Design, Conduct, Analysis.* Oxford University Press, 1982.

[191] ME Schnitzer, D Harel, V Ho, A Koushik, and J Merckx. Identifiability and estimation under the test-negative design with population controls with the goal of identifying risk and preventive factors for sars-cov-2 infection. *Epidemiology*, 32:690–697, 2021.

[192] EG Schouten, JM Dekker, FJ Kok, and S Le Cessie et al. Risk ratio and rate ratio estimation in cardiovascular mortality case-cohort designs: hypertension and cardiovascular mortality. *Stat Med*, 12:1733–1745, 1993.

[193] HE Segaloff, B Cheng, AV Miller, and JG Petrie et al. Influenza vaccine effectiveness in the inpatient setting: evaluation of potential bias in the test-negative design by use of alternate control groups. *Am J Epidemiol*, 189:250–260, 2020.

[194] KJ Sherman, JR Daling, A Stergachis, and NS Weiss et al. Sexually transmitted diseases and tubal pregnancy. *Sexually Transmitted Diseases*, 17:115–121, 1990.

[195] A Sjolander and S Greenland. Ignoring the matching variables in cohort studies - when is it valid and why? *Stat Med*, 32:4696–4708, 2013.

[196] DM Skowronski, C Masaro, TL Kwindt, and A Mak et al. Estimating vaccine effectiveness against laboratory-confirmed influenza using a sentinel physician network: results from the 2005-2006 season of dual a and b vaccine mismatch in canada. *Vaccine*, 25:2842–2851, 2007.

[197] LH Smith and TJ VanderWeele. Simple sensitivity analysis for control selection bias. *Epidemiology*, 31:e44–e45, 2020.

[198] JD Snoep, A Morabia, S Hernández-Díaz, M Hernán, and JP Vandenbroucke. Commentary: a structural approach to berkson's fallacy and a guide to a history of opinions about it. *Int J Epidemiol*, 43:515–521, 2014.

[199] H Song, A Michel, O Nyrén, and AM Ekström et al. A caga-independent cluster of antigens related to the risk of noncardia gastric cancer: associations between helicobacter pylori antibodies and gastric adenocarcinoma explored by multiplex serology. *Int J Cancer*, 134:2942–2950, 2014.

[200] D Spiegelman, CL Rivera-Rodriguez, and S Haneuse. Evaluating public health interventions: 3. the two-stage design for confounding bias reduction-having your cake and eating it two. *Am J Public Health*, 106:1223–1226, 2016.

[201] P Squire. Why the 1936 literary digest poll failed. *The Public Opinion Quarterly*, 52:125–133, 1988.

[202] MJ Stampfer, GA Colditz, WC Willett, and JE Manson et al. Postmenopausal estrogen therapy and cardiovascular disease: ten-year follow-up from the nurses' health study. *New Engl J Med*, 325:756–762, 1991.

[203] K Steenland and JA Deddens. Increased precision using counter-matching in nested case-control studies. *Epidemiology.*, 8:238–242, 1997.

[204] N Stoer, A Salim, K Bokenberger, I Karlsson, and M Reilly. Is the matched extreme case-control design more powerful than the nested case-control design? *Stat Methods Med Res*, 28:1911–1923, 2019.

[205] N Stoer and SO Samuelsen. Inverse probability weighting in nested case-control studies with additional matching—a simulation study. *Stat Med*, 32:5328–5339, 2013.

[206] C Sudlow, J Gallacher, N Allen, and V Beral et al. Uk biobank: An open access resource for identifying the causes of a wide range of complex diseases of middle and old age. *PLoS Medicine*, 12:e1001779, 2015.

[207] S Suissa. The case-time-control design. *Epidemiology*, 6:248–253, 1995.

[208] S Suissa. The quasi-cohort approach in pharmacoepidemiology: upgrading the nested case-control. *Epidemiology*, 22:242–246, 2015.

[209] S Suissa, S Dell'Aniello, S Vahey, and C Renoux. Time-window bias in case-control studies: Statins and lung cancer. *Epidemiology*, 22:228–231, 2011.

[210] SG Sullivan, EJ Tchetgen Tchetgen, and BJ Cowling. Theoretical basis of the test-negative study design for assessment of influenza vaccine effectiveness. *Am J Epidemiol*, 184:345–353, 2016.

[211] Z Sun, B Mukherjee, JP Estes, PS Vokonas, and SK Park. Exposure enriched outcome dependent designs for longitudinal studies of gene-environment interaction. *Stat Med*, 36:2947–2960, 2017.

[212] M-P Sylvestre, E Huszti, and JA Hanley. Do oscar winners live longer than less successful peers? a reanalysis of the evidence. *Ann Intern Med*, 145:361–363, 2006.

[213] RE Tarone. On heterogeneity tests based on efficient scores. *Biometrika*, 72:91–95, 1985.

[214] WL Teh, E Abdin, JA Vaingankar, and E Seow et al. Prevalence of stroke, risk factors, disability and care needs in older adults in singapore: results from the wise study. *BMJ Open*, 8:e020285, 2018.

[215] D Thomas. Addendum to 'methods of cohort analysis: appraisal by application to asbestos mining' by liddell fdk, mcdonald jc, thomas dc. *J R Stat Soc A*, 140:469–491, 1977.

[216] Y Tindberg, C Bengtsson, F Granath, and M Blennow et al. Helicobacter pylori infection in swedish school children: lack of evidence of child-to-child transmission outside the family. *Gastroenterology*, 121:310–316, 2001.

[217] P Tugwell and JA Knottnerus. Is the 'evidence-pyramid' now dead? *J Clin Epidemiol.*, 68:1247–1250, 2015.

[218] H Ury. Efficiency of case-control studies with multiple controls per case: continuous or dichotomous data. *Biometrics*, 31:643–649, 1975.

[219] E van Doorn, M Darvishian, F Dijkstra, and GA Donker et al. Influenza vaccine effectiveness estimates in the dutch population from 2003 to 2014: The test-negative design case-control study with different control groups. *Vaccine*, 35:2831–2839, 2017.

[220] JP Vandenbroucke, EB Brickley, CMJE Vandenbroucke-Grauls, and N Pearce. A test-negative design with additional population controls can be used to rapidly study causes of the sars-cov-2 epidemic. *Epidemiology*, 31:836–843, 2020.

[221] JP Vandenbroucke and N Pearce. Incidence rates in dynamic populations. *Int J Epidemiol*, 41:1472–1479, 2012.

[222] JP Vandenbroucke and N Pearce. Test-negative designs differences and commonalities with other case–control studies with 'other patient' controls. *Epidemiology*, 30:838–844, 2019.

[223] S Wacholder, JK McLaughlin, DT Silverman, and JS Mandel. Selection of controls in case-control studies: I. principles. *Am J Epidemiol*, 135:1019–1028, 1992.

[224] S Wacholder, JK McLaughlin, DT Silverman, and JS Mandel. Selection of controls in case-control studies III design options. *Am J Epidemiol*, 135:1042–1050, 1992.

[225] H Wainer, G Lee, and P Velleman. Visual revelations: giving the finger to dating services. *CHANCE*, 21:59–61, 2008.

[226] C Wang, I Le Ray, B Lee, A Wikman, and M Reilly. Association of blood group and red blood cell transfusion with the incidence of antepartum, peripartum and postpartum venous thromboembolism. *Sci Rep*, 9:13535, 2019.

[227] S Wang, C Linkletter, M Maclure, and D Dore et al. Future cases as present controls to adjust for exposure trend bias in case-only studies. *Epidemiology*, 22:568–574, 2011.

[228] CR Weinberg. Invited commentary: self-control is a virtue. *Am J Epidemiol.*, 185:1184–1186, 2017.

[229] D Westreich. Berkson's bias, selection bias, and missing data. *Epidemiology*, 23:159–164, 2012.

[230] HJ Whitaker, CP Farrington, B Spiessens, and P Musonda. Tutorial in biostatistics: the self-controlled case series method. *Stat Med*, 25:1768–1797, 2006.

[231] S Wickham, M Whitehead, D Taylor-Robinson, and B Barr. The effect of a transition into poverty on child and maternal mental health: a longitudinal analysis of the uk millennium cohort study. *Lancet Public Health*, 2:e141–e148, 2017.

[232] V Wintzell, H Svanström, and B Pasternak. Selection of comparator group in observational drug safety studies: alternatives to the active comparator new user design. *Epidemiology*, 33:707–14, 2022.

[233] M Wolkewitz, J Beyersmann, P Gastmeier, and M Schumacher. Efficient risk set sampling when a time-dependent exposure is present: matching for time to exposure versus exposure density sampling. *Methods Inf Med*, 48:438–443, 2009.

[234] AY Wong, A Root, IJ Douglas, and CS Chui et al. Cardiovascular outcomes associated with use of clarithromycin: population based study. *Brit Med J*, 352:h6926, 2016.

[235] M Woodward. *Epidemiology: Study Design and Data Analysis.* Chapman and Hall/CRC, 2005.

[236] B Woolf. On estimating the relation between blood group and disease. *Ann Hum Genet*, 19:251–253, 1955.

[237] World Health Organization. Global health observatory data repository, July 2018.

[238] World Health Organization. Human papillomavirus (hpv) and cervical cancer. `https://www.who.int/en/news-room/fact-sheets/detail/human-papillomavirus-(hpv)-and-cervical-cancer`, 2019. Accessed: 2020-04-20.

[239] W Ye, AM Ekström, LE Hansson, R Bergström, and O Nyrén. Tobacco, alcohol and the risk of gastric cancer by sub-site and histologic type. *Int J Cancer*, 83:223–229, 1999.

[240] W Ye, M Held, J Lagergren, and L Engstrand et al. Helicobacter pylori infection and gastric atrophy: risk of adenocarcinoma and

squamous-cell carcinoma of the esophagus and adenocarcinoma of the gastric cardia. *J Natl Cancer I*, 96:388–396, 2004.

[241] N Ylitalo, P Sørensen, A Josefsson, and M Frisch et al. Smoking and oral contraceptives as risk factors for cervical carcinoma in situ. *Int J Cancer*, 81:357–365, 1999.

[242] EA Zang and EL Wynder. Reevaluation of the confounding effect of cigarette smoking on the relationship between alcohol use and lung cancer risk, with larynx cancer used as a positive control. *Preventive Medicine*, 32:359–370, 2001.

[243] LP Zhao and S Lipsitz. Designs and analysis of two-stage studies. *Stat Med*, 11:769–782, 1992.

Index